The Biological Bases of Drug Tolerance and Dependence

NEUROSCIENCE PERSPECTIVES

Editor: Peter Jenner
Pharmacology Group
Biomedical Sciences Division
King's College London
Manresa Road
London SW3 6LX

Titles in this series:

Roger Horton and Cornelius Katona (eds), Biological Aspects of Affective Disorders
Trevor Stone (ed), Adenosine in the Nervous System

The Biological Bases of Drug Tolerance and Dependence

edited by

J.A. Pratt

Department of Physiology and Pharmacology, Royal College,
University of Strathclyde, Glasgow, UK

ACADEMIC PRESS

Harcourt Brace Jovanovich, Publishers

London San Diego New York

Boston Sydney Tokyo Toronto

ACADEMIC PRESS LIMITED
24/28 Oval Road,
London NW1 7DX

United States Edition published by
ACADEMIC PRESS INC.
San Diego, CA 92101

This book is printed on acid free paper

A catalogue record for this book
is available from the British Library

ISBN 0-12-564250-4

Typeset by P & R Typesetters Ltd, Salisbury, UK
Printed and Bound in Great Britain by
St Edmundsbury Press,
Bury St Edmunds,
Suffolk

Contents

Contributors

David Ball Reckitt and Colman Psychopharmacology Unit, School of Medical Sciences, University Walk, Bristol BS8 1TD, UK

David J.K. Balfour Department of Pharmacology and Clinical Pharmacology, University Medical School, Ninewells Hospital, Dundee DD1 9SY, UK

Brian M. Cox Department of Pharmacology, F. Edward Hebert School of Medicine, Uniformed Services University of the Health Sciences, Bethesda, MD 20814, USA

Gregory I. Elmer National Institute on Drug Abuse, Addiction Research Centre, Box 5180, Baltimore, MD 21224, USA

Dorothy W. Gallager Neurogen Corporation, 35 Northeast Industrial Road, Branford, CT 06405, USA

Frank R. George Department of Psychology & Center on Alcoholism, Substance Abuse and Addiction, University of New Mexico, North East Albuquerque, New Mexico 871 31-1161, USA

Paul Glue Reckitt and Colman Psychopharmacology Unit, School of Medical Sciences, University Walk, Bristol BS8 1TD, UK

Teresa D. Hernandez Yale University School of Medicine, Department of Psychiatry, Abraham Ribicoff Research Facilities and Connecticut Mental Health Center, New Haven, CT 06508, USA

Hilary J. Litttle Pharmacology Department, The Medical School, University Walk, Bristol BS8 1TD, UK

Rodney J. Marley Yale University School of Medicine, Department of Psychiatry, Abraham Ribicoff Research Facilities and Connecticut Mental Health Center, New Haven, CT 06508, USA

David J. Nutt Reckitt and Colman Psychopharmacology Unit, School of Medical Sciences, University Walk, Bristol BS8 1TD, UK

Roger G. Pertwee Division of Pharmacology, School of Biomedical Sciences, Marischal College, University of Aberdeen, Aberdeen AB9 1AS, UK

Judith A. Pratt Department of Physiology and Pharmacology, Royal College, University of Strathclyde, 204 George Street, Glasgow G1 1XW, UK

Mary C. Ritz National Institute on Drug Abuse, Addiction Research Centre, Box 5180, Baltimore, MD 21224, USA

Linda L. Werling Department of Pharmacology, George Washington University School of Medicine, Washington, DC 20037, USA

Marina E. Wolf Wayne State University School of Medicine, Department of Psychiatry, Cellular and Clinical Neurobiology Program, Lafayette Clinic, 951 East Lafayette, Detroit, Michigan 48207, USA

Francis J. White Wayne State University School of Medicine, Department of Psychiatry, Cellular and Clinical Neurobiology Program, Lafayette Clinic, 951 East Lafayette, Detroit, Michigan 48207, USA

Series Preface

The driving force for the production of this series lies in my own inability to keep up with the advances occurring in those areas of neuroscience in which I am especially interested. So many times I have been frustrated by being unable to find a current review of an important research area. Even when I resort to bothering colleagues who are experts in a particular field, I am told, more often than not, that such an overview does not exist. In my own area of expertise I frequently send away students empty-handed who have asked me to direct them to a definitive article on a well researched topic.

Although regrettable, perhaps this situation is not surprising since the neurosciences are one of the most diverse and rapidly advancing areas in the biological sphere. By definition, research in the neurosciences encompasses anatomy, pathology, biochemistry, physiology, pharmacology, molecular biology, genetics and therapeutics. Indeed, there are few individuals capable of maintaining a grasp of the literature in all these aspects of their own research interests let alone in other fields.

My answer was to establish *Neuroscience Perspectives* and to develop gradually a series of individual edited monographs dealing in depth with issues of current interest to those working in the neuroscience area. Each volume is being designed to bring a multidisciplinary approach to the subject matter by pursuing the topic from the laboratory to the clinic. As a consequence I have asked the editors of the individual volumes to produce a balanced critique of their topic which will be read, understood and enjoyed by as wide an audience as possible within the realm of neuroscience.

The choice of the topics for the series is a difficult matter. In the first instance these were largely dictated by my own interests or by my awareness of important and fundamental work being undertaken by colleagues. More recently, I have been recruiting subject matter and editors through attending a variety of diverse symposia in the neuroscience area. However, the choice of topics should reflect the needs of the audience reached by the series. So I invite you to let me know of areas which you feel are of importance and to give me suggestions for individuals who would be keen to edit a book for *Neuroscience Perspectives*.

Finally, it only remains to thank those individuals at Academic Press who have already worked for several years to develop *Neuroscience Perspectives*. In particular, Dr. Carey Chapman who has the unenviable task of recruiting the editors that I suggest and then harassing them for the completed work. My hope is that the series will fill the gap that I perceive and provide for my colleagues in the neurosciences a collection of interesting books which will become reference volumes in their field. I hope you will enjoy *Neuroscience Perspectives*.

Peter Jenner

Preface

The use and abuse of psychoactive chemicals has been present in many societies since ancient times. In more recent years the increasingly widespread use of these natural, as well as synthetic and semisynthetic psychoactive substances has led to large numbers of individuals becoming dependent on such drugs. The resulting social and medical problems are enormous. However, in general we do not really know how to wean people off drugs of dependence effectively. One of the reasons for this problem is that our knowledge of the neuronal mechanisms underlying the development of drug tolerance and dependence is limited. The main objective of this volume is to bring together reviews from a number of distinguished research groups, in order to provide a comprehensive account of our current understanding of the neuronal adaptive processes that (may) underlie tolerance to and dependence upon a variety of psychotropic drugs of abuse.

The drugs considered include both those that are legally and freely available in Western societies (nicotine and alcohol) and those that are widely used (cannabinoids, psychomotor stimulants, opioids and benzodiazepines) despite their sale and consumption being controlled by legislation.

Throughout this volume the term 'drug dependence' rather than 'addiction' has been used as the meaning of the latter has become imprecise with its popular use. Some features of dependence are common to several classes of psychoactive drugs of abuse despite their disparate psychopharmacological profiles. Often, repeated administration of a drug of dependence leads to tolerance, i.e. after chronic use increasingly larger doses are needed to elicit the same effect as after acute exposure. Physical dependence in which a withdrawal syndrome is elicited by removing the drug is also a common feature. Finally, the ability of a drug to produce psychic craving is an important factor that leads to the continued abuse of drugs. These three features occur with varying degrees for the different drugs of abuse.

The first two chapters of this book are general overviews. Nutt and colleagues discuss the main clinical features associated with drugs of dependence and I have attempted to bring together some of the common neuronal adaptive processes that may contribute to the processes of tolerance and dependence for several drugs of abuse. Each of the subsequent chapters is a detailed review of current research aimed at identifying the cellular and molecular mechanisms underlying tolerance to, and dependence upon, each of the various drug classes. Finally, George and colleagues consider the role of genetics in the vulnerability to drug dependence, an important area but one that is still in its infancy.

One of the challenges for the future is to determine which of the cellular and molecular changes in the brain underlie the behavioural changes in the organism that are critical to the development of drug tolerance and dependence. Only then, will we be in the position to identify pharmacological strategies useful for the treatment of dependent individuals. It is my objective that this volume will provide researchers from various disciplines with a reference book as well as be a stimulus for them to develop a more integrated approach in investigations of the neurobiology of drug dependence.

Judith A. Pratt

CHAPTER 1

PSYCHOTROPIC DRUG TOLERANCE AND DEPENDENCE: COMMON UNDERLYING MECHANISMS?

Judith A. Pratt

Department of Physiology and Pharmacology, Royal College, University of Strathclyde, 204 George Street, Glasgow G1 1XW, UK

Table of Contents

THE BIOLOGICAL BASES OF DRUG TOLERANCE AND DEPENDENCE
ISBN 0-12-564250-4

1.1 Introduction

It is clear that drugs from a wide range of chemical classes that elicit their psychopharmacological effects through differing mechanisms of actions can produce tolerance and dependence. The processes that underlie these phenomena are complex and for many drugs of abuse incompletely understood. A variety of different experimental strategies have been employed to investigate the mechanisms involved. Possible mechanisms of tolerance include changes in the metabolism and distribution of drug in the body and changes in the properties of neuronal receptors in the brain. In addition, the contribution of behavioural variables such as the environment in which the drug is administered can also be important. Research into the relative contributions and significance of these various mechanisms which may underlie tolerance to and dependence upon a particular drug class is still in its infancy (Goudie and Emmett-Oglesby, 1989). However, pharmacodynamic factors would appear to play a particularly important role. The subsequent chapters in this text will focus on the adaptive processes that occur at the cellular and molecular levels in brain following chronic treatment with a wide spectrum of psychotropic drugs. Where appropriate, attempts will be made to correlate changes in neuronal function with behavioural signs of tolerance and dependence. To place this work in a broader context it is preceded by an overview of the clinical features of psychotropic drug tolerance and dependence. Finally, the importance of genetic approaches to the analysis of dependence processes is considered. This comprehensive overview should provide a stimulus for investigators to develop a more intergrated approach to the analysis of the functionally important mechanisms involved in dependence and also provide a rational basis for the identification of new pharmacological strategies useful in its treatment.

This chapter will provide an overview of some of the common mechanisms of psychotropic drug tolerance and dependence, concentrating on drug-induced adaptive changes in the characteristics of neuronal receptors and the neuroanatomical pathways involved.

1.2 Mechanisms of acute actions of psychotropic drugs

Prior to an evaluation of the mechanisms by which tolerance and dependence can occur, it is necessary to first consider the acute mechanisms of action of psychotropic drugs. The interaction of a drug with specific receptors on the neuronal membrane is generally accepted to elicit the cellular changes responsible for the various behavioural properties by which the drug is classed, for example as a sedative or stimulant.

The hypnosedative benzodiazepines and barbiturates are thought to enhance the actions of the inhibitory neurotransmitter γ-aminobutyric acid (GABA) that are mediated by the $GABA_A$ receptor (Olsen and Venter, 1986; Chapter 3). This receptor complex contains an integral transmembrane chloride channel, a GABA recognition site, and a number of allosteric regulatory binding sites (Olsen and Venter, 1986; Chapter 3). Benzodiazepines and barbiturates act at separate allosteric regulatory sites to increase the frequency and duration, respectively, of opening of GABA-dependent chloride channels (Study and Barker, 1981). Ethanol may also elicit some of its actions through an interaction at the $GABA_A$ receptor complex, although the exact mechanism(s) remain unclear (Ticku and Burch, 1980; Chapter 4).

There are at least three opioid receptor subtypes, of which the μ-receptor is most frequently considered as being the site important in dependence. Morphine acts at μ-receptors to produce a membrane hyperpolarization that results from activation of G protein-linked potassium channels (North *et al.*, 1987; Aghajanian and Wang, 1986).

Nicotine is considered to exhibit its central effects through an interaction with nicotinic acetylcholine receptors that contain an integral transmembrane sodium channel. Agonist binding leads to channel opening and depolarization responses (Wonnacott, 1987).

In contrast to the aforementioned drugs, psychostimulants exhibit their actions by elevating the synaptic levels of dopamine and other monoamines. The former effect is of greatest importance for their psychostimulant properties. Hence, cocaine and amphetamine inhibit the dopamine reuptake mechanism which is the primary mechanism for terminating transmitter action (Kuczenski, 1983; Ritz *et al.*, 1987). Amphetamine also stimulates the release of dopamine. Less is known about the action of the psychotropic cannabinoids, but recent evidence points to a receptor-mediated effect (see Chapter 8).

The diverse array of receptor–effector mechanisms involved in eliciting the responses to various psychotropic drugs indicate a multitude of possible processes involved in tolerance and dependence that may differ for each drug class.

1.3 Mechanisms of tolerance

The term tolerance refers to the phenomenon whereby, after repeated exposure, a given dose of a drug produces a decreased effect, or larger doses are required to produce effects similar to those produced after acute exposure.

The distinction between the terms tolerance and desensitization (tachyphylaxis) is not a sharp one. The former is conventionally used to describe gradual decreases in responsiveness to a drug, which may take days or weeks to develop. In contrast, desensitization is generally applied to situations where there is a rapid diminution in response.

When applied to psychotropic drugs of abuse, tolerance can be conveniently divided into a number of forms that give some indication of the mechanisms involved. Pharmacokinetic (dispositional) tolerance results from any change in the absorption, distribution, metabolism or excretion of a drug which leads to a reduction in the concentration of the drug at its site of action. Pharmacodynamic tolerance arises from adaptational processes occurring in the brain. These include changes at the primary site of drug action as well as changes in neurotransmitter function in neuronal pathways downstream from the initial interaction. Behavioural (learned) tolerance is a term applied to the phenomenon whereby the environment in which the drug is repeatedly administered can influence the development of tolerance. An additional feature of tolerance is that of cross-tolerance, in which tolerance to one drug is extended to another of a different chemical class. In direct opposition to tolerance is sensitization (reverse tolerance) in which the effects of a drug increase following repeated administration.

Tolerance is often considered within the context of dependence (see Chapter 2 for definition), but there are situations where they may be separate. The term dependence, rather than addiction, has been used throughout this volume as the latter is an imprecise term with emotional connotations.

1.4 Pharmacodynamic tolerance

1.4.1 Adaptive processes at the level of the drug–receptor interaction

One hypothesis that has been put forward as a possible common mechanism that could explain tolerance to the psychopharmacological effects of drugs of abuse is that chronic drug exposure leads to adaptational processes occurring at the drug–receptor complex such that the receptor becomes less responsive to the effects of the drug or the endogenous ligand for the receptor (for review see Overstreet and Yamamura, 1979; Poste and Crooke, 1985). This is an attractive hypothesis since it can also go some way to explain dependence. Hence one concept that has evolved is that chronic drug administration leads to the initiation of adaptive processes which counter the effects of the drug and that these processes persist after the drug has been cleared from the brain, thereby leaving the opposing processes unopposed (Koob & Bloom, 1988). In this context it is pertinent that the withdrawal syndrome observed after cessation of a drug tends to be opposite to the symptoms produced by acute administration of that drug. For example, anxiety and insomnia occur following withdrawal from benzodiazepines. This, together with other evidence, has led Lader and File (1987) to consider the hypothesis that benzodiazepine tolerance and withdrawal are manifestations of the same dependence mechanism. However, not all evidence supports this. Perceptual disturbances that occur following benzodiazepine withdrawal, for example, do not appear to be opposite to the acute behavioural effects of these drugs. With other drugs of abuse, such as ethanol and the opiates, there is both clinical and experimental evidence (Koob and Bloom, 1988; Chapter 2) that in some circumstances tolerance and dependence may be separated, indicating that each process may occur by a different mechanism.

1.4.1.1 Receptor regulation

At the simplest level, one common mechanism that could regulate the overall responsiveness of neurones to repeated drug exposure is an alteration in receptor number. It has been suggested that chronic exposure to agonists induces a decrease in receptor number (downregulation), whereas prolonged exposure to antagonists evokes an increase in receptor number (for reviews see Poste and Crooke, 1985; Overstreet and Yamamura, 1979). Downregulation, or loss of receptors from the cell surface after repeated occupancy by the ligand, could involve internalization, degradation, and/or changes in the recycling of the receptor.

Whilst downregulation of receptors is often presumed to underlie tolerance to various drugs of abuse, there is limited experimental evidence to support this view. For example, most investigators have found no change in benzodiazepine receptor number after chronic benzodiazepine administration (see Chapter 3). Those studies that did observe a decrease in receptor density generally employed extremely large doses of drugs that are unlikely to be related to the clinical situation (Rosenberg and Chiu, 1981; Tietz *et al.*, 1986).

Following repeated exposure to morphine, while there is evidence that there are selective but modest reductions in μ-receptor density (Werling *et al.*, 1989), other mechanisms are thought to be a more likely explanation of tolerance (see Section 1.4.1.2 and Chapter 7).

Interestingly, chronic nicotine exposure has consistently been shown to increase the density of nicotinic receptors in the brain rather than to decrease them (Marks *et al.*, 1986; Nordberg *et al.*, 1985; Benwell *et al.*, 1988). It has been hypothesized that this apparent paradox may be related to the powerful desensitizing properties of nicotine, observed in isolated tissues, such that on repeated exposure it acts as an antagonist, rather than an agonist (Wonnacott, 1987). At present, the evidence for a causal relationship between the changes in nicotine binding sites and tolerance to the behavioural effects of the drug remains equivocal (see Chapter 5).

The relatively recent identification of cannabinoid receptors has meant that the role of changes in receptor characteristics in tolerance to the psychotropic cannabinoids has yet to be explored (see Chapter 8).

The psychostimulant drugs can be contrasted with other drugs of abuse in that both tolerance and sensitization occur to their behavioural effects after chronic drug exposure. Tolerance is often considered to develop to the euphoric effects of psychostimulants, whereas sensitization occurs to other behaviours, resulting in stereotypy and enhanced locomotor activity. The role of changes in the characteristics of the dopamine reuptake sites in contributing to these diametrically opposed behaviours is unclear. Sensitization appears to result from a number of neuronal adaptations that result in enhanced dopamine release and D_1 dopamine receptor sensitivity (see Chapter 6).

1.4.1.2 Receptor uncoupling

For several psychotropic drugs, there is evidence that chronic drug treatment results in an uncoupling of the receptor from its effector mechanism.

Thus, for the benzodiazepines, the reduced response to GABA observed in electrophysiological studies, and which is proposed to underlie the behavioural tolerance to these drugs (see Chapter 3), is thought to be a result of an allosteric 'uncoupling' of GABA and benzodiazepine recognition sites of the $GABA_A$ receptor. The enhancement of benzodiazepine binding by GABA is reduced following chronic benzodiazepine administration to rodents and following repeated exposure of neuronal cells in culture to benzodiazepines (Roca *et al.*, 1990a, b; Gallager *et al.*, 1984; Mele *et al.*, 1984).

The exact molecular mechanisms underlying the uncoupling process have yet to be fully explored. Possibilities include (a) modification of the $GABA_A$ receptor, such as by phosphorylation, (b) changes in the production of endogenous ligand(s), (c) prolonged conformational change in the receptor, or (d) altered subunit composition of the receptor. Roca *et al.* (1990b) have excluded the possible involvement of cAMP-dependent phosphorylation mechanisms mediating uncoupling, although cAMP-independent mechanisms could be involved. Roca *et al.* (1990b) also argue against alterations in the production of endogenous ligands because of the extensive dialysis procedures used in their experimental protocol. Against the view of changes in the conformational state of the $GABA_A$ recognition site is the evidence that desensitization of the $GABA_A$ receptor occurs within seconds of exposure to GABA (Mierlak and Farb, 1988), whereas the uncoupling takes a much more prolonged period of time to develop. However, it is possible that chronic exposure to an allosteric modulator may evoke changes in the conformational state of $GABA_A$ receptor at a slower rate. Indeed, Gallager and colleagues have produced some evidence to support a conversion from a low-affinity to a high-affinity (desensitized) GABA receptor (Heninger and Gallager, 1988) following chronic diazepam administration to rats, although further experimental evidence is required.

An attractive hypothesis for the mechanism underlying uncoupling is that changes in expression of the various subunits of the $GABA_A$ receptor could have occurred. This is based on the knowledge that the degree of enhancement of benzodiazepine binding by GABA in transfected cells depends upon the particular α-subunit being expressed (Pritchett *et al.*, 1989; Luddens and Wisden, 1991). Indeed, recent findings show reduced levels of mRNA for the α_1- but not β_1-subunit in cerebral cortex after continuous diazepam administration to rats (Heninger *et al.*, 1990; see Chapter 3). Thus it is possible that different α or γ variants become expressed after chronic benzodiazepine exposure, resulting in the strength of coupling between the benzodiazepine and GABA recognition sites being reduced. The availability of probes for the numerous isoforms of the $GABA_A$ receptor subunits will enable a more detailed analysis using *in situ* hybridization techniques. Finally, further evidence to support synthesis of new receptors being involved is that the $t_{1/2}$ for uncoupling is similar to the $t_{1/2}$ for benzodiazepine receptor turnover (Roca *et al.*, 1990b).

Other hypnosedatives which produce an uncoupling effect at the $GABA_A$ receptor complex include the barbiturates and, less convincingly, ethanol. Chronic exposure to barbiturates reduces the coupling between a number of the components of the $GABA_A$ receptor complex; between the barbiturate and benzodiazepine recognition site, between the benzodiazepine and GABA recognition site, and betweeen the GABA recognition site and the chloride channel (Roca *et al.*, 1990b; Morrow *et al.*, 1990). Chronic ethanol exposure reduces GABA receptor-mediated chloride-uptake in cerebral cortical synaptoneurosomes but does not have a consistent effect on benzodiazepine binding although GABA binding is generally reduced (Morrow *et al.*, 1990; see Chapter 4).

It is of particular interest that recent studies have demonstrated that, like benzodiazepines, ethanol evokes a reduction in α_1-subunit mRNA in cerebral cortex following chronic ethanol exposure, although chronic pentobarbitone administration is without effect (Morrow *et al.*, 1990). This does not exclude the possibility that other subunits may be modified by barbiturates. Thus, it is possible that tolerance to hypnosedatives may be associated with the regulation of genes encoding the various $GABA_A$ receptor subunits. It should be borne in mind, however, that altered GABA function is thought to be only one component of several neuronal changes that are thought to be involved in ethanol tolerance and dependence (see Chapter 4).

The adaptive processes underlying opioid tolerance also appear to involve receptor–effector uncoupling. In a neuronal cell line and in tissue from animals receiving chronic administration of morphine, there was a loss in guanyl nucleotide regulation of binding of μ-agonists (Werling *et al.*, 1989; Chapter 7).

In summary, a number of adaptive processes can occur following repeated exposure to psychotropic drugs. In isolated tissues and cells, continuous exposure to some agonists (e.g. nicotine, opiates and GABA) can produce a rapid desensitization. This effect, in which receptors are still present on the membrane surface, could be a result of changes in the conformational state of the receptor, such as through phosphorylation. It is difficult to extrapolate such findings to the *in vivo* situation; nevertheless such studies provide important information about the mechanisms of receptor regulation. In brain tissue dissected from tolerant animals, downregulation of receptors and receptor uncoupling have been observed. The latter effect would appear to be a promising candidate for explaining tolerance to the effects of a number of psychotropic drugs. However, it is likely that no single neuronal adaptive process can account for the behavioural tolerance observed *in vivo*. It is possible that there is a complex interaction between a number of processes; some of these may be necessary before others are initiated. If this is the case it is not surprising that the temporal relationships for tolerance development and certain neuronal adaptive processes do not always correlate. Another critical point is that some neuronal systems may be more critically involved in tolerance development than others (see Sections 1.4.2 and 1.6).

A detailed discussion of the contribution of pharmacokinetic and behavioural variables to the development of drug tolerance is outside the scope of this text. However, these are reviewed briefly in subsequent chapters where appropriate. The relative contributions of pharmacodynamic, pharmacokinetic and behavioural factors to drug tolerance and dependence are summarized in Table 1. It can be observed that pharmacodynamic factors play an important role, whereas pharmacokinetic factors make a significant contribution to drug tolerance only in the case of the barbiturates and ethanol.

1.4.2 Adaptive processes in neuronal pathways consequent on receptor occupation

The behavioural profile of psychotropic drugs is a result of alterations in activity of numerous neuronal systems subsequent to a primary site of action at specific receptor sites. Similarly, each class of psychotropic drug produces

Table 1 Factors contributing to the development of psychotropic drug tolerance and dependence.

	Pharmacodynamic				
	Receptor downregulation	Receptor uncoupling	Changes in other neural systems	Pharmacokinetic	Behavioural
Opiates	+	++	+	–	++
Barbiturates	?	++	?	+	+
Benzodiazepines	?	++	?	–	+
Ethanol	N/A	N/A	++	+	+
Cannabinoids	?	?	+	–	?
Nicotine	–	?	++	–	++

–, absent; +, present; ?, uncertain/unknown; N/A, not appropriate.

a characteristic dependence syndrome. The mechanisms through which changes in activity in the various neuronal systems affected by each class of drug contribute to the processes of tolerance and dependence are complex and difficult to study experimentally.

In considering the neuronal processes underlying dependence liability at least two factors are important: firstly, the extent to which drugs exhibit 'rewarding' properties, and secondly, the degree of severity of the withdrawal syndrome. The first is thought to be a result of a drug's ability to affect dopamine secretion in the mesolimbic pathway and has been associated with craving for the drug (see Section 1.5). The second factor is thought to be a result of adaptive changes in neuronal function after chronic drug treatment. These changes not only may be attributed to changes at the primary site of drug action (i.e. the receptor) but may also be due to changes in activity of neuronal pathways downstream from the initial interaction at the receptor. Withdrawal symptoms may be a result of activity of neuronal pathways specifically affected by each drug class, or of pathways commonly affected by different classes of drug.

Some examples of the role of 'downstream' events in the tolerance and dependence processes are considered below. In identifying such pathways it is first ncessary to consider how drugs may affect a variety of neuronal systems after acute administration.

Nicotine can evoke a variety of behaviours ranging from a locomotor stimulant to a 'tranquillizing' effect. The consequences of occupation of nicotinic acetylcholine receptors are to increase the turnover of noradrenaline (NA) and dopamine (DA) and to reduce the turnover of 5-hydroxytryptamine (5-HT). Such changes in monoamine turnover may underlie the various behavioural effects of nicotine. Changes in DA and NA turnover appear to be a result of an action of nicotine on acetylcholine receptors in cell body regions of dopamine- and noradrenaline-containing neurones (e.g. ventral tegmental area and locus coeruleus) rather than an action at the terminals (see Chapter 5). Chronic infusions of nicotine result in a reduced effect of nicotine on DA turnover in the striatum but results in enhanced DA release in the mesolimbic system (Kirch *et al.*, 1987; Fung, 1989). It has been suggested that the increased DA levels in the mesolimbic system may be associated with the enhanced locomotor responses to nicotine that occur following chronic nicotine exposure and possibly with the coping mechanisms involved after exposure to aversive environments (see Chapter 5). In contrast, the changes evoked by nicotine on hippocampal 5-HT systems appear unrelated to effects on locomotor activity. Balfour has hypothesized that nicotine interacts with the processes by which animals habituate to stressful environments and that this may involve hippocampal 5-HT. Such interactions may contribute to the dependence process.

Benzodiazepines, like nicotine, also exhibit a diverse range of behavioural effects. Whilst this is considered to result from an initial interaction at benzodiazepine receptors, altered activity in other neuronal systems is likely because of the widespread distribution of these receptors in the brain and their location in numerous neuroanatomical circuits. Benzodiazepines have been shown to reduce the turnover of a variety of monoamine transmitters. The one that has attracted the most attention is 5-HT. Considerable evidence has accumulated to suggest that benzodiazepines reduce 5-HT turnover (for reviews see Pratt *et al.*, 1985; Iversen, 1984) and it has been argued repeatedly that this may be related to their anxiolytic effects although not all evidence supports this view. Moreover, it is unclear at present how changes in 5-HT neuronal function that can occur after chronic benzodiazepine treatment contribute to the processes of tolerance and dependence (Johnston and File, 1986; Nutt, 1986). Based on clinical findings, Nutt (1986) has proposed that there may be an increase in monoamine function during withdrawal from benzodiazepines.

For drugs such as ethanol and cannabinoids, that are highly lipophilic, some of their effects on neuronal membrane function may be brought about by non-receptor-mediated processes. For example, cannabis and ethanol can induce changes in membrane phospholipids. The consequences of these initial interactions will be to modify neurotransmitter release and alter firing in neuronal pathways. Acutely, cannabinoids affect the turnover of a variety of neurotransmitters, especially monoamines. Tolerance develops to some of these effects. Cross-tolerance occurs with some hypnosedatives. This is probably because there are common pathways affected, downstream from the drug's initial primary effects on the neuronal membrane (see Chapter 8). Such pathways could therefore have a significant role in tolerance and dependence.

Another proposed action of ethanol is a primary action at the lipid–protein interface surrounding receptors within the membrane (see Chapter 4). This may account for why ethanol, in relatively small concentrations, can affect $GABA_A$ and N-methyl-D-aspartate (NMDA) receptor function. Both receptors contain a variety of allosteric sites which may be affected to a considerable degree if the lipid–protein interface is perturbed. It is possible that these transmitters are involved in the tolerance and dependence process although accumulating evidence is emerging that neuronal calcium channels may be critically involved (for review see Littleton *et al.*, 1988; Chapter 4). Changes in calcium channel function may be consequent on the changes in neuronal excitability evoked by ethanol's ability to enhance excitatory and reduce inhibitory amino acid function.

With respect to the clinical situation, it is of interest to note that some symptoms, such as tremor, anxiety and hyperthermia, are shared by opiates, barbiturates, benzodiazepines and ethanol, indicating recruitment of common dependence pathways. However, ethanol fails to relieve opiate withdrawal symptoms and vice versa, although ethanol can partially alleviate the symptoms of hypnosedative withdrawal. Perhaps this is not surprising as it is known that ethanol, barbiturates and benzodiazepines all modify $GABA_A$ receptor function and are thus likely to affect common neuroanatomical pathways consequent on receptor occupation.

1.4.3 Partial agonists versus subtype-specific ligands and tolerance development

The recent advances in the molecular biology of neurotransmitter receptors have provided a challenge for scientists to develop compounds that bind more selectively to one particular receptor subtype than another. It is anticipated that certain compounds would exhibit their desired clinical effect (e.g. anxiolysis, analgesia) without producing unwanted effects such as tolerance and dependence. A completely different approach is the development of partial agonists. This approach exploits differences in receptor reserve in the different neuronal systems that are responsible for the various behavioural effects of a drug.

At present, the benzodiazepine and opiate receptors are the subject of debate in these matters. Two subtypes for the neuronal benzodiazepine receptor have been proposed on the basis of results from radioligand binding studies. However, at present the experimental evidence for the proposal that one type mediates sedation and the other anxiolysis is lacking (Nutt, 1990). Recent advances in the molecular biology of the $GABA_A$ receptor may mean that some ligands may be designed which will bind preferentially to a particular subunit composition, thereby enabling them to exert a restrictive profile of action (Luddens and Wisden, 1991). Haefely argues that partial agonists for the benzodiazepine receptor can also elicit a restricted profile of action (Haefely, 1988; Haefely *et al.*, 1990) with less potential for tolerance and dependence than benzodiazepine receptor full agonists. Partial agonists exhibit anxiolytic and anticonvulsant actions at low percentage occupation and cannot evoke sedative-like effects even at 100% receptor occupation. Moreover, such compounds display reduced ability to evoke tolerance and dependence when compared to full agonists. Haefely *et al.* (1990) propose that the neuronal systems mediating anticonvulsant and anti-anxiety effects have a higher receptor reserve than neuronal systems mediating unwanted effects. With present knowledge, it is difficult to explain whether the lack of sedation and tolerance of a new benzodiazepine ligand is attributable to partial agonist properties or to inactivity at hypothetical receptor subtypes mediating unwanted effects. Clearly this will be an area of intensive research in future years, not only for benzodiazepines but also for other drugs of abuse.

1.5 The comparative ability of psychotropic drugs to modulate activity of the mesolimbic reward pathway

A variety of drugs of abuse have been shown to have positive rewarding properties in a number of paradigms. They are readily self-administered in a variety of species, display conditioned place preference behaviour, and are able to lower reinforcement thresholds for brain stimulation reward (see Chapters 5, 6 and 7). The neuroanatomical pathways mediating the reinforcing effects of drugs of abuse have been the focus of much investigation. In particular, the mesolimbic and, to a lesser extent, the mesocortical DA pathway have been proposed to be critically involved in the expression of reinforcement reward (see Chapters 6 and 7).

1.5.1 Psychostimulants and opiates

There is substantial evidence that the mesolimbic (and also the mesocortical) dopaminergic pathways are important for the rewarding properties of cocaine and amphetamine. Hence, DA antagonists attenuate the rewarding effects of psychostimulants. Similarly, 6-hydroxydopamine lesions of mesolimbic, but not nigro-striatal, DA neurones block rewarding responses to these drugs (Koob and Bloom, 1988; Chapter 6). The mesolimbic DA pathway is also implicated in the rewarding properties of opiates. As with amphetamine, rats will self-administer morphine directly into the nucleus accumbens, although morphine has a more pronounced effect when injected into the ventral tegmental area (VTA) (Bozarth and Wise, 1981). However, the involvement of DA in the rewarding responses to opiates has recently come under scrutiny because 6-hydroxydopamine lesions of the accumbens have minimal effect on the intravenous administration of heroin (Pettit *et al.*, 1984; Dworkin *et al.*, 1988). Nevertheless, cell body lesions of the nucleus accumbens block self-administration of both opiates and psychostimulants, indicating the importance of this structure *per se*. Similar effects are observed following cell body lesions of the ventral pallidum (Hubner and Koob, 1990). These findings have led Koob and colleagues to propose that the nucleus accumbens–ventral pallidum circuit may be a common pathway for both stimulant and opiate reinforcement. It would therefore appear that whilst psychostimulants evoke changes in DA release through an action at the level of the terminals of the mesolimbic pathway, the opiates would appear to exert at least some of their reinforcing effects through an action at opiate receptors postsynaptic to the DA terminals within the accumbens. Nevertheless, an action at the level of opiate receptors in the VTA to evoke an increase in mesolimbic DA cell firing is also considered to be important in the rewarding effects (for review see Wise, 1990). Both classes of drug are able to increase the extracellular

Table 2 Comparative ability of psychotropic drugs to increase dopamine concentrations *in vivo* in the mesolimbic and the nigrostriatal systems of the rat.

	% of Basal dopamine release		Peak effect (minutes post-drug)		
Drug (dose)	Accumbens	Caudate	Accumbens	Caudate	Ref.
Amphetamine					
1 mg/kg s.c.	1000	550	60	60	1
0.75–3.0 mg/kg i.p.	350–1000	350–1000	20	20	4
Cocaine					
5 mg/kg s.c.	350	250	90	90	1
	300	ND	100	ND	3
Morphine					
0.05–10 mg/kg s.c.	140–200	100–180	60–180	60–100	1
Ethanol					
1.0 g/kg i.p.	190	130	40	40	1
Nicotine					
0.6 mg/kg s.c.	220	140	30	40	1
Δ^9-THC					
1.0 mg/kg i.p.	150	ND	40	ND	2

Data are expressed as approximate percentages of baseline dopamine concentrations from: 1, Di Chiara and Imperato (1988); 2, Chen *et al.* (1990); 3, Hurd *et al.* (1989); 4, Robinson and Camp (1990).

concentration of DA in the nucleus accumbens as determined by microdialysis in freely moving rats (Table 2) (Di Chiara and Imperato, 1988; Robinson and Camp, 1990; Hurd *et al.*, 1989; Sharp *et al.*, 1987).

1.5.2 Other drugs

In addition to the opiates and psychostimulants, other drugs of abuse are able to stimulate the release of DA in the nucleus accumbens (Table 2). Nicotine facilitates DA release *in vitro* and *in vivo* (Rowell *et al.*, 1987; Imperato *et al.*, 1986) and this occurs to a greater degree in the accumbens than in the caudate (Imperato *et al.*, 1986). The site of action of nicotine appears to be at the level of the VTA (Mereu *et al.*, 1987; see Chapter 5).

There are few reports dealing with the reinforcing properties of benzodiazepines, but in a place preference paradigm lesions of the mesolimbic dopaminergic terminals in the accumbens attenuate the effect of diazepam (Spyraki and Fibiger, 1988), suggesting an involvement of brain DA systems in the rewarding effects of benzodiazepines. The exact locus of action is unclear. Whilst a GABAergic pathway descends from the nucleus accumbens to the VTA (Walaas and Fonnum, 1980), it seems that an action on VTA neurones is most likely. Thus, O'Brien and White (1987) propose that benzodiazepines act directly on non-DA cells in the VTA to produce disinhibition of DA neurones. In other brain structures, however, systemic administration of benzodiazepines reduces DA turnover (Wood, 1982).

Recently, Chen *et al.* (1990) have demonstrated that, in addition to Δ^9-tetrahydrocannabinol (THC) augmenting brain stimulation reward, it too can enhance DA release in the nucleus accumbens *in vivo*. These effects were antagonized by naloxone, indicating an involvement of endogenous opioids.

In a recent comparative study involving a variety of drugs of abuse (opiates, cocaine, amphetamine, nicotine and ethanol), Di Chiara and Imperato (1988) demonstrated a relatively greater drug-induced increase in DA concentrations in the accumbens, as compared to the caudate nucleus, using the technique of brain microdialysis. Drugs not abused by humans (imipiramine and atropine) were without effect. The authors propose that the preferential stimulation of DA transmission in the mesolimbic system might be a fundamental property of drugs that are abused, irrespective of the pharmacological class to which they belong. However, other groups, whilst supporting a role for the mesolimbic system in reward, do not demonstrate a preferential increase in DA secretion in the accumbens following psychostimulant administration (Sharp *et al.*, 1987; Robinson and Camp, 1990). Indeed, as the data in Table 2 illustrate, there are in general only modest differences in the ability of psychotropic drugs to evoke increases in DA secretion in the mesolimbic, as compared to the nigro-striatal, system.

In addition, Di Chiara and Imperato (1988), whilst acknowledging that the mesolimbic dopaminergic system contributes to the rewarding effects as well as to the psychomotor activating effect of psychotropic drugs, argue that the motor activation does not appear to be essential for reward since ethanol and barbiturates retain their rewarding properties at doses that depress motor behaviour.

In summary, despite drugs of abuse acting through separate distinct primary mechanisms, it would appear that many secondarily activate final common pathway(s), such as the mesolimbic DA pathway, which mediate their rewarding properties.

1.5.3 Reward and craving

The relationship between the rewarding properties of a drug and its ability to induce 'craving' has been the subject of much discussion. One proposal, for psychostimulants, is that craving is a correlate of DA depletion that results from prolonged drug use such that the motivational factor to continue drug use is an effort to re-elevate synaptic concentrations of DA (for reviews see Dackis and Gold, 1985; Wise, 1990). However, there is considerable evidence that repeated psychostimulant administration results in sensitization to motor behaviours which are associated with an enhancement of stimulant-induced DA release in the striatum and the nucleus accumbens (see Chapter 6). If this is the case, then the rewarding properties of psychostimulants would also be expected to display sensitization. Indeed, the results of some groups are supportive of psychostimulant sensitization in self-administration and conditioned place preference studies (Piazza *et al.*, 1989; Lett, 1989). Clearly these latter studies are against the generally accepted view that tolerance develops to the euphoric effects of psychostimulants. One possible explanation is that drug users may increase the dose of psychostimulants because of the desire to attain more intensive 'highs' rather than because they are tolerant to the euphoric effects (Robinson, 1991). Indeed there is some experimental evidence in support of this. Using a self-administration paradigm, Hurd *et al.* (1989) demonstrated that the ability of cocaine to elevate DA levels within the nucleus accumbens was reduced in rats repeatedly exposed to the drug. It is possible that these rats were sensitized to cocaine such that lower levels of synaptic DA were able to maintain reinforcement (see Chapter 6). In contrast, others have found increases in the extracellular concentrations of cocaine and dopamine after chronic cocaine administration and suggest that behavioural sensitization may be a result of a reduction in the metabolism of the drug (Pettit *et al.*, 1990).

1.5.4 Reward and other neurotransmitters

It has been suggested that DA is not the only neurochemical substrate mediating reward (Hurd *et al.*, 1989). In a conditioned place preference paradigm, lesions of 5-HT-containing neurones of the nucleus accumbens attenuate the rewarding properties of morphine, but not cocaine (Spyraki *et al.*, 1988). These data suggest that 5-HT neurones are a functional component of the circuitry involved in the rewarding properties of some, but not all, drugs of abuse.

Cholecystokinin (CCK) is co-localized with DA in a subset of mesolimbic DA neurones (Hokfelt *et al.*, 1980). There is accumulating evidence that CCK and DA can interact at pre- and postsynaptic levels in the accumbens as well as at the levels of the VTA (Crawley, 1988; Wang, 1988). The potential importance of CCK in reward processes is demonstrated by the finding that infusion of CCK into the VTA can potentiate amphetamine-conditioned place preferences (Pettit and Mueller, 1989).

1.5.5 Other roles of the mesolimbic dopamine pathway

Exposure to certain environmental stressors and anxiogenic drugs can activate the mesocortical and mesolimbic DA system (Scatton *et al.*, 1988; Roth *et al.*, 1988). Whilst it has been argued that such responses occur preferentially in the mesocortical system (Roth *et al.*, 1988), nevertheless increases in accumbens DA metabolism have been reported following immobilization stress and following administration of the anxiogenic agent methyl-β-carboline carboxylate (βCCM) to rats. It has been suggested that such responses may reflect a heightened attention of the animal in an attempt to cope with the stressor (Scatton *et al.*, 1988). The role of DA in reward processes, and in responses to stress, may be critically important to the dependence liability of some drugs of abuse. The addictive properties of nicotine, for example, appear to be enhanced if the drug is administered during exposure to stressful stimuli (see Chapter 5).

1.6 Metabolic mapping of functional activity in neuronal pathways during drug dependence

It is evident from the preceding discussion that a knowledge of the brain structures and pathways involved in psychotropic drug tolerance and withdrawal reactions is critical to our understanding of dependence processes.

A number of approaches have been employed to identify such structures in dependent animals. These include: (i) lesioning of discrete neuronal pathways combined with behavioural analyses; (ii) electrophysiological recordings from neurones in discrete brain regions; and (iii) regional analysis of changes in receptor properties using autoradiographic or radioligand binding techniques. The first two approaches give insight into important structures, but do not identify other interconnected structures that may be of greater functional relevance. The third approach has limitations in that any regional changes identified may not be of functional importance in the behavioural expression of tolerance and withdrawal.

A different experimental strategy which has only been applied to a limited extent in the elucidation of the neuroanatomical pathways involved in drug dependence is to employ the 2-deoxyglucose autoradiographic technique for mapping local rates of cerebral glucose use (LCGU) in the conscious animal (Sokoloff *et al.*, 1977). Changes in glucose use following a particular pharmacological or physiological stimulus reflect changes in activity predominantly in nerve terminals and so the technique provides a complete neuroanatomical map of the structures functionally affected as a consequence of receptor occupation. This technique can be particularly powerful when changes in LCGU are correlated with a specific behavioural event.

1.6.1 Reward and psychostimulants

In self-stimulation experiments, in which rats responded for rewarding electrical stimulation to the VTA, Eposito *et al.* (1984) reported marked increases in glucose utilization in specific neuronal projection fibres as well as in selective terminal sites such as the nucleus accumbens, mediodorsal thalamic nucleus and medial prefrontal cortex. These findings reiterate the importance of the VTA–accumbens pathway in rewarding brain stimulation and extend our knowledge of the neural substrates of reward from the level of a single neuronal pathway to the level of integrated neuronal networks. Moreover, the increases in glucose use in structures involved in reward processes are augmented after morphine and cocaine administration (Kornetsky *et al.*, 1989).

It is of obvious interest to extend such studies to drug abusers. The [^{14}C]2-deoxyglucose (2-DG) method has been adopted for use in humans by positron emission tomography (PET) for visualization and measurement of radioactivity in brain regions after administration of short-lived radioactive tracers such as [^{18}F]2-DG. Whilst current PET instrumentation lacks the spatial resolution to visualize structures such as the accumbens, projection areas such as the limbic cortex can be visualized.

In an attempt to determine cerebral metabolism correlates of cocaine-induced euphoria, London *et al.* (1990a) used [^{18}F]2-DG to investigate the effects of cocaine hydrochloride on regional cerebral metabolism in polydrug abusers. Cocaine evoked reductions in glucose use in virtually all brain regions

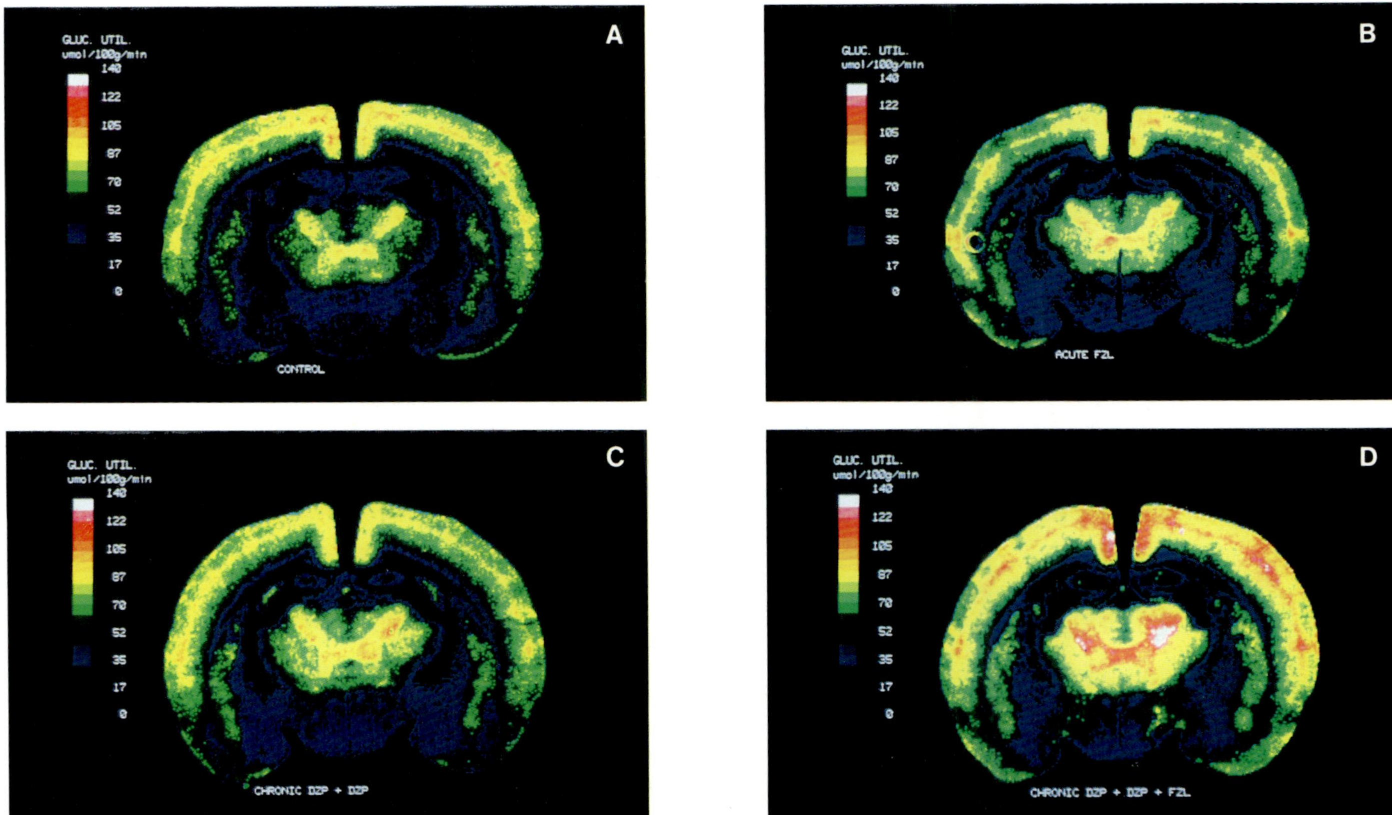

Figure 1 Autoradiograms prepared from coronal sections of rat brain showing the effect of flumazenil-precipitated withdrawal from diazepam on LCGU. A, control; B, 'acute' flumazenil (5 mg/kg); C, chronic diazepam (5 mg/kg i.p. daily for 28 days); D, chronic diazepam (5 mg/kg i.p. daily for 28 days) + flumazenil (5 mg/kg). Note that acute flumazenil does not evoke changes in LCGU compared to controls but precipitates marked increases in glucose use in the anterior thalamus and posterior cingulate cortex following chronic diazepam (Laurie and Pratt, 1990, 1991).

investigated (neocortex, basal ganglia and thalamus) with the exception of the pons and the cerebellum. Interestingly these findings contrast with those from animal data in which cocaine is generally found to stimulate LCGU in drug-naive rats (Porrino *et al.*, 1988; London *et al.*, 1986). The reasons for these differences are at present unclear.

In animal studies, cocaine evokes different patterns of LCGU depending on the dose employed (Porrino *et al.*, 1988). At doses of 0.5 mg/kg, changes in glucose use are restricted to the prefrontal cortex and nucleus accumbens, whereas 5.0 mg/kg produces widespread increases in glucose use, particularly in the extrapyramidal system. A decrease in glucose use, however, occurs in the lateral habenula. The psychostimulant amphetamine derivative methylenedioxymethamphetamine (MDMA, 'ecstasy') also evokes marked stimulation of glucose use in the extrapyramidal motor system and a decrease in glucose use in the lateral habenula. However, some other limbic structures display an increase in glucose use (Wilkerson and London, 1989). The authors conclude that some of the effects of MDMA upon glucose use resemble those previously described with cocaine, amphetamine and phencyclidine, implicating some common mechanism in the action of these drugs. Interestingly, in a recent study McBean *et al.* (1990) found that repeated administration of methylenedioxyamphetamine (MDA) produced profound increases in glucose use in the hippocampus and globus pallidus despite measuring cerebral metabolism several weeks after the last treatment. Such changes may be related to the known ability of this drug to destroy 5-HT nerve terminals. The significance of these findings to human drug abusers is presently unknown but clearly MDA can induce long-lasting alterations in cerebral functional activity.

1.6.2 Acute and chronic effects of psychotropic drugs

The acute effects of psychotropic drugs upon LCGU does not necessarily resolve which brain areas are associated with a particular psychopharmacological response to a drug. Many drugs evoke several different behavioural responses and these are mutually superimposed upon acute administration. London *et al.* (1988) reported increases in glucose use in selective structures of the limbic system, and in the basal ganglia and cerebellum, following acute administration of nicotine. They postulate that these changes may underlie the ability of nicotine to act as a reinforcer, to modulate memory and mood and to influence locomotor activity. Benzodiazepines and opiates evoke widespread reductions in LCGU (Beck *et al.*, 1989; Kelly *et al.*, 1986; Laurie and Pratt, 1989; Foster *et al.*, 1987) when administered acutely to animals or humans. The response in rats to morphine is less widespread if the drug is administered via pellets implanted subcutaneously (Kimes and London, 1989) rather than if administered intraperitoneally.

In summary, acute administration of several different drugs of abuse evokes widespread alterations in LCGU. These data are consistent with many neuronal systems being involved in the various acute psychopharmacological responses to a drug and the widespread distributions of nicotine, opiate and benzodiazepine receptors throughout the brain.

A strategy to identify the neuronal systems involved in the ability of a drug to modify a particular behavioural response is to perform the 2-DG technique in animals undergoing a behavioural task (e.g. rewarding brain stimulation) and evaluate the ability of drugs to modify activity in the affected neuronal systems (see above). An alternative strategy which has been employed in our laboratories to investigate the neuronal systems involved in benzodiazepine tolerance is to capitalize upon the knowledge that tolerance to the various effects of benzodiazepines proceeds at distinguishable rates. Tolerance to benzodiazepine-induced sedation occurs rapidly (within 3–5 days) whereas tolerance to the anxiolytic effect is not apparent until at least 2 weeks (for review see File, 1985). Using the 2-DG technique we have been able to functionally discriminate between neuronal structures and pathways involved in tolerance to diazepam-induced sedation and those involved in tolerance to its other effects. Following tolerance to the sedative effect (3 days pretreatment), structures of the auditory and visual pathways, together with some brainstem nuclei (e.g. locus coeruleus) and some target cortical areas, exhibited tolerance to the depressant effects of diazepam upon glucose use (Laurie and Pratt, 1989). By one month of treatment, tolerance had also occurred in some limbic structures such as the mammillary body and the subiculum, although glucose use remained depressed in hippocampal layers and in structures that provide inputs to the hippocampus. These data suggest that the outflow of neuronal activity from the hippocampus to the mammillary body is restored after chronic treatment and may implicate these pathways in tolerance to the anxiolytic effects of diazepam (Laurie and Pratt, 1989).

There have been very few studies that have investigated the chronic effects of other drugs of abuse upon LCGU and the relationship of any changes in glucose use with tolerance to specific behavioural effects.

London *et al.* (1990b) reported that animals receiving nicotine subcutaneously twice daily for 10 days displayed tolerance to the effects of a nicotine challenge upon glucose use in the VTA, some components of the visual pathway, the cerebellum and the vestibular nuclei. Interestingly, no regions showed sensitization despite some evidence of locomotor stimulation in these animals. In a different experimental design in which rats received nicotine by continuous infusion, Grunwald *et al.* (1988) demonstrated that both acute and chronic exposure to nicotine resulted in increases in glucose use in a few components of the visual and limbic system. However, in the globus pallidus and septal nucleus, nicotine evoked increases in LCGU only after chronic exposure. An obvious difference between the findings of the two studies is in the treatment protocols. Clearly further insights into the neural bases of nicotine-induced tolerance and dependence will be gained in future studies aimed at investigating temporal changes in psychopharmacological responses and correlating these with associated temporal changes in cerebral metabolism.

Chronic ethanol treatment has been shown to evoke a general depression of cerebral glucose use in thalamic, extrapyramidal and limbic structures (Nobrega *et al.*, 1987) although no correlations with behavioural responses were made. Using PET with [^{18}F]2-DG as the tracer, Volkow *et al.* (1990) found that acute ethanol inhibited cortical and cerebellar glucose metabolism but had little effect in the basal ganglia in alcoholics and normal volunteers. The inhibition was more pronounced in the alcoholics than in the controls.

1.6.3 Withdrawal from psychotropic drugs

A few studies have attempted to identify the neuronal systems functionally affected during withdrawal from psychotropic drugs in dependent animals, using quantitative 2-DG autoradiography.

A comparison of the patterns of LCGU responses evoked during withdrawal from phenobarbitone, diazepam and morphine is summarized in Table 3. Clearly the responses differ for the different drugs but in general the direction of the changes in glucose use are in the opposite direction to those occurring after acute drug administration. Withdrawal from phenobarbitone evokes marked increases in glucose use in motor, cortical and auditory and visual system structures with less effect in the limbic system (Marietta *et al.*, 1989). In contrast, naloxone-precipitated morphine withdrawal affects limbic system structures primarily (Kimes and London, 1989). Flumazenil-precipitated withdrawal from diazepam produces only modest rises in glucose use in some limbic, motor, auditory and visual system structures. However, pronounced increases occur in components of the Papez circuit (Figure 1) (Laurie and Pratt, 1990, 1991). This circuit would also appear to be important in diazepam tolerance and in the anxiogenic effects of the benzodiazepine receptor partial inverse agonist FG 7142 (Pratt *et al.*, 1988; Laurie and Pratt, 1989). It is noteworthy that withdrawal from phenobarbitone and morphine also evokes marked increases in LCGU in the Papez circuit. This circuit contains the subiculum, mammillary body, anterior thalamic nuclei and cingulate cortex and has been proposed as the neural substrate of emotion (Papez, 1937). Changes in this circuitry could therefore underlie some of the emotional responses related to anxiety during drug withdrawal. Interestingly, only morphine withdrawal evokes marked increases in LCGU in the mesolimbic reward pathway. Such changes could be associated with the craving for the drug during withdrawal.

Table 3 Function-related changes in glucose use during withdrawal from psychotropic drugs.

	Limbic system							
Drug withdrawal	Papez circuit	Septohippocampal formation	Other limbic	Mesolimbic 'reward' pathway	Basal ganglia and cerebellum	Auditory/visual system	Cerebral cortex	Ref.
Phenobarbitone (spontaneous)	↑↑	–	↑	–	↑↑	↑↑	↑↑	1
Diazepam (flumazenil precipitated)	↑↑	↑	↑	↑	↑	↑	–	2
Morphine (naloxone precipitated)	↑↑	↑↑	↑↑	↑↑	↑	↑	↑	3

↑, significant increases in LCGU compared to the vehicle and/or chronic drug-treated group; –, no significant effect.
Refs: 1, Marietta *et al.* (1989); 2, Laurie and Pratt (1990, 1991); 3, Kimes and London (1989).

Overall, it would appear that both common and separate neuronal systems are involved in withdrawal from psychotropic drugs of abuse. However, some caution should be made in drawing further conclusions because of the differences in the methods employed for inducing withdrawal (spontaneous or antagonist precipitated) and the differences in the severity of the behavioural syndromes induced by the different treatment regimes. Future research directed at correlating behavioural withdrawal responses with changes in LCGU will aid in our understanding of the neuronal systems involved and provide a rational basis for the development of drugs that might be useful in the treatment of the dependence process.

1.7 Strategies for the pharmacological treatment of drug dependence

Rational treatment for psychotropic drug tolerance and dependence rely upon the knowledge of (1) the critically important adaptive pharmacodynamic responses that occur after continued drug administration, (2) the neuroanatomical pathways important in the 'rewarding' effects of the drug, and (3) the neuroanatomical circuits important in the physical withdrawal symptoms. For many drugs of abuse this knowledge is incomplete. Any pharmacological treatment(s) must also take into account the relative contributions of the withdrawal distress, manifest in physical symptoms, as compared to the distress marked by craving, to the continuation of drug-taking behaviour. This will vary for each drug of abuse. Moreover, the treatment should not itself possess any rewarding properties, otherwise it will possess no advantages over current substitution therapies (e.g. methadone for morphine dependence).

For the opiate drugs, Bozarth and Wise (1984) have provided evidence that separate neural systems are involved in mediating the reinforcing effects of opiates versus the physical dependence-inducing effects. Drug-naive rats readily learned to self-administer morphine into the VTA. However, naloxone does not precipitate signs of physical dependence. In contrast, dependence is observed following morphine infusions into the periventricular grey region (PVG). Bozarth and Wise (1984) propose that the primary rewarding properties of morphine are independent of the drug's ability to produce physical dependence. However, Koob and Bloom (1988) argue that the nucleus accumbens is involved both in the aversive stimulus effects of withdrawal and in reward.

There is now good evidence for a role of the locus coeruleus in the expression of opiate withdrawal symptoms. It is speculated that the increased firing rate of locus coeruleus neurones demonstrated in morphine-dependent animals undergoing withdrawal may be a consequence of an initial action at the level of the PVG (see Chapter 7). The α_2-agonist clonidine can inhibit the changes in locus coeruleus activity during morphine withdrawal and suppress some of the symptoms of withdrawal (see Chapter 7). The pharmacological basis for this pharmacological approach to the treatment of opiate withdrawal is that α_2-adrenoceptors are coupled to the same potassium channels as opiate receptors in the locus coeruleus. However, if reward and physical dependence are mediated by distinct neuronal systems, attention should also be given to the treatment of the rewarding properties of drugs which lead to craving on withdrawal.

Another possible pharmacological strategy for the treatment of drug dependence is to prevent the adaptive pharmacodynamic responses that occur following repeated drug exposure. For example, intermittent administration of the benzodiazepine antagonist flumazenil during chronic benzodiazepine treatment appears to 're-set' the $GABA_A$ receptor, thereby reducing tolerance and attenuating withdrawal behaviours (see Chapter 3). Similarly, administration of calcium channel-blocking drugs during chronic ethanol treatment prevents the upregulation of calcium channel binding sites that occurs following chronic ethanol treatment (see Chapter 4). Whether such treatments prove useful in the clinic remains to be fully evaluated. One obvious problem is that they have to be administered concurrently with the psychotropic drug in questions. However, such drugs may be of benefit in the prevention of relapse (see Chapter 4).

Of critical importance to the treatment of drug dependence is to identify pharmacological agents that can prevent psychotropic drug craving. With the knowledge that the rewarding properties of a variety of drugs of abuse are associated with an alteration in the activity of the mesolimbic DA pathway, this system is an obvious drug target. 5-HT_3 antagonists have been reported to inhibit the enhancement of DA release from the nucleus accumbens evoked by drugs of abuse and to prevent conditioned place preference induced by morphine and nicotine (Imperato and Angelucci, 1989; Carboni *et al.*, 1989). Interestingly, these drugs are also able to prevent the behavioural suppression that occurs after withdrawal from chronic treatment with nicotine, ethanol, cocaine, and benzodiazepines (Costall *et al.*, 1990). Whether these effects translate to a useful effect in the clinic remains to be demonstrated. The recent findings that selective CCK_B antagonists can attenuate the behavioural signs of diazepam withdrawal (Hughes *et al.*, 1990), together with the knowledge that CCK can modify mesolimbic DA function (Marshall *et al.*, 1990), raise the possibility of the potential usefulness of CCK ligands in the treatment of drug dependence.

1.8 Concluding comments

This chapter has sought to provide an overview of the cellular and molecular adaptive processes that may underlie tolerance to and dependence upon a variety of drugs of abuse. In particular, any common mechanisms have been highlighted. In general it has not been possible to correlate changes in receptor density after chronic drug treatment with tolerance to the behavioural effects of a drug. Changes in receptor coupling and in activity of neuronal pathways downstream from the initial drug–receptor interaction are proposed to be a more likely explanation of tolerance and dependence. However, it is likely that no single neuronal adaptive process can account for the behavioural signs of tolerance and withdrawal and that there is a complex interaction between a number of processes; some of these may be necessary before others are initiated. One common feature of the majority of drugs of abuse is their ability to modulate activity of the mesolimbic reward pathway, albeit through differing mechanisms. Changes in activity of this pathway may relate to the 'craving' that occurs during drug withdrawal. However, many other neuronal pathways are likely to be recruited during tolerance and withdrawal. It is activity in these pathways that is responsible for the characteristic dependence syndrome observed for each drug class. Some of the neuronal systems affected may be common to several drugs of abuse. Information on the functionally important neuronal pathways, together with the critically important adaptive processes that occur at the receptor level, is crucial to our further understanding of drug tolerance and dependence. The success of future strategies for the treatment of drug dependence will depend on the integrated approach of neuroscientists employing a variety of experimental approaches in the identification of these mechanisms.

Acknowledgements

I would like to take this opportunity to thank Dr D. Laurie and Dr R. Brett for their contribution to the 2-deoxyglucose experiments concerning benzodiazepine tolerance and dependence reported in this chapter. These investigations were supported by the Wellcome Trust.

References

Aghajanian, G.K. & Wang, Y.Y. (1986) *Brain Res.* **371**, 390–394.
Beck, T., Wenzel, J., Kuschinsky, K. & Krieglstein, J. (1989) *Brain Res.* **497**, 205–213.

Benwell, M.E.M., Balfour, D.J.K. & Anderson, J.M. (1988) *J. Neurochem.* **50**, 1243–1247.

Bozarth, M.A. & Wise, R.A. (1981) *Life Sci.* **28**, 551–555.

Bozarth, M.A. & Wise, R.A. (1984) *Science* **224**, 516–517.

Carboni, L., Acquas, E., Leone, P. & Di Chiara, G. (1989) *Psychopharmacology* **97**, 175–178.

Chen, J.P., Paredes, W., Li, J., Smith, D., Lowinson, J. & Gardner, E.L. (1990) *Psychopharmacology* **102**, 156–162.

Costall, B., Jones, B.J., Kelly, M.E., Naylor, R.J., Onaivi, E.S. & Tyers, M.B. (1990) *Pharmacol. Biochem. Behav.* **36**, 339–344.

Crawley, J.N. (1988) *Ann. N.Y. Acad. Sci.* **537**, 380–396.

Dackis, C.A. & Gold, M.S. (1985) *Neurosci. Biobehav. Rev.* **9**, 469–477.

Di Chiara, G. & Imperato, A. (1988) *Proc. Natl Acad. Sci. USA* **85**, 5274–5278.

Dworkin, S.I., Guerin, G.F., Co, C., Goeders, N.E. & Smith, J.E. (1988) *Pharmacol. Biochem. Behav.* **30**, 1051–1057.

Eposito, R.U., Porrino, L.J., Seeger, T.F., Crane, A.M., Everist, H.D. & Pert, A. (1984) *Proc. Natl Acad. Sci. USA* **81**, 635–639.

File, S.E. (1985) *Neurosci. Biobehav. Rev.* **9**, 113–121.

Foster, N.L., Van Der Spek, F.L., Aldrich, M.S., Berent, S., Hichwa, R.H., Sakellares, J.C., Gilman, S. & Agranoff, B.W. (1987) *J. Cereb. Blood Flow Metab.* **7**, 415–420.

Fung, Y.K. (1989) *J. Pharm. Pharmacol.* **41**, 66–68.

Gallager, D.W., Lakoski, J., Gonsalves, S. & Rauch, S. (1984) *Nature* **308**, 74–77.

Goudie, A.J. & Emmett-Oglesby, M.W. (eds) (1989) *Psychoactive Drugs: Tolerance and Sensitization.* Clifton, New Jersey, Humana Press.

Grunwald, F., Schrock, H., Theilen, H., Biber, A. & Kuschinsky, W. (1988) *Brain Res.* **456**, 350–356.

Haefely, W. (1988) In *Chloride Channels and their Modulation by Neurotransmitters and Drugs* (eds Biggio, G. & Costa, E.), pp 275–292. New York, Raven Press.

Haefely, W., Martin, J.R. & Schoh, P. (1990) *Trends Pharmacol. Sci.* **11**, 452–456.

Heninger, C. & Gallager, D.W. (1988) *Neuropharmacology* **27**, 1073–1076.

Heninger, C., Saito, N., Tallman, J.F., Garrett, K.M., Vitek, M.P., Duman, R.S. & Gallager, D.W. (1990) *J. Mol. Neurosci.* **2**, 101–107.

Hokfelt, T., Skirboll, L., Rehfeld, J.F., Goldstein, H., Markey, K. & Dann, O. (1980) *Neuroscience* **5**, 2093–2124.

Hubner, C.B. & Koob, G.F. (1990) *Brain Res.* **508**, 20–29.

Hughes, J., Boden, P., Costall, B., Domeney, A., Kelly, E., Horwell, D.C., Hunter, J.C., Pinnock, R.D. & Woodruff, G.N. (1990) *Proc. Natl Acad. Sci. USA* **87**, 6728–6732.

Hurd, Y.L., Weiss, F., Koob, G.F., And, N.-E. & Ungerstedt, U. (1989) *Brain Res.* **498**, 199–203.

Imperato, A. & Angelucci, L. (1989) *Neurosci. Lett.* **101**, 214–217.

Imperato, A., Mulas, A. & Di Chiara, G. (1986) *Eur. J. Pharmacol.* **175**, 211–214.

Iversen, S..D. (1984) *Neuropharmacology* **23**, 1553–1560.

Johnston, A.L. & File, S.E. (1986) *Pharmacol. Biochem. Behav.* **24**, 1467–1470.

Kelly, P.A., Ford, I. & McCulloch, J. (1986) *Neuroscience* **19**, 257–265.

Kimes, A.S. & London, E.D. (1989) *J. Pharmacol. Exp. Ther.* **248**, 538–545.

Kirch, D.G., Gerhardt, G.A., Shelton, R.C., Freedman, R. & Watt, R.J. (1987) *Clin. Neuropharmacol.* **10**, 376–383.

Koob, G.F. & Bloom, F.E. (1988) *Science* **242**, 715–723.

Kornetsky, C., Lyons, D., Bain, G., Sokoloff, L. & Porrino, L.J. (1989) *J. Cereb. Blood Flow Metab.* **9**, Suppl. 1, S334.

Kuczenski, R. (1983) In *Stimulants: Neurochemical, Behavioural and Clinical Perspectives* (ed. Creese, I.), pp 31–61. New York, Raven Press.
Lader, M.H. & File, S.E. (1987) *Psychol. Med.* **17**, 539–547.
Laurie, D.J. & Pratt, J.A. (1989) *Brain Res.* **504**, 101–111.
Laurie, D.J. & Pratt, J.A. (1990) *Br. J. Pharmacol.* **99**, 134P.
Laurie, D.J. & Pratt, J.A. (1991) *Psychopharmacology*. Submitted.
Lett, B.T. (1989) *Psychopharmacology* **98**, 357–362.
Littleton, J., Harper, J., Hudspith, M., Pagonis, C., Dolin, S.J. & Little, H.J. (1988) *Psychopharmacology of Addiction* (ed. Lader, M.), pp 60–72. Oxford University Press, Oxford.
London, E.D., Wilkerson, G., Goldberg, S.R. & Risner, M.E. (1986) *Neurosci. Lett.* **68**, 73–78.
London, E.D., Connolly, R.J., Szikszay, M., Wamsley, J.K. & Dam, M. (1988) *J. Neurosci.* **8**, 3920–3928.
London, E.D., Cascella, N.G., Wong, D.F., Phillips, R.L., Dannals, R.F., Links, J.M., Herning, R., Grayson, R., Jaffe, J.H. & Wagner, H.N. (1990a) *Arch. Gen. Psychiatry* **47**, 567–574.
London, E.D., Fanelli, R.J., Kimes, A.S. & Moses, R.L. (1990b) *Brain Res.* **520**, 208–214.
Luddens, H. & Wisden, W. (1991) *Trends Pharmacol. Sci.* **12**, 49–51.
Marietta, C.A., Wixan, H.N., Weight, F.F. & Eckardt, M.J. (1989) *Brain Res.* **496**, 173–179.
Marks, M.J., Romm, E., Gaffney, D.K. & Collins, A.C. (1986) *J. Pharmacol. Exp. Ther.* **237**, 809–819.
Marshall, F.H., Barnes, S., Pinnock, R.D. & Hughes, J. (1990) *Br. J. Pharmacol.* **99**, 845–848.
McBean, D.E., Sharkey, J., Ritchie, I.M. & Kelly, P.A. (1990) *Neuroscience* **38**, 271–275.
Mele, L., Sagratella, S. & Massotti, M. (1984) *Brain Res.* **323**, 93–102.
Mereu, G., Yoon, K.-W.P., Boi, V., Gessa, G.L., Naes, L. & Westfall, T.C. (1987) *Eur. J. Pharmacol.* **141**, 395–399.
Mierlak, D. & Farb, D.H. (1988) *J. Neurosci.* **8**, 814–820.
Morrow, A.L., Montpied, P., Lingford-Hughes, A. & Paul, S.M. (1990) *Alcohol* **7**, 237–244.
Nobrega, J.N., Toepell, A.P. & Rakoff, V. (1987) *Exp. Neurol.* **95**, 303–312.
Nordberg, A., Wahlstrom, G., Arnelo, U. & Larsson, C. (1985) *Drug Alcohol Depend.* **16**, 9–17.
North, R.A., Williams, J.T., Suprenant, A. & Christie, M.J. (1987) *Proc. Natl Acad. Sci. USA* **84**, 5487–5491.
Nutt, D. (1986) *Trends Pharmacol. Sci.* **7**, 457–460.
Nutt, D. (1990) In *Current Aspects of the Neurosciences*, Vol. 2 (ed. Osborne, N.N.), pp 259–293. Macmillan Press, London.
O'Brien, D.P. & White, F.J. (1987) *Eur. J. Pharmacol.* **142**, 343–354.
Olsen, R. & Venter, J. (eds) (1986) *Benzodiazepine-GABA Receptors and Chloride Channels: Structural and Functional Properties*. New York, Alan R. Liss.
Overstreet, D.H. & Yamamura, H.I. (1979) *Life. Sci.* **25**, 1865–1878.
Papez, J.W. (1937) *Arch. Neurol. Psychiatr.* **38**, 725–743.
Pettit, H.O. & Mueller, K. (1989) *Psychopharmacology* **99**, 423–426.
Pettit, H.O., Ettenberg, A., Bloom, F.E. & Koob, G.F. (1984) *Psychopharmacology* **84**, 167–173.
Pettit, H.O., Par, H.-T., Parsons, L.H. & Justice, J.B. (1990) *J. Neurochem.* **55**, 798–804.

Piazza, P.V., Deminiere, J., Le Moal, M. & Simon, H. (1989) *Science* **245**, 1511–1513.
Porrino, L.J., Domer, F.R., Crane, A.M. & Sokoloff, L. (1988) *Neuropsychopharmacology* **1**, 109–118.
Poste, G. & Crooke, S.T. (1985) *Mechanisms of Receptor Regulation*. New York, Plenum Press.
Pratt, J.A., Jenner, P. & Marsden, C.D. (1985) *Neuropharmacology* **24**, 59–68.
Pratt, J.A., Laurie, D.J. & McCulloch, J. (1988) *Brain Res.* **475**, 218–231.
Pritchett, D.B., Luddens, H. & Seeburg, P.H. (1989) *Science* **245**, 1389–1392.
Ritz, M.C., Lamb, J., Goldberg, S.R. & Kuhar, M.J. (1987) *Science* **237**, 1219–1223.
Robinson, T.E. (1991) In *The Biological Basis of Substance Abuse* (eds Barchas, J. & Korenman, S.) Oxford University Press, New York. In press.
Robinson, T.E. & Camp, D.M. (1990) *Neuropsychopharmacology* **3**, 163–173.
Roca, D.J., Rozenberg, I., Farrant, M. & Farb, D.H. (1990a) *Mol. Pharmacol.* **37**, 37–43.
Roca, D.J., Schiller, G.D., Friedman, L., Rozenberg, I., Gibbs, T.T. & Farb, D.H. (1990b) *Mol. Pharmacol.* **37**, 710–719.
Rosenberg, H.C. & Chiu, T.H. (1981) *Eur. J. Pharmacol.* **70**, 453–460.
Roth, R.H., Tam, S.-Y., Yoshishige, I., Yang, J.-X. & Deutch, A.Y. (1988) *Ann. N.Y. Acad. Sci.* **537**, 138–147.
Rowell, P.P., Carr, L.A. & Garner, A.C. (1987) *J. Neurochem.* **49**, 1449–1454.
Scatton, B., D'Angio, M., Driscoll, P. & Serrano, A. (1988) *Ann, N.Y. Acad. Sci.* **537**, 124–137.
Sharp, T., Zetterstrom, T., Ljungberg, T. & Ungerstedt, U. (1987) *Brain Res.* **401**, 322–330.
Sokoloff, L., Reivich, M., Kennedy, C., Des Rosiers, M.H., Patlak, C.S., Pettigrew, K.D., Sakurada, O. & Shinohara, M. (1977) *J. Neurochem.* **28**, 897–916.
Spyraki, C. & Fibiger, H.C. (1988) *Psychopharmacology* **94**, 133–137.
Spyraki, C., Nomikos, G.G., Galanopoulo, P. & Daifotis, Z. (1988) *Behav. Brain Res.* **29**, 127–134.
Study, R.E. & Barker, J.L. (1981) *Proc. Natl Acad. Sci. USA* **78**, 7180–7184.
Ticku, M.K. & Burch, T. (1980) *J. Neurochem.* **34**, 417–423.
Tietz, E.I., Rosenberg, H.C. & Chiu, T.H. (1986) *J. Pharmacol. Exp. Ther.* **236**, 284–292.
Volkow, N.D., Hitzemann, R., Wolf, A.P., Logan, J., Fowler, J.S. & Christman, D. (1990) *Psychiatry Res.* **35**, 39–48.
Walaas, I. & Fonnum, F. (1980) *Neuroscience* **5**, 63–72.
Wang, R.Y. (1988) *Ann. N.Y. Acad. Sci.* **537**, 362–379.
Werling, L.L., McMahon, P.N. & Cox, B.M. (1989) *Proc. Natl Acad. Sci. USA* **86**, 6393–6397.
Wilkerson, G. & London, E.D. (1989) *Neuropharmacology* **28**, 1129–1138.
Wise, R.A. (1990) In *Psychotropic Drugs of Abuse* (International Encyclopedia of Pharmacology and Therapeutics—section 130) (ed. Balfour, D.J.K.), pp 23–58. New York, Pergamon Press.
Wonnacott, S. (1987) *Hum. Toxicol.* **6**, 343–353.
Wood, P.L. (1982) *J. Pharmacol. Exp. Ther.* **222**, 674–679.

CHAPTER 2

CLINICAL FEATURES OF DRUG TOLERANCE AND DEPENDENCE

David J. Nutt, Paul Glue and David Ball

Reckitt and Colman Psychopharmacology Unit, School of Medical Sciences, University Walk, Bristol BS8 1TD

Table of Contents

2.1 Introduction

This chapter will provide an overview of clinical aspects associated with use or abuse of psychotropic drugs, concentrating on tolerance, dependence and withdrawal. It is beyond the scope of this chapter to describe in detail economic, epidemiological or anthropological aspects of drug use; however, it is salutary to mention such issues, to place them in perspective. Firstly, the use of drugs which produce psychological effects is almost universal. In Western cultures, it would be unusual to find people who have never once used coffee, alcohol, or tobacco. In non-Western cultures, the prevalence of fermented drinks and use of naturally occurring psychotropics, such as khat, coca leaves, or hallucinogenic plants, is common (Ghodse, 1989). Secondly, use of psychotropics is not confined to man. Other mammalian species in the wild are known to seek out and self-administer substances which subsequently alter

THE BIOLOGICAL BASES OF DRUG TOLERANCE AND DEPENDENCE
ISBN 0-12-564250-4

their behaviour. There are supporting data from many research groups world-wide, who have shown that under laboratory conditions mammalian species from rodents to monkeys will self-administer drugs. Perhaps a feature of mammalian species is the capability and the desire to experience the effects of mind-altering drugs.

2.1.1 Definition of terms

Tolerance is perhaps the easiest of the terms to define. It is a state whereby repeated exposure to a drug produces smaller effects, or larger doses are required to produce similar effects to those produced after initial administration. It may be caused by changes in the rate in which the drug is distributed or metabolized in the body, or by adaptational processes occurring in the brain (see also Chapter 1). Although tolerance may occur over different time-courses (e.g. acute tolerance occurring within minutes to hours versus chronic tolerance developing after prolonged drug administration), the latter phenomenon is more important clinically and will be discussed here. Another important feature of tolerance is that of cross-tolerance. If tolerance to one type of drug (e.g. depressants) occurs, tolerance to other, chemically dissimilar depressants will usually also be present. This has been clearly demonstrated for alcohol, benzodiazepines, barbiturates and other hypnosedative drugs, and forms the basis for substitution treatment of dependency.

Drug dependence and drug abuse are terms whose definitions are more problematic, due to the interactive nature of the various components (behavioural, cognitive, physiological and social) that appear to contribute to them. Dependence has been defined by the World Health Organization (1981) as 'a state, psychic and sometimes also physical, resulting from the interaction between a living organism and a drug, characterized by behavioural and other responses that always include a compulsion to take the drug on a continuous or periodic basis in order to experience psychic effects, and sometimes to avoid the discomfort of its absence. Tolerance may or may not be present'. Clearly this definition includes several different constructs, some psychic and some physical. Alternatives which emphasize clinical factors are those of Edwards (1982), and the rather similar DSM-III-R (American Psychiatric Association, 1987) diagnostic criteria for Psychoactive Substance Dependence. Important features include:

(i) a subjective awareness or compulsion to use a drug, often related to unsuccessful efforts to reduce drug intake;
(ii) continued drug use despite awareness of harmful effects to (e.g.) physical health, social functioning, etc.;
(iii) priority of drug taking or obtaining drugs over other activities, limiting normal social or work roles;

(iv) the development of tolerance and withdrawal symptoms;
(v) after abstinence, dependence may recur rapidly with reuse of the drug.

In the above definitions, a distinction is made between physical and psychological dependence. This often causes confusion, which stems from a dualist approach to mind and body, which is unhelpful. Although psychological dependence may not manifest physical or structural changes in the body, we must assume that changes have occurred in the brain at a molecular or receptor level.

Central to the definition of psychological dependence is the compulsion to repeatedly take a drug. Clinically, this may be manifest by craving. Although this is a difficult construct to define, there are two components to this phenomenon. One component involves a dysphoric mood state related to inability to get access to a desired drug, and the other involves a pleasurable state of anticipation prior to taking it. Both components may be motivating factors, and individuals may experience both states at different times, or they may alternate over a short period of time.

In contrast, physical dependence is only seen in the relative absence of a drug, when a range of physical and psychic symptoms, a withdrawal state, is present. The ease and degree to which withdrawal symptoms develop defines the liability of a particular drug to produce physical dependence. As a generalization, the withdrawal syndrome seen after cessation of a drug tends to be opposite to the symptoms produced by acute administration of that drug (e.g. anxiety, insomnia and arousal seen after withdrawal of hypnosedatives; depression and lethargy after withdrawal of stimulants). Physical and psychological dependence may be distinguished clinically; for instance, abrupt cessation of tricyclic antidepressants produces a hyperautonomic state, with no evidence of psychological dependence, whereas nicotine withdrawal produces predominantly psychological changes, with minimal physical symptoms.

The major difference between drug abuse and drug dependence is quantitative. The DSM-III-R (American Psychiatric Association, 1987) uses the former term to describe people who have a maladaptive pattern of drug use of insufficient severity to qualify them for a diagnosis of drug dependence. In practice, it is difficult to clearly distinguish abusers and those who are dependent. It might be argued that for illegal drugs, use of a single dose could be considered abuse, in that social or occupational problems (e.g. arrest) could arise by virtue of the drug's illegality. For legally available drugs, such as alcohol, levels below the present legal limit to drive have been shown to impair psychophysiological testing (Baloh *et al.*, 1979). This would make it difficult to set a limit distinguishing use and abuse.

Tolerance and dependence are commonly assumed to occur together, but there are circumstances where they may be separated. For instance, after administration of very long acting opioid agonists, tolerance may be seen without a particularly marked withdrawal syndrome (physical dependence). This is presumably due to the rate of clearance of the drug being sufficiently slow to allow recovery from the central adaptation of receptors. Tolerance and dependence have also been distinguished pharmacologically. Studies that have shown the involvement of monoamine neurotransmitters in tolerance development to alcohol have demonstrated no effect on the alcohol withdrawal syndrome (for review see Nutt and Glue, 1986).

In discussing dependence, it is clear that pharmacological factors alone cannot account for this complex state. Personality, cognitive, environmental and other influences are important in the development and maintenance of dependency. Although a comprehensive discussion of the role of these factors is outside the scope of this chapter, they will be briefly mentioned below.

2.1.2 Predisposing factors

Much has been written on aspects of personality, relationships, and social environment that might predispose to dependency, the majority in relation to non-prescription drugs and alcohol. For instance, amongst a possibly representative sample of US narcotic addicts, 93% had another psychiatric diagnosis in addition to substance abuse, most commonly depression (56%) or personality disorder (65%) (Khantzian and Treece, 1985). The category of personality disorder noted in narcotic addicts was noted to be heterogeneous, with a predominance of antisocial personality disorder (Khantzian and Treece, 1985; Rounsaville *et al.*, 1982). In a large prospective study from the US looking at marijuana and cocaine use, it was noted that factors associated with starting to take drugs and persistent drug taking in adult life were similar. These included being part of a social group where drug taking was accepted, and participating in delinquent behaviour (Kandel and Raveis, 1989). Studies looking at premorbid personality characteristics in alcoholics suggest that a range of aggressive, impulsive and antisocial features are seen in boys or young men prior to adult alcoholism (Jones, 1968; McCord *et al.*, 1962; Vaillant, 1983). The importance of economic factors on rates of alcoholism has also been demonstrated (Kendell, 1979; Kendell *et al.*, 1983).

There are fewer studies looking at factors associated with dependence on nicotine and caffeine, and prescribed psychotropics. In a large prospective study, it was reported that subjects who subsequently started smoking had higher neuroticism scores on the Maudsley Personality Inventory (Cherry and Kiernan, 1978). Older studies have generally shown that established smokers have higher neuroticism scores (review: Warburton, 1988).

Although tentative, it is possible to describe two broad personality groups that are associated with drug dependency. The first type has antisocial

Table 1

Drug	Tolerance	Psychological dependence (abuse/craving)	Physical dependence (withdrawal)
Hypnosedatives			
alcohol	++	++	++
benzodiazepines (high dose)	++	+	+
benzodiazepines (therapeutic dose)	?+	0	+?
barbiturates	++	+	++
Opiates	++	++	++
Psychostimulants	++	++	++
Caffeine	+	?+	+
Nicotine	+	++	+

0, absent; +, present; ?, uncertain.

personality features, and the second is marked with traits of personal anxiety and dependence (Ashton, 1989; Tyrer, 1989).

Genetic factors have been less explored, although this situation is now being rectified in the light of recent evidence that alcoholism may be inherited. Scandinavian adoption studies have revealed different subtypes of the disease, some of which are highly heritable (Cloninger *et al.*, 1989). The high incidence in certain racial groups (e.g. American Indians) may also suggest genetic predisposition, although environmental factors are hard to rule out. Similar studies would be possible, although harder to perform, for other forms of substance abuse. Environmental factors are involved in drug tolerance and withdrawal. This issue has been well evaluated by a number of groups (Siegel, 1988).

The remainder of this chapter examines clinical aspects of tolerance to and dependence in the range of commonly used psychoactive substances. A summary of this is given in Table 1.

2.2 Hypnosedatives

2.2.1 Alcohol

Abuse of alcohol, with its multiple physical and social consequences, is one of the great medical problems of today. It is well established that there is a close relationship between intake and indices of physical damage, and that in a population, intake is determined predominantly by cost (Kendell, 1979). Nevertheless, even in societies where alcohol is severely restricted or expensive, abuse and dependence are still recognized, reflecting the enormous attraction of alcohol. This attraction develops in the face of adverse actions, such as nausea, vomiting, and hangover, and in part develops as tolerance to these side-effects is manifest. However, tolerance also develops to the reinforcing properties and dosage escalation is usual.

The reasons why people use alcohol vary. A wide spectrum of motivating factors can be identified. At one end there is anxiety reduction; hence alcohol abuse and dependence is frequently seen in patients with anxiety disorders. The routine use of alcohol in social gatherings such as parties is partly indicative of its anxiolytic properties. At the other extreme, alcoholics drink for oblivion, a state not dissimilar to anaesthesia. In between lie the euphoriant effects of alcohol, which have some similarities with those produced by opioids and stimulants (Nutt, 1988).

Alcohol dependence has been well described (Edwards, 1982). Core features include increasing importance of alcohol in daily activities, narrowing of drinking repertoire, constriction of social activities to fit in with access to alcohol, and impairment of work and social performance. In parallel, other features such as tolerance development, withdrawal, and relief drinking practices to suppress withdrawal symptoms are seen. Subjective compulsion to drink is usually present, but may be hard to elicit, since denial is actively practised. Approaches to such craving are in their infancy, although drugs such as lithium (Clarke and Fawcett, 1989) and alcohol dehydrogenase inhibitors (Antabuse and Abstem) have been tried with mixed results. More recently research has focused upon a possible role for 5-HT in craving, based on data that 5-HT reuptake inhibitors can reduce intake in heavy social drinkers (Naranjo and Sellers, 1989).

Although alcohol withdrawal symptomatology has been described for many years, (Isbell *et al.*, 1955; Victor and Adams, 1953), it is only recently that the relationship has been established between the development of withdrawal symptoms and absent or reduced levels of alcohol in the body. Withdrawal symptoms do not develop unless there is a prolonged and heavy history of alcohol intake, and they tend to become more severe as drinking continues (Ballenger and Post, 1978). Alcohol withdrawal symptoms occur at particular times after stopping or reducing alcohol intake, rather than occurring randomly or simultaneously (Victor and Adams, 1953). For instance, symptoms such as anxiety, tremor and sweating, which are associated with increased sympathetic drive, tend to be maximal 24 hours after stopping drinking. Seizures occur most commonly 24–48 hours after the last drink. Delirium tremens, a state of vivid hallucinations, autonomic overactivity, severe agitation and delirium, is seen 48–72 hours after the cessation of drinking (Victor and Adams, 1953). The mechanisms underlying withdrawal have become better understood in the last decade (Glue and Nutt, 1990).

2.2.2 Benzodiazepines

Benzodiazepine dependence is a subject of much controversy at present, with imminent law suits against doctors and drug companies from patients claiming they have been seriously affected by inappropriate prescribing of these drugs. Putting aside the legal situation, what evidence is there that benzodiazepines cause dependence? This has to be assessed from two viewpoints, high-dose and normal-dose usage. While it is known that very high doses administered for weeks or months will lead to physical withdrawal (Hollister *et al.*, 1961) there is little evidence that these drugs are used in this fashion. Indeed, in a series of careful studies performed on drug-experienced volunteers, Griffiths *et al.* (1980, 1984) have demonstrated that benzodiazepines are perceived as less rewarding than similar compounds such as the barbiturates. However, there is a 'black market' in some benzodiazepines, especially diazepam, and it appears that the reinforcing properties of this and certain other benzodiazepines, such as triazolam, may reflect their pharmacokinetic profile of rapid brain entry. Overall the 'street value' of benzodiazepines is low in comparison with other abused drugs, which confirms a relative lack of 'buzz'. These issues are well discussed in the definitive review by Woods *et al.* (1987).

Interestingly, certain preparations of temazepam have become more abused recently as addicts of other harder drugs have discovered that they can aspirate the benzodiazepine/propylene glycol contents of the capsules and directly intravenously inject them. This has led to these preparations being replaced by others with a solid core.

In the clinical situation a relatively small percentage of users escalate their dosage beyond what is normally considered the therapeutic maximum (for anxiety) of 30 mg diazepam equivalents/day (Dunbar *et al.*, 1989). Those who do appear to be either those with previous addictions (including alcoholism) or those with severe anxiety, especially panic disorder. In the latter case we suspect that the need for high doses reflects the resistance of this illness to conventional doses, perhaps because of an underlying abnormality of benzodiazepine receptor function that attenuates the action of agonist benzodiazepines (Nutt *et al.*, 1990). Almost certainly, the addict is using higher doses to offset the tolerance that develops to the 'buzz'.

Normal dose dependence was first reported in the late 1970s, and this led to much of the present concern with the prolonged clinical use of benzodiazepines (Petursson and Lader, 1981a, b, 1984). Studies from several centres have revealed that a proportion of patients, who had been on standard therapeutic doses of benzodiazepines for months or years, develop withdrawal symptoms on stopping. At first these findings were criticized as merely revealing the recrudescence of the original anxiety (Merz and Ballmer, 1983). However, the emergence of new symptoms such as visual illusions and seizures argued against that being the sole explanation (Petursson and Lader, 1984; Nutt, 1986). In addition it is possible to detect signs of mild withdrawal in volunteers who have been on high 'therapeutic' doses for several weeks (Brosan *et al.*, 1986). Thus a short-lasting withdrawal reaction does seem to have been established, although most authorities agree that it is only problematic in about a third of chronic users. This is thought to reflect underlying personality traits (Tyrer *et al.*, 1983; Tyrer, 1989; Ashton, 1989), although it may be an indication of inherited differences in benzodiazepine receptor function, as has been shown in animals (Nutt and Lister, 1988). Moreover it should be pointed out that there has not yet been a controlled study of long-term use in a patient population that has been fully assessed at the outset of treatment, so we cannot be certain what influence premorbid psychology and illness has on the likelihood of developing new symptoms in withdrawal. Many of the symptoms thought to be unique to benzodiazepine withdrawal have recently been shown to be surprisingly common in a general population (Rodrigo and Williams, 1986). One exception is, of course, seizures.

The contribution that mild/subclinical withdrawal makes to perpetuating 'normal dose dependence' is also unclear. It has been suggested that recurrent mini-withdrawals might be self-medicated and thus lead to a vicious cycle of repeated medication. Testing such a theory in a population with an illness that is as chronic as anxiety may be impossible. Similar problems apply to understanding the actions of benzodiazepines in epilepsy where tolerance is seen in many cases and rebound seizures can also occur (Haigh and Feely, 1988).

2.2.3 Barbiturates

The addictive potential of barbiturates and similar compounds such as meprobamate is substantially greater than that of the benzodiazepines. This observation, coupled with a lesser ratio of safety in overdose, led to the virtual extinction of the barbiturate class of drugs as treatments of psychological illness, particularly anxiety (Tyrer, 1982). Laboratory studies have confirmed these clinically derived observations, as barbiturates are better liked and given a higher 'street value' by drug-experienced volunteers (Griffiths *et al.*, 1980). This is probably a consequence of their pharmacokinetic and pharmacodynamic properties, with fast brain entry and high efficacy both contributing.

Physical dependence is well recognized and a withdrawal syndrome similar to that reported for benzodiazepines, but generally more severe, has long been apparent (Isbell *et al.*, 1950). Why chronic barbiturate users should not complain about the long-term sequelae of use, as seemingly some benzodiazepine users do, is a mystery. Sadly, the concern and publicity about benzodiazepines has led to some prescribers reverting to barbiturates in the misguided belief that they may be safer.

2.3 Opiates

These are the classically addictive drugs of pushers and poets! It would appear that both groups use them for their ability to promote visions of better places, as an escape from the mundanity of the real world. However, there has been a tendency for the target of users to evolve from transcendental inspiration towards the more immediate 'buzz' or 'rush'. Thus means of accelerating the entry of opiate into the brain have been devised which include intravenous injections and smoking ('chasing the dragon'). To perhaps a greater extent than with any of the other abused drugs the cultural aspects of opiate use have major impacts on the rewards of their use. Thus in some environments needle sharing, despite the attendant risks of AIDS, is an essential part of the pleasure. However, there are addicts who have become addicted as a result of therapeutically administered analgesics. These, now only a small proportion of registered addicts, and an even smaller fraction of total users, persist in taking opiates on account of physical dependence, i.e. they are unable to cope with withdrawal. For the majority, though unpleasant, withdrawal is not the main reason why users find it so hard to desist. Rather it is the sense of pleasure and escape that these drugs offer, coupled with great peer-group pressure and intense situational craving. The latter would appear to be a conditioned experience in which visual or auditory stimuli associated with previous 'highs' can evoke a surge of pleasurable memories. These memories, and the contrast between them and the usual more mundane state of the user, naturally accentuate the desire to experience them yet again (O'Brien *et al.*, 1986).

There are thus at least three factors controlling opiate usage: the 'high' or reinforcing action, craving and the fear/fact of withdrawal. Opiates are reinforcing via an action at μ-receptors (Martin, 1967). Tolerance to this action is common and results in an escalation of usage so that a single addict may generate a habit of up to a gram a day. The fact that the opiate 'high' is produced by activation of central μ-receptors is the basis of treatments with opiate antagonists such as naloxone, or more usually its long-acting relative naltrexone. Blockade of μ-receptors prevents their occupation by agonists such as morphine or heroin and thus these cease to be reinforcing (Mello *et al.*,

1981). Extinction of drug-taking behaviour should then ensue since the act of administration is not associated with any pleasurable consequences. In practice this approach works but there are problems. Naltrexone has to be taken regularly, generally under supervision; it can lead to side-effects such as hepatitis and depression; it is generally not liked, due in part to its completely preventing any pleasurable experiences with agonists and in part to its intrinsic anhedonic properties.

Several alternative options to naltrexone are under investigation. One possibility is the development of long-acting antagonists that could perhaps be given only once weekly or less. A second is the use of substitutes such as methadone. This replacement of a 'street' drug with one of similar potency given orally, that can only be obtained from a clinic, has some appeal. However, it can be construed by addicts and society as encouraging drug taking for pleasure, and methadone can be sold to other addicts if its use is not properly supervised. The third option is the use of partial μ-agonists such as buprenorphine. This compound binds very tightly to the μ-receptor and thus has the ability to prevent full agonists accessing it (Cowan *et al.*, 1977). Hence the reinforcing properties of agonists are blocked, as with naltrexone. However, the intrinsic partial μ-activity may improve patient compliance by providing some partial reinforcement, and perhaps avoiding the depressant actions of naltrexone. Studies with buprenorphine reveal it to be a very effective suppressor of heroin self-administration (Mello *et al.*, 1981, 1982) and, of course, it will be much safer in overdose, since it is intrinsically less capable of producing respiratory depression. However, even a weak partial agonist like buprenorphine can give a 'buzz' when given intravenously, and the solubility of buprenorphine has led to some diversion of analgesic supplies for this purpose (Lewis, 1985). A possible solution lies in an appropriate combination with naltrexone. When taken orally, the buprenorphine will predominate and the naltrexone will not be noticed. However, if given intravenously the naltrexone will have preferential access to the CNS, will precipitate withdrawal if other opiates are present, and will block the reinforcing actions of buprenorphine. Such an approach is still only theoretical, but could readily be examined in the clinic. Impetus to such a development is given by the unexpected finding that when used to treat heroin addicts, buprenorphine, but not methadone, markedly reduced cocaine usage as well (Kosten *et al.*, 1989a, b). Since mixtures of opiates and cocaine (speedballs) are in common use, a compound that blocked the actions of both drugs would be of especial benefit.

Opiate withdrawal is now well characterized in animal models and appears to be due to a rebound release of inhibition, particularly in the noradrenergic cells of the locus coeruleus (Taylor *et al.*, 1988). This explains the efficacy of the α_2-agonist clonidine in suppressing withdrawal (Gold *et al.*, 1978, 1980), since it also inhibits firing of these neurones (see Chapter 7). Clinical regimes based on a short tapering course of clonidine are now well established, and there are standardized regimes for covering accelerated withdrawal produced by opiate antagonist precipitation (Ghodse, 1989).

A clinical problem that has emerged with the use of naltrexone maintenance therapy is that of conversion from agonist to antagonist without precipitation of withdrawal, and the therapeutic penalty that this would entail. The unusual properties of buprenorphine have offered a solution to this common difficulty (Bickel *et al.*, 1988; Kosten and Kleber, 1988). The transfer from heroin or other agonists, including methadone, to buprenorphine can be completed without withdrawal due to the partial agonism and slow receptor kinetics of buprenorphine. After a period of several days on buprenorphine to allow elimination of heroin etc., naltrexone can be introduced. Again the high affinity of buprenorphine for the μ-receptor prevents significant displacement by the antagonist, and so precipitated withdrawal is not observed. Moreover the long half-line of buprenorphine means that spontaneous withdrawal is also not problematic. These observations of applied pharmacology having the ability to overcome areas of great difficulty in opiate dependence augur well for future pharmacological interventions in other aspects of opiate addiction.

2.4 Psychostimulants

2.4.1 Amphetamine and cocaine

This class of drugs includes a chemically diverse group of compounds, which have common clinical features of producing euphoria, increased energy and arousal. The most commonly abused drugs are amphetamine and cocaine, though others include methylphenidate, pemoline, and various appetite suppressants. Recently MDMA (Ecstasy) has been added to this list. Part of the reason for the recent increase in use of these drugs is that they have become more available in the USA and UK, and the price of cocaine in particular has fallen. Concurrently there has also been a change in the method of administration, with smoking of free-base forms of cocaine ('crack') and amphetamine ('ice') gaining prominence. This reflects the recent 'technological' development of an easy way of producing a free-base by suppliers, and addicts' demands for a more rapidly absorbed drug to give a bigger rush. The entry of cocaine into the brain appears to be as fast after smoking crack as after intravenous cocaine. The faster peak and more rapid clearance of crack probably contributes to its greater dependence liability compared with other forms of cocaine.

There is a complex pattern of tolerance development to psychostimulants. Tolerance occurs to some, but not all, of the psychological effects of cocaine. For instance, during a cocaine binge, retrospective reports suggest that users experience less cocaine-induced euphoria later on, compared with that experienced at the beginning of a binge (Gawin and Kleber, 1986). The reduced euphoriant effect cannot be restored by increasing the dose of cocaine. Very large doses do produce some euphoria, but additional anxiety, paranoia, and unpleasant arousal are also reported (Gawin and Kleber, 1986). Clinically this is important, as it can masquerade as other psychiatric disorders, and is commonly self-medicated with alcohol or opioids. One of the great dangers of cocaine is its cardiovascular toxicity. This is exacerbated by the fact that tolerance does not develop to this action (Ambre *et al.*, 1988; Foltin *et al.*, 1988), in contract to the tolerance to the psychological effects. Thus, as addicts use larger doses to maintain a 'high', they increase their cardiovascular risk.

In contrast to the reduced euphoric effects that are seen with tolerance, sensitization, the reverse of tolerance, can be demonstrated by enhanced behavioural effects after repeated administration. In several animal species, including monkeys, increased locomotor and stereotypic behaviour, and increased susceptibility to developing seizures, have been seen after chronic cocaine (for reviews see Johanson and Fischman, 1989; Chapter 6). It has been suggested that the paranoid schizophrenia-like psychoses seen after prolonged administration of cocaine or amphetamine in man may be due to this mechanism (Post and Weiss, 1988; Snyder, 1973).

After cessation of cocaine use, a withdrawal syndrome develops, although the precise phenomenology and time-course have not been fully established. There are clinical observations from a number of authors suggesting that symptoms such as tiredness, low mood, and sleep disturbance (e.g. insomnia and hypersomnia) commonly occur for days or weeks after stopping cocaine. The only carefully documented prospective study of cocaine withdrawal to date (Gawin and Kleber, 1986) described a sequence of three sets of symptoms: the 'crash', 'withdrawal' and 'extinction' phases. It seems likely that this phenomenon reflects relative underfunctioning of brain noradrenergic processes, since the reuptake blocker desipramine has been shown to be of value (Gawin and Kleber, 1984). Other pharmacological approaches to cocaine addiction involve the use of dopamine antagonists such as flupenthixol (Gawin *et al.*, 1989), since cocaine is though to act by releasing dopamine. Additionally, the opioid agonist–antagonist buprenorphine has been shown to reduce cocaine use in subjects in a heroin detoxification programme (Kosten *et al.*, 1989a, b). Supportive animal work revealing that buprenorphine will almost completely suppress cocaine self-administration in monkeys has recently been published (Mello *et al.*, 1989).

2.4.2 Nicotine

The commonest method of nicotine intake is tobacco smoking. Therefore most of the literature refers to this behaviour. Despite well-recognized health risks, largely because of the method of delivery, 33% of the adult population continue to smoke (General Household Survey, 1986).

Nicotine is the active component of the various tobacco preparations. This is suggested by several lines of evidence. The average cigarette contains 10 mg of nicotine of which 1–2 mg will be rapidly absorbed from the large alveolar surface area of the lungs. The result is a bolus of nicotine delivered to the brain within seconds (Milhorn, 1989). Studies using radiolabelled nicotine have demonstrated high-affinity binding sites in the rat brain (London *et al.*, 1985; Clarke *et al.*, 1985). Metabolism studies employing deoxy-glucose indicate that these sites are functionally significant (London *et al.*, 1985).

Tobacco use itself is controlled by nicotine levels. Various manipulations of such levels have been shown to produce compensatory changes in tobacco use and nicotine extraction. Reducing the nicotine content of cigarettes and increasing renal excretion of nicotine by manipulation of the urinary pH increases cigarette smoking (Ashton *et al.*, 1979; Benowitz and Jacob, 1985). Increasing the nicotine content of cigarettes and providing alternative sources of nicotine reduce smoking behaviour (Ashton *et al.*, 1979; Henningfield *et al.*, 1983). Whilst the elimination half-life of nicotine is 2 h the redistribution half-life of 8 min is probably more important in determining the time-course of action (Jones, 1987). This rapid redistribution allows the smoker to control the central effects of nicotine accurately.

Nicotine has been shown to act as a positive reinforcer in both animal and human subjects, but does so under a more limited range of circumstances than other drugs of abuse (Henningfield and Nemeth-Coslett, 1988; Henningfield and Goldberg, 1983, 1988a, b). There is some debate as to whether nicotine acts as a euphoriant or not (Henningfield and Nemeth-Coslett, 1988; Warburton, 1988). In support of the euphoriant theory, some of the neurochemical systems that are implicated in pleasure or reward are affected by nicotine (see Chapter 5). Nicotine induces dopamine release in the mesolimbic system (Rowell *et al.*, 1987). Research demonstrating a possible opioid mechanism, i.e. reduced smoking after naloxone (Karras and Kane, 1980), has yet to be replicated.

Other theories on nicotine dependence emphasize social and interpersonal factors. There is a positive association between smoking and both neurotic (Cherry and Kiernan, 1978) and extrovert traits (Eysenck, 1963). Environmental stress is also an important determinant of smoking behaviour and the common observation that smoking increases during examination periods is verified by rigorous clinical studies. Smoking has been shown to reduce irritability, aggression, and the autonomic nervous system reactivity to stress, whilst increasing pain tolerance. Contentment and relaxation have been shown to increase in a puff by puff fashion in parallel with plasma nicotine levels (review: Warburton, 1988). Nicotine may have beneficial effects and can improve performance on psychological testing in both smokers and non-smokers alike (Henningfield and Nemeth-Coslett, 1988; Jones, 1987; Warburton, 1988).

Different factors are important in initiating and maintaining dependence during a smoking career. Initiation of smoking occurs mainly during adolescence and rarely after the age of 20, and at this stage social, cultural and psychological pressures predominate (Jones, 1987; Mann *et al.*, 1986; Silvis and Perry, 1987). Once the learning process has been accomplished, pharmacological factors add to these, including smoking for the effects of nicotine and/or avoidance of withdrawal symptoms. In addition, smoking becomes associated with a vast variety of external cues. Fifteen years of smoking 20 cigarettes a day, each inhaled 10 times, results in more than one million conditioning trials!

Acute tolerance to many effects of nicotine, for example cardiovascular responses, occurs even during the time taken to smoke a cigarette (Benowitz *et al.*, 1982). The evidence to support the development of chronic tolerance is more speculative. For instance, other autonomic symptoms that trouble the novice smoker disappear over time, and intake increases until it stabilizes at approximately 20–30 cigarettes per day (Henningfield and Nemeth-Coslett, 1988).

Nicotine withdrawal occurs on abrupt cessation of all types of nicotine formulations (Henningfield and Goldberg, 1988a, b). The DSM-III-R (American Psychiatric Association, 1987) criteria for nicotine withdrawal include: craving for nicotine; irritability, frustration, or anger; anxiety; difficulty with concentration; restlessness; decreased heart rate; and increased appetite or weight gain. These withdrawal symptoms occur within hours of stopping smoking, and are relieved by smoking. They decline after 1–3 weeks (Milhorn, 1989).

Nicotine replacement, in the form of chewing gum or more recently skin patches, is the primary pharmacological treatment to aid detoxification. This, combined with psychological techniques, for example behavioural techniques, cognitive therapy and group work (Fisher *et al.*, 1988; Milhorn, 1989), produces a long-term abstinence rate of approximately 30% in motivated subjects (Jarvis *et al.*, 1982; Lam *et al.*, 1987). Other pharmacological approaches requiring further verification include nicotinic blockade with mecamylamine (Jarvik and Henningfield, 1988), clonidine to improve withdrawal (Glassman *et al.*, 1984) and the use of silver acetate gum which provides an aversive stimulus on contact with sulphides in tobacco smoke (Jarvik and Henningfield, 1988).

2.4.3 Caffeine

Caffeine is the most widely used behaviourally active drug in the world (Gilbert, 1984). In the UK and the USA the daily per capita consumption is 444 mg and 211 mg respectively. Behavioural animal techniques and human studies have shown that tolerance to caffeine can occur within days. Tolerance at the level of individual reticular neurones has been demonstrated following 2 weeks of chronic caffeine exposure in rats (Chou *et al.*, 1985). Studies in human subjects have likewise noted tolerance to many of the effects of caffeine. For example, cardiovascular and biochemical responses to caffeine show almost complete development of tolerance after regular administration over 4 days (Ammon *et al.*, 1983; Robertson *et al.*, 1981, 1984).

In contrast to cocaine and amphetamine, caffeine is not consistently self-administered. Similarly it is not consistently euphoric and indeed can be dysphoric, producing symptoms of anxiety and nervousness (Griffiths and Woodson, 1988). One explanation may be that the positive reinforcing effects of caffeine are related to an ongoing state of physical dependence. Following overnight abstinence, heavy users report pleasant and desirable effects after caffeine, in contrast to coffee abstainers who report unpleasant or undesirable effects (Goldstein and Kaizer, 1969; Goldstein and Whitby, 1969). Further support for this explanation comes from the demonstration under double-blind conditions that 94% of subjects who drink caffeinated coffee prefer caffeinated coffee. Subjects who drink decaffeinated coffee show no preference for caffeinated over decaffeinated coffee (Griffiths *et al.*, 1986).

Adenosine, an endogenous neuromodulator, is implicated in caffeine dependence. Adenosine agonists produce sedation and are anticonvulsant whilst caffeine acts as a competitive antagonist (Snyder *et al.*, 1981; Phillis and Kostopoulos, 1975). Chronic administration of caffeine increases brain adenosine receptors, shifts A_1 adenosine receptors to a high-affinity state and increases functional sensitivity to adenosine (Green and Stiles, 1986; Chou *et al.*, 1985). Such a receptor-mediated response could account for caffeine dependence and withdrawal states.

Adrenergic mechanisms have also been suggested as a mechanism of caffeine dependence. Caffeine produces downregulation of adrenoceptors in rat brain (Green and Stiles, 1986), whilst a recent study in mice has demonstrated that monoamine utilization is affected in various brain areas, including limbic structures (Hadfield and Milio, 1989). Benzodiazepine theories have also been considered. Caffeine antagonizes diazepam-induced impairment of psychomotor and cognitive skills (Mattila and Nuotto, 1983; Roache and Griffiths, 1987). However, *in vivo* and *in vitro* studies of caffeine and benzodiazepine interactions at a receptor level have, as yet, proved inconclusive.

A caffeine withdrawal syndrome has been described (Griffiths and Woodson, 1988). In animals it is characterized by reduced locomotor activity. Human case reports and studies, some of which were performed under double-blind conditions, define the most common symptoms of withdrawal as headache and fatigue with a variety of other symptoms occurring at a lower frequency. Severity of withdrawal symptoms ranged from mild to incapacitating with onset occurring at 12–24 h, peaking at 20–48 h and lasting approximately one week.

Caffeine detoxification may be clinically important, particularly in anxiety disorders. Amelioration of anxiety symptoms has been shown to occur on caffeine withdrawal (Bruce and Lader, 1989) and increased caffeine sensitivity has been demonstrated in panic patients (Charney *et al.*, 1985; Lee *et al.*, 1988). Griffiths and Woodson suggest that the initial management of caffeine dependency is one of abrupt withdrawal in a supportive therapeutic context. Should significant withdrawal symptoms be experienced then replacement, dose tapering and supportive measures (e.g. aspirin for headache) can be employed. However, these authors caution that each case should be considered individually (Griffiths and Woodson, 1988).

2.5 Conclusions

Mankind uses and abuses a variety of drugs. The acute effects of the varying classes of compounds range from profound sedation and tranquillity, through euphoria, to activation and stimulation. However, tolerance and dependence appear to be common features. These occur in different ways; initially there is the loss of aversive side-effects, such as nausea (e.g. opioids, nicotine, and alcohol) and ataxia/sedation (hypnosedatives). Subsequently pleasurable effects may attenuate, leading to dosage escalation, often with secondary physical complications. For most drugs, withdrawal reflects the adaptive changes that underlie tolerance, although in the case of the psychostimulants, transmitter depletion may be the primary pathology. Drug usage is maintained by a complex interaction of pleasurable drug effects, and the desire to avoid withdrawal. Pharmacological approaches to drug dependence therapy can be directed towards either or both phenomena, but are still in their infancy.

References

Ambre, J.L., Belknap, S.M., Nelson, J., Ruo, T.I., Shin, S.G. & Atkinson, A.J. (1988) *Clin. Pharmacol. Ther.* **44**, 1–8.

American Psychiatric Association (1987) *Diagnostic and Statistical Manual*, 3rd edn., Washington, D.C., American Psychiatric Association.

Ammon, H., Bieck, P., Mandalaz, D. & Verspohl, E. (1983) *Br. J. Clin. Pharmacol.* **15**, 701–706.

Ashton, H. (1989) *Br. Med. J.* **298**, 103–104.

Ashton, H., Stepney, R. & Thompson, J. (1979) *Br. Med. J.* **2**, 357–360.

Ballenger, J.C. & Post, R.M. (1978) *Br. J. Psychiatry* **133**, 1–14.

Baloh, R.W., Sharma, S., Moskowitz, H. & Griffith, R. (1979) *Aviat. Space Envir. Med.* **50**, 18–23.

Benowitz, N. & Jacob, P. (1985) *J. Pharmacol. Exp. Ther.* **234**, 153–155.

Benowitz, N., Jacob, P., Jones, R. & Rosenberg, J. (1982) *J. Pharmacol. Exp. Ther.* **221**, 368–372.

Bickel, W.K., Stitzer, M.L., Bigelow, G.E., Liebson, I.A., Jasinski, D.R. & Johnson, R.E. (1988) *Clin. Pharmacol. Ther.* **43**, 72–78.

Brosan, C., Broadbent, D.E., Nutt, D.J. & Broadbent, M. (1986) *Psychol. Med.* **16**, 561–571.

Bruce, M.S. & Lader, M. (1989) *Psychol. Med.* **19**, 211–214.

Charney, D.S., Heninger, G.R. & Jatlow, P.I. (1985) *Arch. Gen. Psychiatry* **42**, 233–243.

Cherry, N. & Kiernan, K. (1978) In *Smoking Behaviour; Physiological and Psychological Influences* (ed. Thornton, R.), p 12. Edinburgh, Churchill Livingstone.

Chou, D., Khan, S., Forde, J. & Hirsh, K. (1985) *Life Sci.* **36**, 2347–2358.

Clarke, D.C. & Fawcett, J. (1989) In *Recent Developments in Alcoholism*, Vol. 7 (ed. Galanter, M.), p 315. New York, Plenum.

Clarke, P., Schwartz, R., Paul, S., Pert, C. & Pert, A. (1985) *J. Neurosci.* **110**, 391–392.

Cloninger, C.R., Sigvardsson, S., Gilligan, S.B., von Knorring, A., Reich, T. & Bohman, M. (1989) In *Alcohol Research from Bench to Bedside* (eds Gordis, E., Tabakoff, B. & Linnoila, M.), p 3. New York, Haworth.

Cowan, A., Lewis, J.W. & Macfarlane, I.R. (1977) *Br. J. Pharmacol.* **60**, 537–545.

Dunbar, G.C., Perera, M.H. & Jenner, F.A. (1989) *Br. J. Psychiatry* **155**, 836–841.

Edwards, G. (1982) *The Treatment of Drinking Problems.* London, Grant McIntyre.

Eysenck, H. (1963) *Life Sci.* **3**, 777–792.

Fisher, E., Bishop, D., Goldmuntz, J. & Jacobs, A. (1988) *Chest* **93**, (Suppl.), 69S–78S.

Foltin, R.W., Fischman, M.W., Pedroso, J.J. & Pearlson, G.D. (1988) *Drug Alcohol Depend.* **22**, 169–177.

Gawin, F.H. & Kleber, H.D. (1984) *Arch. Gen. Psychiatry* **41**, 903–909.

Gawin, F.H. & Kleber, H.D. (1986) *Arch. Gen. Psychiatry* **43**, 107–113.

Gawin, F.H., Allen, D. & Humblestone, B. (1989) *Arch. Gen. Psychiatry* **46**, 322–325.

General Household Survey (1988) *Smoking: 1977–1986*, p 159. London, HMSO.

Ghodse, H. (1989) *Drugs and Addictive Behaviour.* Oxford, Blackwell Scientific Publications.

Gilbert, R. (1984) In *The Methylxanthine Beverages and Foods: Chemistry, Consumption and Health Effects* (ed. Spiller, G.), p 185. New York, Liss.

Glassman, A., Jackson, W., Walsh, B. & Roose, S. (1984) *Science* **226**, 864–866.

Glue, P. & Nutt, D.J. (1990) *Br. J. Psychiatry* **157**, 491–499.

Gold, M.S., Redmond, D.E. & Kleber, H.D. (1978) *Lancet* **II**, 599–602.

Gold, M.S., Pottash, A.C., Sweeney, D.R. & Kleber, H.D. (1980) *J.A.M.A.* **243**, 343–346.
Goldstein, A., & Kaizer, S. (1969) *Clin. Pharmacol. Ther.* **10**, 477–488.
Goldstein, A. & Whitby, O. (1969) *Clin. Pharmacol. Ther.* **10**, 489–497.
Green, R. & Stiles, G. (1986) *J. Clin. Invest.* **77**, 222–227.
Griffiths, R.R. & Woodson, P.P. (1988) *Psychopharmacology* **94**, 437–451.
Griffiths, R.R., Bigelow, G.E., Liebsin, I. & Kaliszak, J.E. (1980) *J. Pharmacol. Exp. Ther.* **215**, 649–661.
Griffiths, R.R., McLeod, D.R., Bigelow, G.E., Liebson, I. & Roache, J.D. (1984) *Psychopharmacology* **84**, 147–154.
Griffiths, R.R., Bigelow, G.E. & Liebson, I.A. (1986) *J. Pharmacol. Exp. Ther.* **239**, 416–425.
Hadfield, M. & Milio, C. (1989) *Life Sci.* **45**, 2637–2644.
Haigh, J.R.M. & Feely, M. (1988) *Trends Pharmacol. Sci.* **9**, 361–366.
Henningfield, J. & Goldberg, S. (1983) *Pharmacol. Biochem. Behav.* **19**, 989–992.
Henningfield, J. & Goldberg, S. (1988a) *Pharmacol. Biochem. Behav.* **30**, 217–220.
Henningfield, J. & Goldberg, S. (1988b) *Pharmacol. Biochem. Behav.* **30**, 221–226.
Henningfield, J. & Nemeth-Coslett, R. (1988) *Chest* **93** (Suppl.), 37S–55S.
Henningfield, J., Miyasato, K. & Jasinski, D. (1983) *Pharmacol. Biochem. Behav.* **19**, 887–890.
Hollister, I.E., Motzenbecker, F.P. & Degan, R.O. (1961) *Psychopharmacologia* **2**, 63–68.
Isbell, H., Altschul, S., Kornetsky, C.H., Eisenman, A.J., Flanary, H.G. & Fraser, H.F. (1950) *Arch. Neurol. Psychiatry* **64**, 1–28.
Isbell, H., Fraser, H.F., Wikler, A. *et al.* (1955) *Q. J. Studies Alcohol* **16**, 1–33.
Jarvik, M. & Henningfield, J. (1988) *Pharmacol. Biochem. Behav.* **30**, 279–294.
Jarvis, M., Raw, M., Russell, M. & Feyerabend, C. (1982) *Br. Med. J.* **285**, 537–540.
Johanson, C. & Fischman, M.W. (1989) *Pharmacol. Rev.* **41**, 3–52.
Jones, M.C. (1968) *J. Consult. Clin. Psychol.* **32**, 2–12.
Jones, R. (1987) In *Psychopharmacology: The Third Generation of Progress* (ed. Meltzer, H.), p 1589. New York, Raven Press.
Kandel, D.B. & Raveis, V.H. (1989) *Arch. Gen. Psychiatry* **46**, 109–116.
Karras, A. & Kane, J. (1980) *Life Sci.* **27**, 1541–1545.
Kendell, R.E. (1979) *Br. Med. J.* **i**, 367–371.
Kendell, R.E., de Ronmanie, M. & Ritson, E.B. (1983) *Br. J. Addict.* **78**, 365–379.
Khantzian, E.J. & Treece, C. (1985) *Arch. Gen. Psychiatry* **42**, 1067–1071.
Kosten, T.R. & Kleber, H.D. (1988) *Life Sci.* **42**, 635–641.
Kosten, T.R., Kleber, H.D. & Morgan, C. (1989a) *Life Sci.* **44**, 887–892.
Kosten, T.R., Kleber, H.D. & Morgan, C. (1989b) *Biol. Psychiatry* **26**, 637–639.
Lam, W., Sze, P., Sacks, H. & Chalmers, T. (1987) *Lancet* **ii**, 27–30.
Lee, M.A., Flegel, P., Greden, J.F. & Cameron, O.G. (1988) *Am. J. Psychiatry* **145**, 632–635.
Lewis, J.W. (1985) *Drug Alcohol Depend.* **14**, 363–372.
London, E., Waller, S. & Wamsley, J. (1985) *Neurosci. Lett.* **53**, 179–184.
Mann, L., Johnson, R. & Levine, D. (1986) *Psychosomatics* **27**, 713–718.
Martin, W.R. (1967) *Pharmacol. Rev.* **19**, 463–521.
Mattila, M. & Nuotto, E. (1983) *Med. Biol.* **61**, 337–343.
McCord, J., McCord, W. & Thurber, E. (1962) *J. Abnorm. Social Psychology* **64**, 361–369.
Mello, N.K., Mendelson, J.H., Kuehnle, J.C. & Sellers, M.S. (1981) *J. Pharmacol. Exp. Ther.* **216**, 45–54.

Mello, N.K., Mendelson, J.H. & Kuehnle, J.C. (1982) *J. Pharmacol. Exp. Ther.* **223**, 30–39.
Mello, N.K., Mendelson, J.H., Bree, M.P. & Lukas, S.E. (1989) *Science* **245**, 859–862.
Merz, W.A. & Ballmer, U. (1983) *J. Psychoactive Drugs* **15**, 71–83.
Milhorn, H. (1989) *Am. Family Physician* **39**, 214–224.
Naranjo, C.A. & Sellers, E.M. (1989) In *Recent Developments in Alcoholism*, Vol. 7 (ed. Galanter, M.), p 255. New York, Plenum.
Nutt, D.J. (1986) *Trends Pharmacol. Sci.* **7**, 457–460.
Nutt, D.J. (1988) *Current Opinion Psychiatry* **1**, 330–334.
Nutt, D.J. & Glue, P. (1986) *Br. J. Addict.* **81**, 327–338.
Nutt, D.J. & Lister, R.L. (1988) *Psychopharmacology* **94**, 435–436.
Nutt, D.J., Glue, P. & Lawson, C.W. (1990) *Prog. Neuropsychopharm. Biol. Psychiatry* **14**, 737–752.
O'Brien, C.P., Ehrman, R.N. & Ternes, J.W. (1986) In *Behavioural Analysis of Drug Dependence* (eds Goldberg, S.R. & Stolerman, I.P.), p 329. Orlando, Academic Press.
Petursson, H. & Lader, M.H. (1981a) *Br. J. Addict.* **76**, 133–145.
Petursson, H. & Lader, M.H. (1981b) *Br. Med. J.* **283**, 643–645.
Petursson, H. & Lader, M.H. (1984) *Dependence on Tranquillizers*. London, Oxford University Press.
Phillis, J. & Kostopoulos, G. (1975) *Life Sci.* **17**, 1085–1094.
Post, R.M. & Weiss, S.R.B. (1988) In *Mechanisms of Cocaine Abuse and Toxicity* (eds Clouet, D., Asghar, K. & Brown, R.), p 217. Washington DC, US Government.
Roache, J.D. & Griffiths, R.R. (1987) *Pharmacol. Biochem. Behav.* **26**, 801–812.
Robertson, D., Wade, D., Workman, R. & Woosley, R. (1981) *J. Clin. Invest.* **67**, 1111–1117.
Robertson, D., Hollister, A., Kincaid, D. *et al.* (1984) *Am. J. Med.* **77**, 54–60.
Rodrigo, E.K. & Williams, P. (1986) *Psychol. Med.* **16**, 467–472.
Rounsaville, B.J., Weissman, M.M., Kleber, H.D. & Wilber, C. (1982) *Arch. Gen. Psychiatry* **39**, 161–166.
Rowell, P., Carr, L. & Garner, A. (1987) *J. Neurochem.* **49**, 1449–1454.
Siegel, S. (1988) In *The Psychopharmacology of Addiction* (ed. Lader, M.), p 73. Oxford, Oxford University Press.
Silvis, G. & Perry, C. (1987) *Pediatr. Clin. North Am.* **34**, 363–379.
Snyder, S.H. (1973) *Am. J. Psychiatry* **130**, 61–67.
Snyder, S.H., Katims, J.J., Annau, Z., Bruns, R.F. & Daly, J.W. (1981) *Proc. Natl Acad. Sci. USA* **78**, 3260–3264.
Taylor, J.R., Elsworth, J.D., Garcia, E.J., Grant, S.J., Roth, R.H. & Redmond, D.E. Jr (1988) *Psychopharmacology* **96**, 121–134.
Tyrer, P. (1982) *Drugs in Psychiatric Practice*. London, Butterworths.
Tyrer, P. (1989) *Br. Med. J.* **298**, 102–105.
Tyrer, P., Owen, R. & Dawling, S. (1983) *Lancet* **i**, 1402–1406.
Vaillant, G. (1983) *The Natural History of Alcoholism*. Harvard University Press, Boston.
Victor, M. & Adams, R.D. (1953) *Res. Publ. Assoc. Res. Nerv. Ment. Dis.* **32**, 526–573.
Warburton, D. (1988) In *The Psychopharmacology of Addiction* (ed. Lader, M.), p 27. Oxford University Press, Oxford.
Woods, J.H., Katz, J.L. & Winger, G. (1987) *Pharmacol. Rev.* **39**, 251–419.
World Health Organization (1981) *Bull. WHO* **59**, 225–242.

CHAPTER 3

BIOCHEMICAL AND ELECTROPHYSIOLOGICAL MECHANISMS UNDERLYING BENZODIAZEPINE TOLERANCE AND DEPENDENCE

Dorothy W. Gallager[1], Rodney J. Marley[2] and Theresa D. Hernandez[2]

[1] *Neurogen Corporation, 35 Northeast Industrial Road, Branford, Connecticut 06405, USA*

[2] *Yale University School of Medicine, Department of Psychiatry, Abraham Ribicoff Research Facilities and Connecticut Mental Health Center, New Haven, Connecticut 06508, USA*

Table of Contents

3.1 Introduction

Prolonged exposure to benzodiazepine agonists is accompanied by a time-dependent decrease in responsivity, or 'tolerance', to the therapeutic usefulness

THE BIOLOGICAL BASES OF DRUG TOLERANCE AND DEPENDENCE
ISBN 0-12-564250-4

of these agents as anticonvulsants, sedative-hypnotics and antipanic agents (Savic *et al.*, 1991; Nutt, 1986; Woods and Charney, 1988; Gallager *et al.*, 1989). Accumulating evidence also indicates that physical dependence and the development of a withdrawal syndrome upon drug discontinuation occurs following long-term benzodiazepine use, even at low to moderate doses (Rickles *et al.*, 1988; Marks, 1985; Nutt, 1986). Although the basis for decreases in drug responsivity and physical dependence is not well understood, present knowledge indicates that tolerance to benzodiazepines is not primarily due to pharmacokinetic differences (Gallager *et al.*, 1985; Greenblatt and Shader, 1986; Haigh *et al.*, 1986). Since a functional alteration in the CNS response to benzodiazepines is postulated to occur with chronic exposure, it seems important to first discuss the acute mechanism of action of the benzodiazepines in naive animals. This chapter will then focus on the functional and neurochemical mechanisms that may underlie benzodiazepine tolerance and dependence.

3.2 Mechanisms of acute actions of the benzodiazepines

Preclinical studies indicate that many of the pharmacological actions of benzodiazepines are mediated by a selective facilitation of the actions of the major inhibitory neurotransmitter, γ-aminobutyric acid (GABA) (Schoch *et al.*, 1985; Haefely and Polc, 1986; Tallman and Gallager, 1985). Binding to a high-affinity benzodiazepine recognition site on the $GABA_A$ receptor (Mohler and Okada, 1977; Squires and Braestrup, 1977) is significantly correlated with *in vivo* activity in a number of behavioural and clinical tests predictive of benzodiazepine potency (Braestrup and Nielsen, 1983; Paul *et al.*, 1979; Tallman *et al.*, 1980). Blockade of this site with a competitive antagonist prevents all of the therapeutic actions of the benzodiazepines (Hunkeler *et al.*, 1981; Haefely and Hunkeler, 1988). Inverse agonists produce a reduction of the inhibitory actions of GABA via their interactions at the benzodiazepine modulatory site and can cause anxiogenic and/or proconvulsant effects (Braestrup *et al.*, 1984; Dorow *et al.*, 1983). A large literature supports the existence of a complex of proteins associated with postsynaptic GABA responses as a major site of action for the benzodiazepines (Olsen and Tobin, 1990; Schofield, 1989). The existence of the GABA–benzodiazepine–ionophore complex suggests a means by which such compounds, which are structurally unrelated to GABA, could allosterically modify responses to this inhibitory neurotransmitter. Electrophysiological and chloride flux studies have shown that many agents, including benzodiazepines, barbiturates, picrotoxin and some steroids, can modulate GABA activity at the $GABA_A$

receptor (Polc, 1988; Peters *et al.*, 1988; Olsen and Venter, 1986; Farrant and Webster, 1989). Fluctuation analysis of GABA responses in the presence of benzodiazepines suggests that benzodiazepine agonists increase the frequency of channel opening in response to GABA without significantly altering the mean duration of channel opening (Polc, 1988; Barker and Owen, 1986). Patch-clamp analyses are consistent with this benzodiazepine-induced increase in GABA efficacy; in the presence of diazepam, GABA-activated chloride currents are potentiated two-fold (Bormann and Sakmann, 1984; Bormann, 1988). Binding studies also support a close association between GABA and benzodiazepine actions. It has been shown that benzodiazepines enhance GABA binding to its receptor (Costa *et al.*, 1978; Johnston and Skerritt, 1983). Conversely, GABA enhances benzodiazepine binding (Tallman *et al.*, 1978). These reciprocal interactions demonstrate a close association between GABA and benzodiazepine binding sites which is supported by their co-solubilization and immunoprecipitation (for review see Stephenson, 1988).

Structurally, the $GABA_A$ receptor complex is a heteroligomeric, transmembrane acidic glycoprotein (Czajkowski *et al.*, 1989; Sweetman and Tallman, 1986; Mamalaki *et al.*, 1987) with binding (recognition) sites for benzodiazepines and GABA in association with a chloride ion channel and binding sites for drugs closely linked to the channel (Olsen and Tobin, 1990; Schofield, 1989). Major subunits for the $GABA_A$ receptor complex have been cloned and sequenced (Schofield, 1989). Using cDNA probes to screen a variety of libraries, different subunits have been identified, including six α-subunits (Olsen and Tobin, 1990; Schofield, 1989; Lolait *et al.*, 1989b; Wisden *et al.*, 1989), three β-subunits (Ymer *et al.*, 1989; Lolait *et al.*, 1989a), and at least two γ-subunits (Pritchett *et al.*, 1989b); evidence for additional δ- and ε-subunits also exists (Shivers *et al.*, 1989; Schofield, 1989). These results were not anticipated from biochemical studies, as subunits of affinity-purified $GABA_A$ receptor were electrophoretically resolved into only two bands. Apparently the bands are heterogeneous, including varieties of α-, β-, γ-, δ- and ε-subunits (Pritchett *et al.*, 1989b; Sieghart, 1989). Based on sequence information, complementary RNAs for these subunits have been shown to code for electrophysiologically active GABA receptors which retain many of their pharmacological characteristics when reconstituted into expression systems (Verdoorn *et al.*, 1990; Sigel *et al.*, 1990). While α- and β-subunits alone and in combination can reconstitute GABA-gated and barbiturate-modulated chloride channels (Schofield *et al.*, 1987; Levitan *et al.*, 1988), responses to the actions of benzodiazepines also require the presence of the γ_2-subunit (Pritchett *et al.*, 1989a, b; Sigel *et al.*, 1990). While the *in vivo* stoichiometry is not yet known, co-expression of α-, β- and γ-subunits in transfected mammalian cells yields a GABA-gated ion channel with appropriate benzodiazepine pharmacology (Pritchett *et al.*, 1989b; Verdoorn *et al.*, 1990;

Sigel *et al.*, 1990). Since the size of the non-aggregated monomeric form of the purified bovine or rat receptor is 230–290 kDa (Mamalaki *et al.*, 1987; Stephenson, 1988; Olsen and Tobin, 1990) and the individual subunits are 50–53 and 55–59 kDa, a tetrameric or pentameric subunit structure may be a core structure of this receptor complex. Sigel *et al.* (1990) identified the combination of subunits of $\alpha_5\beta_2\gamma_2$ as the minimal requirement for reproducing consensus properties of the vertebrate $GABA_A$ receptor channel in a reconstituted (*Xenopus* oocyte) expression system.

It is still not clear which subunits carry the binding sites for benzodiazepines, GABA or the chloride ion channel associated sites. Affinity-purified receptor protein studies using labelled specific agonists ([^{3}H]muscimol, [^{3}H]flunitrazepam) indicated that the β-subunit carries the GABA recognition site (Deng *et al.*, 1986; Cavalla and Neff, 1985; Casalotti *et al.*, 1986), while the α-subunit contains the recognition site for benzodiazepines (Mohler *et al.*, 1980; Thomas and Tallman, 1981). Now, using various translation systems, it is not clear whether the GABA, benzodiazepine or barbiturate/convulsant binding sites are coded for by the α-, β-, γ-, δ-, or ε-subunit or a combination of these subunits. *In situ* hybridization studies suggest that the γ_2-unit is encoded within neurones known to contain high-affinity benzodiazepine binding sites (Pritchett *et al.*, 1989b; Siegel, 1988). Similar analysis of δ-subunit mRNA localization shows a good correlation with the distribution of high-affinity muscimol binding sites (Shivers *et al.*, 1989).

Despite these limitations in our knowledge of the exact structure of the complex *in vivo*, it seems clear that the benzodiazepines function at the $GABA_A$ receptor. The existence of multiple subunits and their heterogeneous distribution make it likely that the function of the $GABA_A$ receptor in different regions of the brain may be regulated independently and may have different responses to benzodiazepines both acutely and chronically (Schofield, 1989; Olsen and Tobin, 1990; Sigel *et al.*, 1990). Any search for mechanisms underlying the development of tolerance/dependence must therefore address this molecular diversity.

3.3 Mechanisms of tolerance/dependence following chronic benzodiazepine agonist exposure

3.3.1 Functional changes

Since the primary site of action of the benzodiazepines is at a recognition site associated with the $GABA_A$ receptor complex, a number of laboratories have examined components of the $GABA_A$ complex following treatment producing tolerance to and physical dependence on benzodiazepines (for review see Gallager *et al.*, 1989). Functional studies have been carried out to examine the ability of the GABAergic system to adapt to chronic occupation of the benzodiazepine site within the functional $GABA_A$ receptor complex. Electrophysiological studies on cerebellar Purkinje cells (Waterhouse *et al.*, 1984), in spinal cell culture (Farb *et al.*, 1984; Sher *et al.*, 1983), on dorsal raphe neurones (Gallager *et al.*, 1984a; Gonsalves and Gallager, 1987) and on substantia nigra pars reticulata (SNr) neurones (Wilson and Gallager, 1987; Tietz and Rosenberg, 1988) have shown that *chronic* administration of benzodiazepines *reduces* their ability to enhance GABA-mediated inhibition. Such actions represent tolerance to the selective facilitation of GABAergic inhibition when tested in a naive system, as described above.

Direct electrophysiological evidence for decreased postsynaptic sensitivity to GABA has been reported for dorsal raphe neurones after prolonged benzodiazepine exposure (Gallager *et al.*, 1984a). Rats exposed to a benzodiazepine agonist, diazepam, show a decrease in sensitivity of dorsal raphe neurones to iontophoretically applied GABA and a loss in the ability of benzodiazepines to enhance sensitivity to GABA in this nucleus. This change is selective since 5-HTergic sensitivity of these same neurones is not significantly altered by chronic diazepam exposure. A behaviourally measurable reduction in sensitivity to a GABA agonist after prolonged benzodiazepine exposure has also been reported (Tietz and Rosenberg, 1988). Electrophysiological studies in out laboratory have shown that administration of the benzodiazepine antagonist Ro15-1788 to chronic diazepam-treated rats reverses GABAergic subsensitivity in dorsal raphe neurones (Gallager *et al.*, 1984a; Gonsalves and Gallager, 1985). Since it has been shown that tolerance to benzodiazepines develops as a result of the interaction of a benzodiazepine with its receptor (File, 1982; Gallager *et al.*, 1984a), such data support the critical role of the benzodiazepine site in mediating the shift in GABA sensitivity. In addition, we have documented a temporal relationship between the onset of changes in GABAergic sensitivity in dorsal raphe neurones and the development of tolerance to the anticonvulsant effects of diazepam following chronic exposure to diazepam (Gonsalves and Gallager, 1987). These data suggest a fundamental change in neuronal sensitivity to GABA related to the duration of benzodiazepine exposure. A biochemical technique to measure GABA-stimulated $^{36}Cl^-$ uptake into brain membrane vesicles has been described as an additional functional measure of the GABA complex (Harris and Allan, 1985; Olsen *et al.*, 1984). Using this system, GABA-stimulated $^{36}Cl^-$ flux has been reported to be acutely modulated by benzodiazepine receptor ligands (agonists, inverse agonists) in a concentration-dependent and pharmacologically appropriate manner (Obata and Yamamura, 1986). Such studies carried out in our laboratory indicate that the ability of GABA to stimulate the influx of $^{36}Cl^-$ was reduced in cortical membrane preparations from rats treated chronically with diazepam (Marley and Gallager, 1989). These results are in agreement with those of Miller *et al.* (1988), who found that chronic lorazepam treatment also resulted in a decrease in muscimol-stimulated chloride uptake in cortical synaptoneurosome preparations. Subsensitivity to GABA-stimulated $^{36}Cl^-$ influx observed in membrane vesicles prepared from cerebral cortices of chronic diazepam-treated animals were thus consistent with electrophysiological evidence for a decrease in the functional responsivity of GABA receptors (Gallager *et al.*, 1989).

3.3.2 Biochemical alterations

To investigate whether receptor alterations accompany the physiologically measurable changes in GABA sensitivity, components of the $GABA_A$ receptor complex were examined using radioligand binding procedures. For a wide variety of drug receptor systems, long-term administration of an agonist produces an apparent decrease or downregulation in drug receptor number (Overstreet and Yamamura, 1979). Although a number of conflicting reports suggest alterations in benzodiazepine binding following various chronic dose regimens (Rosenberg and Chiu, 1981; Miller *et al.*, 1988), our findings (Gallager *et al.*, 1984a) and those of others (Braestrup and Nielsen, 1983; Nutt, 1986; Stephens and Schneider, 1985; Hawkins *et al.*, 1988) indicate that chronic diazepam treatment does not significantly alter the number or affinity of benzodiazepine receptors. Thus, neither agonist ([^{3}H]flunitrazepam) nor antagonist ([^{3}H]Ro15-1788) binding in cerebral cortical membranes was altered (Gallager *et al.*, 1985) following a chronic diazepam regimen which reduces GABAergic responsivity in dorsal raphe neurones and produces anticonvulsant tolerance. Other studies in our laboratory have also shown a lack of change in the number of t-butyl-bicyclo(2,2,2)phosphothionate (TBPS) or bicuculline binding sites following chronic agonist administration (Gallager *et al.*, 1984b; Heninger and Gallager, 1988). TBPS binds to a site in or adjacent to the chloride ion channel, providing a measure of this element of the $GABA_A$ complex (Squires *et al.*, 1983), while bicuculline binds to the μM affinity, functionally significant recognition site for GABA (Olsen and Snowman, 1983).

While not affecting the number of sites available to bind the various components of the GABA–benzodiazepine–chloride ionophore directly, chronic diazepam has been found to significantly alter the allosteric modulation between the various binding sites and GABA. Thus chronic diazepam treatment decreased the ability of GABA to enhance benzodiazepine agonist binding (Gallager *et al.*, 1984a; Hawkins *et al.*, 1988; Massotti *et al.*, 1980; Mele *et al.*, 1984; Schiller and Farb, 1986) (not observed by Stephens and

Schneider (1985)) and to decrease inverse agonist (DMCM) binding in cortical membranes (Heninger and Gallager, 1988).

A number of studies have suggested that the effects of GABA on benzodiazepine binding are associated with a low-affinity component of the GABA recognition site (Olsen, 1982; Olsen *et al.*, 1984; Gallager *et al.*, 1984b). Direct evidence for the involvement of micromolar GABA affinity sites has been provided by the expression of mRNAs for the α- and β-subunits of the GABA receptor in vertebrate cells (Levitan *et al.*, 1988); depending on which of the three α-subunits is expressed with β, half-maximal responses to GABA are obtained at concentrations of approximately 1, 10 or 40 μM. However, different GABA sensitivities are obtained when the γ_2-subunit is co-expressed with α and β, suggesting that the *in vivo* situation may represent additional combinations (Pritchett *et al.*, 1989a; Verdoorn *et al.*, 1990; Sigel *et al.*, 1990). Physiologically, actions of GABA seem to require a micromolar affinity state of the receptor (Krespan *et al.*, 1984; Hamill *et al.*, 1983). The low-affinity component of the GABA recognition site can be assessed by means of tritiated bicuculline binding in the presence of thiocyanate (Gallager *et al.*, 1984b; Olsen and Snowman, 1983). In our studies, we observed a significant increase in the affinity of GABA for the low-affinity site following chronic benzodiazepine exposure (Gallager *et al.*, 1985; Heninger and Gallager, 1988). Other laboratories have reported an increase in high-affinity GABA sites measured with [^{3}H]muscimol after chronic benzodiazepines (Marangos and Crawley, 1982; Abbracchio *et al.*, 1983). These data may be indicative of a preferential conversion to a higher affinity form of the GABA recognition site following chronic diazepam exposure. In the case of the acetylcholine receptor, conversion to a high-affinity state leads to a desensitized and hence non-functional form of the receptor (Changeux *et al.*, 1984). Such a desensitization mechanism would be consistent with the decreased ability of GABA to affect benzodiazepine ligand (agonist and inverse agonist) binding and with the reduced physiological sensitivity to GABA.

The molecular mechanisms underlying subsensitivity of the receptor to GABA and benzodiazepines remain unknown. However, studies in our laboratory suggest that chronic diazepam treatment may be accompanied by an alteration in the mRNA levels for at least one of the subunits of the GABA receptor complex (Heninger *et al.*, 1990). Northern blot and solution hybridization analysis has demonstrated a small (20%) but significant decrease in mRNA for the α_1- but not the β_1-subunit of the GABA receptor complex. Additional studies with more probes will be required to determine if this change is truly selective for the α_1-subunit.

All of our data are consistent with the hypothesis that the functional activity of GABA at the $GABA_A$ receptor complex is reduced. As seen in Table 1, by behavioural, electrophysiological, biochemical and molecular biological

Table 1

Measurement	Measured change after chronic diazepam	Functional effect
Bicuculline seizure threshold	↓ Seizure threshold (loss of anticonvulsant effect)	↓ GABA function
Electrophysiological measurement of GABA sensitivity (dorsal raphe)	↑ Dose of GABA required (↑ IT_{50})	↓ GABA function
Chloride flux	↓ Ability of GABA to stimulate chloride flux	↓ GABA function
Receptor binding changes (cerebral cortex)	↓ Ability of GABA to enhance BZ binding (uncoupling)	
		↓ GABA function
	↑ Affinity of low-affinity GABA recognition site for GABA	
mRNA (α_1 probe)	↓ mRNA by Northern blot analysis	↓ GABA function

techniques we have indications that, at least in certain areas, there is a decrease in the function of GABA.

3.4 Benzodiazepine ligand efficacy and tolerance development

Numerous compounds appear to interact with the benzodiazepine site in the $GABA_A$ complex to alter GABAergic function. When interactions between various benzodiazepine ligands and GABA are analysed by electrophysiological, behavioural and biochemical techniques, it is clear that a whole spectrum of pharmacological agents of this chemical class exist which potentiate, decrease, or have no effect on GABAergic neurotransmission (Richards *et al.*, 1987; Braestrup *et al.*, 1984). These are termed agonists, inverse agonists and antagonists, respectively. Data described in the preceding sections have been obtained using full agonists which cause maximum positive modulation of GABA. However, compounds interacting with the benzodiazepine receptor may also possess partial agonistic properties, combining both agonistic and competitive antagonistic actions. The possible differences in tolerance/dependence liability between these compounds has only recently begun to be explored.

3.4.1 Chronic partial agonist and antagonist effects

The development of tolerance is not uniform across all benzodiazepines (Frey *et al.*, 1984; Gent *et al.*, 1985; Garratt *et al.*, 1988) and, in some instances, does not seem to occur. Chronic exposure to the pyrazoloquinoline CGS 9896, a partial agonist at the benzodiazepine recognition site, does not appear to produce tolerance to its anticonvulsant properties (Boast and Gerhardt, 1987) in experimental animals. More recently it has been reported that chronic treatment of mice with the partial agonist Ro16-6028 (Haefely, 1984) did not produce anticonvulsant (Haigh and Feely, 1988) or anxiolytic (Miller *et al.*, 1990) tolerance or physical dependence as tested by benzodiazepine antagonist precipitation of withdrawal (Moreau *et al.*, 1990). These data suggest that partial agonists, by possessing both agonist and antagonist properties, may circumvent the development of changes associated with tolerance and physical dependence as seen after chronic agonist administration. Our laboratory therefore began an investigation of the effects of chronic occupation of the benzodiazepine binding site *in vivo* by benzodiazepine ligands of differing intrinsic activity. In our study, we measured GABA sensitivity in dorsal raphe neurones, bicuculline-induced seizure threshold and parameters of binding to the $GABA_A$ receptor complex following a 3-week exposure to the partial agonist Ro16-6028. Effects following this partial agonist were compared with alterations seen after chronic agonist (diazepam) and chronic antagonist, Ro15-1788 (flumazenil), exposure (Hernandez *et al.*, 1989).

Our studies demonstrated that chronic exposure to the benzodiazepine antagonist Ro15-1788 did not alter functional or binding measures of the $GABA_A$ complex, nor did it alter the anticonvulsant potency of subsequently administered active benzodiazepine ligands. Thus chronic occupation of the benzodiazepine binding site is not sufficient to produce the biochemical and functional changes observed after chronic agonist (diazepam) exposure. These data therefore provide support for a hypothesis that benzodiazepine tolerance development requires an *active* interaction with the benzodiazepine recognition site. The amount of change (shown in a variety of GABA sensitivity measures, including GABA subsensitivity in dorsal raphe neurones and alterations in affinity for GABA of the GABA recognition site) following chronic benzodiazepine ligands used in our studies in rats, including diazepam, Ro16-6028 and Ro15-1788, could be directly correlated with agonist efficacy: full agonist > partial agonist ≫ antagonist (Hernandez *et al.*, 1989). Such changes suggest that differences in efficacy between these benzodiazepine ligands contribute to differences in tolerance liability and changes in GABA sensitivity and affinity. Thus a comparison of chronic *in vivo* exposure to benzodiazepine ligands of differing efficacy demonstrated that the magnitude of change in various measures of GABA sensitivity can be correlated with agonist efficacy (Figure 1). The magnitude of these changes could also be correlated with increasing potential for tolerance development following chronic exposure to these benzodiazepines. Recently, some physical dependence liability (Martin *et al.*, 1990) and tolerance to the antiseizure effects (Fleischhacker, 1988) to the partial agonist Ro16-6028 has been reported in primates, consistent with our findings in the rat. Such data may suggest a species difference between mice and rats or primates in susceptibility to tolerance/dependence liability for this class of compounds.

3.4.2 Chronic inverse agonist effects

The acute administration of a benzodiazepine inverse agonist such as FG7142 has been shown to result in clinical anxiety (Dorow *et al.*, 1983). Studies in experimental animals show that FG7142 has anxiogenic (Petersen *et al.*, 1982; Corda *et al.*, 1983; File and Pellow, 1984) and proconvulsant activity (Little *et al.*, 1984; Braestrup *et al.*, 1984). These effects are believed to result from a reduction in the inhibitory actions of GABA (Farb *et al.*, 1984; Bormann *et al.*, 1985; Obata and Yamamura, 1986). A number of laboratories have evaluated the effects of chronic *intermittent* exposure to FG7142, which leads

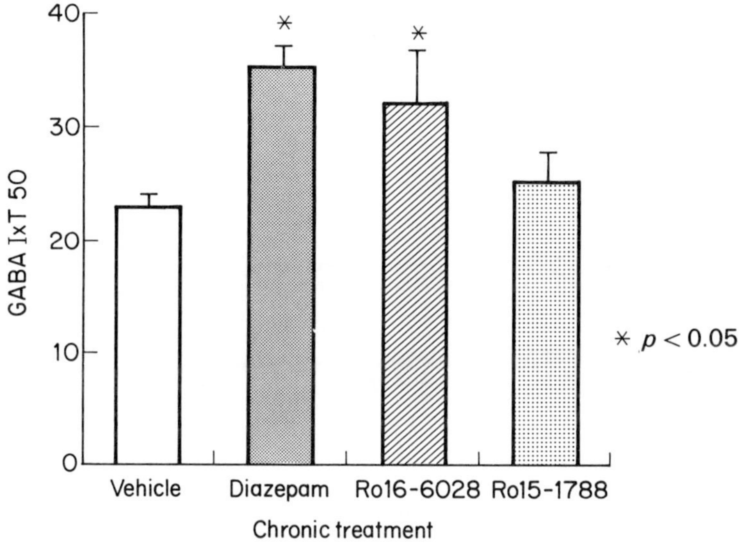

Figure 1 Effects of chronic exposure to benzodiazepine ligands of different efficacy on GABA sensitivity of dorsal raphe neurones. The $I \times T_{50}$ value (nanoCoulombs) is the product of the microiontophoretic current (nAmps) and the time (s) required to inhibit cell firing by 50%. This provides a quantative measure of neuronal sensitivity to GABA. The data was obtained from at least 3 dorsal raphe cells in 6–9 different animals receiving continuous *in vivo* treatments as indicated for 3 weeks. Adapted from Hernandez *et al.* (1989).

to increased seizure susceptibility and kindling (Little *et al.*, 1984; Biggio *et al.*, 1989). Our laboratory has recently evaluated parameters of the $GABA_A$ receptor complex following chronic *continuous* administration of the inverse agonist FG7142. Because of the short half-life of this compound in rodents (Little *et al.*, 1984; Gallager *et al.*, unpublished), we used an osmotic mini-pump (Alzet) to ensure continuous presence of FG7142 in the brain (Marley *et al.*, 1991). Using $^{36}C^-$ flux measurements and bicuculline seizure threshold determinations to evaluate the functional state of the GABA receptor complex, our studies suggest that chronic inverse agonist exposure leads to an apparent increase in GABAergic function (Marley *et al.*, 1991) TBPS binds to a site in or adjacent to the chloride ion channel, providing a measure of this element of the $GABA_A$ complex. We found that TBPS binding in brain membranes from chronically treated animals is also altered in opposite ways by continuous versus intermittent exposure to FG7142 (Thomsen *et al.*, 1991). Consistent with altered functional and biochemical changes following continuous exposure

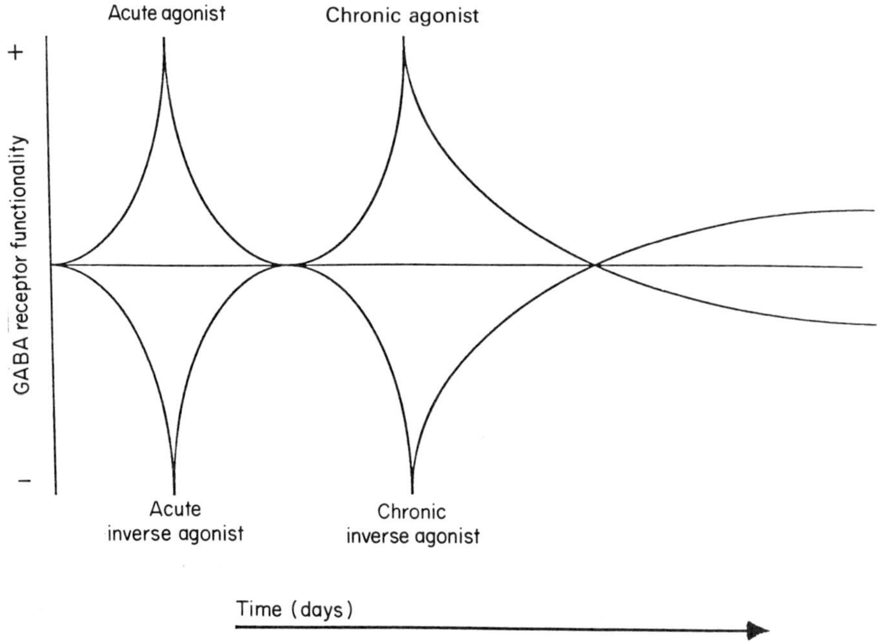

Figure 2 Exposure to acute or chronic benzodiazepine agonist contrasted with effects following acute or chronic exposure to an inverse agonist on GABA receptor function.

to the inverse agonist FG7142, $GABA_A$ subunit mRNA is altered in a manner opposite to that with continuous agonist (diazepam) exposure (Primus and Gallager, 1991). Such findings have led us to postulate that continuous occupation of the benzodiazepine modulatory site of the $GABA_A$ receptor complex results in compensatory effects in GABAergic function which appear to counteract the acute effects of these drugs. A schematic of this hypothesis is shown in Figure 2.

3.5 Regional heterogeneity

Attempts to generalize GABAergic subsensitivity to brain structures other than the raphe using identical techniques have not yielded similar findings. In the substantia nigra zona reticulata (SNr), chronic diazepam treatment failed to alter the sensitivity of reticulata neurones to GABA (Wilson and Gallager, 1987, 1989). Even after chronic exposure, the continued presence of diazepam was able to potentiate reticulata responses to iontophoretically applied GABA, indicating the lack of tolerance development to this effect of diazepam. An additional distinction was that administration of the antagonist Ro15-1788 after chronic diazepam treatment increased GABA sensitivity of dorsal raphe neurones to the level of the controls (Gallager *et al.*, 1984a), whereas Ro15-1788 decreased GABA sensitivity in SNr neurones after chronic diazepam exposure (Wilson and Gallager, 1988, 1989). Thus, neurones of the SNr and the dorsal raphe nucleus appear to respond quite differently to the same chronic diazepam treatment in terms of their sensitivity to iontophoretically applied GABA and their responses to benzodiazepine antagonist administration (Gallager and Wilson, 1988). We also found that chronic diazepam treatment had no effect on GABA-stimulated $^{36}Cl^-$ influx in membrane vesicles prepared from rat cerebellum (Marley and Gallager, 1989). Further evidence for lack of change in GABA/benzodiazepine receptor complex in cerebellum was provided by the observation that in cerebellar Purkinje cells, sensitivity to iontophoretically applied GABA was not decreased by chronic benzodiazepine exposure (Waterhouse *et al.*, 1984). Such data are consistent with electrophysiological evidence for regional differences in GABA sensitivity following chronic diazepam exposure (Gallager and Wilson, 1988). In addition, tolerance to the depressant effects of diazepam on local cerebral glucose use occurs at different rates in different brain regions (Laurie and Pratt, 1989; Chapter 1). Finally, data evaluating levels of mRNA for various $GABA_A$ receptor complex subunits show regionally selective changes (Heninger *et al.*, 1990). Decreases in subunit mRNA were seen in cerebral cortical but not hippocampal or cerebellar tissue. Taken together, these data provide evidence for regionally specific changes occurring at the $GABA_A$ receptor complex following chronic benzodiazepine exposure. Such regional differences may suggest that the development of tolerance to the benzodiazepines could include changes which are intrinsic to various brain areas, changes associated with the neural inputs to those areas (Gallager and Wilson, 1988; Gallager and Tallman, 1990) or differences in vulnerability based on heterogeneous $GABA_A$ receptor subunit composition (Gallager and Tallman, 1990; Schofield, 1989; Olsen and Tobin, 1990).

3.6 Possible pharmacological interventions for preventing or reversing tolerance/physical dependence

3.6.1 Periodic benzodiazepine antagonist exposure

In the process of establishing the role of the benzodiazepine site in mediating the shifts in GABA sensitivity during chronic benzodiazepine agonist exposure, we demonstrated that administration of the benzodiazepine antagonist Ro15-1788 (flumazenil) to diazepam-tolerant rats immediately reversed the GABAergic subsensitivity in doral raphe neurones (Gallager *et al.*, 1984a). We were surprised, however, to find that this reversal was persistent, lasting far beyond the period of expected antagonism of the Ro15-1788 (Gonsalves and Gallager, 1985, 1988). Behavioural experiments also indicated a restoration of anticonvulsant effects of the agonist diazepam following a single exposure to Ro15-1788 in tolerant animals (Gonsalves and Gallager, 1988). This latter experiment was particularly interesting in that it demonstrated that Ro15-1788 was not present in amounts sufficient for antagonizing the anticonvulsant actions of diazepam. Similar data were obtained with the pyrazoloquinoline benzodiazepine antagonist CGS 8216 (Yokoyama *et al.*, 1982), suggesting that the reversal phenomenon could be a general feature of benzodiazepine antagonists (Gonsalves and Gallager, 1988). Additional studies using *in vitro* electrophysiological techniques (Hernandez *et al.*, 1990) and $^{36}Cl^{-}$ flux measurements (Marley *et al.*, unpublished) have supported the normalization of GABAergic function. Increased GABAergic function following continuous inverse agonist exposure is also normalized by antagonist exposure (Gallager, unpublished). Behavioural data from other laboratories support this reversal phenomenon. Thus Nutt and Costello (1987, 1988) report that a single injection of flumazenil in mice resets tolerance to the hypothermic effects of lorazepam. Griffiths and colleagues (Sannerud *et al.*, 1989) describe incomplete reversal of midazolam tolerance in baboons. After flumazenil, midazolam produced a statistically significant increase in signs of ataxia but no reduction in tolerance to other signs of sedation. The ability of flumazenil to reverse tolerance to benzodiazepines has recently been assessed clinically (Savic *et al.*, 1991). In these studies epileptic patients with complex partial seizures, who had developed tolerance to the antiseizure effects of clonazepam, were given a single i.v. injection of flumazenil during their clonazepam treatment. Following the flumazenil treatment, patients were reported to be seizure-free for 6 to 21 days and to show significant reductions in epileptic discharges as monitored by EEG recordings. Such data provide a rationale for improving antiseizure therapy. However, not all signs of tolerance appear to be reversed by antagonist exposure. Thus Ro15-1788 did not change the degree of tolerance to sedation, muscle relaxation or ataxia in diazepam-dependent baboons (Sannerud *et al.*, 1989), nor to the depressant effects of diazepam on acoustic startle responses in rats (Davis and Gallager, 1988). Such discrepancies have been hypothesized to be based on differences in time-course for tolerance development (Gallager *et al.*, 1989). Thus for measures of benzodiazepine tolerance which develop slowly, reversibility would be more readily apparent.

Reversibility of physical dependence by exposure to the antagonist in agonist-dependent animals has also been demonstrated in a number of different species and laboratories. Reductions in symptoms of withdrawal have been shown following repeated injections of antagonist during the course of agonist treatment in baboons (Lamb and Griffiths, 1985; Sannerud *et al.*, 1989) and rhesus monkeys (Gallager *et al.*, 1986). The increased anxiety seen in rats abruptly withdrawn from chronic chlordiazepoxide was found to be reversed by a single injection of flumazenil (File and Baldwin, 1987; Baldwin and File, 1988). In mice, Nutt and Costello (1988) report that a single exposure to flumazenil abolished chronic agonist-induced sensitization to an inverse agonist, a measure they use as an index of dependence.

Taken together, these data indicate that antagonist exposure reverses the altered GABA and benzodiazepine sensitivities associated with prolonged benzodiazepine ligand exposure to their normal functional states (Table 2).

Electrophysiological studies indicate that reversal by the antagonist is rapid, suggesting that allosteric or biochemical changes are involved. Since all of our studies have suggested that a functional alteration in the $GABA_A$ complex occurs with chronic benzodiazepine agonist and inverse agonist resets the $GABA_A$ receptor complex back to its drug-naive state (Gonsalves and Gallager, 1985). In the clinical study demonstrating the ability of flumazenil to reverse anticonvulsant tolerance in epileptic patients (Savic *et al.*, 1991), the authors were able to monitor receptor occupancy using positron emission tomography. Based on these measurements, Savic *et al.* (1991) speculate that the reversal could be due to a rapid conformational change in the $GABA_A$ receptor complex. However, the mechanisms by which chronic occupation of a modulatory site could lead to decreased function of the neurotransmitter and how antagonist occupation of this site could reverse such a process remain elusive. We have postulated that a conformational change and/or a change in phosphorylation of the receptor complex could underlie such effects (Gonsalves and Gallager, 1985; Gallager and Tallman, 1990). Such a hypothesis is made more plausible by the identification of consensus sequences for sites of phosphorylation in the $GABA_A$ receptor complex (Schofield *et al.*, 1987; Pritchett *et al.*, 1989b). More directly, endogenous phosphorylation experiments have provided evidence that the benzodiazepine photolabelled subunit of the $GABA_A$ complex is phosphorylated by an endogenous protein kinase (Sweetman *et al.*, 1988). Direct phosphorylation data are also available for the β-subunit (Browning *et al.*, 1990). Based on new knowledge of molecular biology (Schofield, 1989; Olsen and Tobin, 1990; Sigel *et al.*, 1990), we should be able to determine whether the changes we have observed in the subunit composition of $GABA_A$ receptor complex from tolerant animals could be related to alterations in receptor response. We should ultimately be able to determine, at the molecular level, how changes resulting from acute and chronic occupation of the benzodiazepine site could result in functionally

Table 2

Measurement	Effect of RO15-1788 exposure to tolerant system	Interpretation	Functional effect
Bicuculline seizure Threshold (up to 7 day pretreatment)	Anticonvulsant effects of diazepam re-emerge	Tolerance reversal	Normalize GABA function
Electrophysiology			
in vivo			
acute	Immediate reversal of GABA subsensitivity	Reset to normal GABA sensitivity	Normalize GABA function
i.p. dose during chronic treatment	Single exposure sufficient to normalize GABA sensitivity	Reversal is persistent	Normalize GABA function
in vitro	Reversal of GABA subsensitivity	Reset localized to midbrain	Normalize GABA function
Chloride flux (24 h, i.p.)	Single exposure normalizes GABA sensitivity	Reset to normal GABA sensitivity	Normalize GABA function
Bicuculline binding	Affinity of GABA recognition site normalized	Reverse desensitization	Normalize GABA function
Withdrawal symptoms in primates	Greatly attenuated withdrawal syndrome with periodic exposure to antagonist	Prevent development of physical dependence	Normalize GABA function
Epileptic discharges in patients tolerant to clonazepam	Antiepileptic effects of clonazapam re-emerge	Tolerance reversal	Normalize benzodiazepine sensitivity

opposite responses and how such changes could be regionally specific (Gallager and Tallman, 1990; Gallager *et al.*, 1991).

3.6.2 Pharmacological interventions at other (non-$GABA_A$ complex) sites

There are now reports in the literature of drugs unrelated to the $GABA_A$ system which have been shown in some systems to decrease benzodiazepine withdrawal symptoms. One study evaluated the hypothesis that voltage-sensitive calcium channels might be involved in the development of the withdrawal syndrome after chronic exposure to benzodiazepines (Zharkovsky *et al.*, 1989). These investigators reported significant effects of the calcium channel antagonists, verapamil and nifedipine, in suppressing signs of spontaneous and benzodiazepine antagonist-precipitated withdrawal in diazepam-dependent rats. Calcium channel antagonists have been reported to suppress abstinence signs induced by chronic morphine and ethanol (Bongiani *et al.*, 1986; Little *et al.*, 1986, Chapter 4), suggesting that these agents may have utility in treating general symptoms of withdrawal.

The $5\text{-}HT_{1A}$ agonist anxiolytic, buspirone, has been examined for its effectiveness in treating benzodiazepine withdrawal, both clinically (Schweizer and Rickels, 1986) and in experimental animals (Costall *et al.*, 1989). Buspirone failed to reverse diazepam withdrawal phenomena in either paradigm. In contrast, Costall *et al.* (1989) have reported that the $5\text{-}HT_3$ receptor antagonist, ondansetron, prevented the behavioural suppression and weight loss in diazepam-dependent rodents seen following flumazenil-precipitated withdrawal or spontaneous withdrawal from diazepam. Other studies indicate that ondansetron is able to prevent behavioural suppression which occurs after withdrawal from chronic treatment with nicotine, ethanol or cocaine, suggesting a more general action, perhaps on mesolimbic reward systems (Costall *et al.*, 1989).

The anticonvulsant carbamazepine has been tested for efficacy in attenuating benzodiazepine withdrawal symptoms. Preliminary clinical reports suggest that benzodiazepine (including alprazolam) discontinuation with carbamazepine was more rapid and better tolerated than gradual discontinuation of benzodiazepine treatment alone (Klein *et al.*, 1986; Ries *et al.*, 1989). Since there is little evidence to date that carbamazepine has significant activity at the $GABA_A$ receptor complex (Post, 1987), the mechanism for its efficacy in attenuating benzodiazepine withdrawal symptoms is not yet understood. However, the use of this anticonvulsant in treatment of alcohol withdrawal suggests that it too may have general utility as an anti-withdrawal medication.

Based on the clinical success of clonidine in blocking opiate withdrawal symptoms (Gold *et al.*, 1978), the actions of this α_2 adrenergic-agonist were also tested on diazepam withdrawal symptoms in rats (Kunchandy and Kulkarni, 1986; Baldwin *et al.*, 1989), monkeys (Redmond and Roth, personal communication) and people (Goodman *et al.*, 1986). While clonidine was found to be effective against some of the autonomic symptoms seen during withdrawal (Kunchandy and Kulkarni, 1986; Redmond and Roth, personal communication), this treatment was unable to block the increased anxiety observed during spontaneous withdrawal from benzodiazepine (Baldwin *et al.*, 1989; Goodman *et al.*, 1986) or to block seizures produced by antagonist-precipitated withdrawal (Redmond and Roth, personal communication).

Since the benzodiazepine withdrawal syndrome may be expressed through multiple neurotransmitter systems (Baldwin *et al.*, 1989), it is possible that there will be many agents which are effective against certain withdrawal components. However, if tolerance/dependence to the benzodiazepines is due to changes originating within the $GABA_A$ receptor complex, then agents reversing alterations at this locus are likely to be the most efficacious. This may underlie the success of the recent clinical experiment (Savic *et al.*, 1991). Precise knowledge of the molecular mechanism underlying tolerance and physical dependence should lead to improved therapies using agents acting on this important receptor complex.

Acknowledgements

This work was supported by PHS Grants NS-23321, MH-14276, MH-25642 and the State of Connecticut.

References

Abbracchio, M.P., Balduini, W., Coen, E., Lombardelli, G., Peruzzi, G. & Cattabeni, F. (1983) In *Benzodiazepine Recognition Site Ligands: Biochemistry and Pharmacology* (ed. Biggio, G. & Costa, E.), pp 227–237. New York, Raven Press.

Baldwin, H. & File, S. (1988) *Brain Res. Bull* **20**, 603–606.

Baldwin, H., Hitchcott, P. & File, S. (1989) *Pharmacol. Biochem. Behav.* **34**, 931–933.

Barker, J.L. & Owen, D.G. (1986) In *Benzodiazepine/GABA Receptors and Chloride Channels: Structural and Functional Properties* (eds Olsen, R.W. & Ventor, J.C.), pp 135–165. New York, Alan R. Liss, Inc.

Biggio, G., Giorgi, O., Concas, A. & Corda, M.G. (1989) In *Allosteric Modulation of Amino Acid Receptors: Therapeutic Implications* (eds Barnard, E. & Costa, E.), pp 71–89. New York, Raven Press Ltd.

Boast, C.A. & Gerhardt, S.C. (1987) *Biochem. Behav.* **26**, 601–606.

Bongiani, F., Carla, V., Morono, F. & Pellegrini-Giempieto, D. (1986) *Br. J. Pharmacol.* **88**, 561–567.

Bormann, J. (1988) *Trends Neurosci.* **11**, 112–116.

Bormann, J. & Sakmann, B. (1984) *IUPHAR 9th Int. Congr. Pharmacol. Abstr.* **1984**, 13–14.
Bormann, J., Ferrero, P., Guidotti, A. & Costa, E. (1985) *Regul. Pept.* **4**, 33–38.
Braestrup, C. & Nielsen, M. (1983) In *Handbook of Psychopharmacology* (eds Iversen, S.I.L. & Snyder, S.), pp 285–384. New York, Plenum Press.
Braestrup, C., Honore, T., Nielsen, M., Petersen, E.N. & Jensen, L.H. (1984) *Biochem. Pharmacol.* **33**, 1763–1768.
Browning, M., Bureau, M., Barnes, E. & Olsen, R. (1990) *Proc. Natl Acad. Sci. USA* **87**, 1315–1318.
Casalotti, S., Stephenson, F. & Barnard, E. (1986) *J. Biol. Chem.* **261**, 15013–15016.
Cavalla, D. & Neff, N. (1985) *J. Neurochem.* **44**, 916–921.
Changeux, J.-P., Devillers-Thiery, A. & Chemouilli, P. (1984) *Science* **225**, 1335–1345.
Corda, M., Blaker, W., Mendelson, W., Guidotti, A. & Costa, E. (1983) *Proc. Natl Acad. Sci. USA* **80**, 2072–2076.
Costa, E., Guidotti, A. & Toffano, G. (1978) *Br. J. Pharmacol.* **133**, 239–248.
Costall, B., Jones, B., Kelly, M.E., Naylor, R., Oakley, N., Onaivi, E. & Tyers, M. (1989) *Pharmacol. Biochem. Behav.* **34**, 769–778.
Czajkowski, C., Gibbs, T. & Farb, D. (1989) *Mol. Pharmacol.* **35**, 75–84.
Davis, M. & Gallager, D.W. (1988) *Eur. J. Pharmacol.* **150**, 23–33.
Deng, L., Ransom, R. & Olson, R. (1986) *Biochem. Biophys. Res. Commun.* **138**, 1308–1314.
Dorow, R., Horowski, R., Paschelke, G., Amin, M. & Braestrup, C. (1983) *Lancet,* July 9, 98–99.
Farb, D.H., Borden, L.A., Chan, C.Y., Czajkowski, C.M., Gibbs, T.T. & Schiller, G.D. (1984) *Ann. N. Y. Acad. Sci.* **435**, 1–31.
Farrant, M. & Webster, R. (1989) In *Drugs as Tools in Neurotransmitter Research* (eds Boulton, A., Baker, G. & Juorio, A.), pp 161–219. Clifton, Humana Press Inc.
File, S.E. (1982) *Psychopharmacology* **77**, 284–288.
File, S.E. & Baldwin, H.A. (1987) *Lancet,* July 11, 106–107.
File, S. & Pellow, S. (1984) *Br. J. Pharmacol.* **82** (Suppl.), 240.
Fleischhacker, W.W. (1988) *Lancet,* August 27, 504.
Frey, H., Philippin, H. & Scheuler, W. (1984) *Eur. J. Pharmacol.* **104**, 27–38.
Gallager, D. & Tallman, J. (1990) *Neurochem. Res.* **14**, 113–118.
Gallager, D.W. & Wilson, M.A. (1988) In *Chloride Channels and their Modulation by Neurotransmitters and Drugs* (eds Biggio, G. & Costa, E.), pp 325–336. New York, Raven Press.
Gallager, D.W. Lakoski, J.M., Gonsalves, S.F. & Rauch, S.L. (1984a) *Nature* **308**, 74–76.
Gallager, D.W., Rauch, S.L. & Malcolm, A.B. (1984b) *Eur. J. Pharmacol.* **98**, 159–160.
Gallager, D.W., Malcolm, A.B., Anderson, S.A. & Gonsalves, S.F. (1985) *Brain Res.* **343**, 26–36.
Gallager, D.W., Heninger, K. & Heninger, G. (1986) *Eur. J. Pharmacol.* **132**, 31–38.
Gallager, D.W., Heninger, C. & Wilson, M.A. (1989) In *Allosteric Modulation of Amino Acid Receptors: Therapeutic Implications* (eds Barnard, E.A. & Costa, E.), pp 91–107. New York, Raven Press.
Gallager, D.W., Jacobs, A.A., During, M.J. & Hernandez, T.D. (1991) In *Transmitter Amino Acid Receptors: Structures, Transduction and Models for Drug Development* (eds Barnard, E.A. & Costa, E.), New York, Raven Press.
Garratt, J.C., Gent, J.P., Feely, M. & Haigh, J.R.M. (1988) *Eur. J. Pharmacol.* **145**, 75–80.
Gent, J.P., Feely, M.P. & Haigh, J.R.M. (1985) *Life Sci.* **37**, 849–856.

Gold, M.S., Redmond, D.E. & Kleber, H.D. (1978) *Lancet* **2**, 599–602.
Gonsalves, S.F. & Gallager, D.W. (1985) *Eur. J. Pharmacol.* **110**, 163–170.
Gonsalves, S.F. & Gallager, D.W. (1987) *Brain Res.* **405**, 94–99.
Gonsalves, S.F. & Gallager, D.W. (1988) *J. Pharmacol. Exp. Ther.* **244**, 79–83.
Goodman, W.K., Charney, D.S., Price, L.H., Woods, S.W. & Heninger, G.R. (1986) *Am. J. Psychiatry* **143**, 900–903.
Greenblatt, D.J. & Shader, R.I. (1986) *Psychopharmacol. Bull.* **22**, 416–423.
Haefely, W. (1984) *Clin. Neuropharmacol.* **7**, 670–671.
Haefely, W. & Hunkeler, W. (1988) *Eur. J. Anaesthesiol.* **2**, 3–14.
Haefely, W. & Polc, P. (1986) In *Benzodiazepine-GABA Receptors and Chloride Channels* (eds Olsen, R.W. & Venter, J.C.), pp 97–133. New York, Alan R. Liss.
Haigh, J.R.M. & Feely, M. (1988) *Eur. J. Pharmacol.* **147**, 283–285.
Haigh, J.R.M., Pullar, T., Gent, J.P., Dailley, C. & Geely, M. (1986) *J. Pharm. Pharmacol.* **38**, 931–934.
Hamill, D.P., Bormann, J. & Sakmann, B. (1983) *Nature* **305**, 805–808.
Harris, R.A. & Allan, A.M. (1985) *Science* **228**, 1108–1110.
Hawkins, M., Pravica, M. & Radulovacki, M. (1988) *Pharmacol. Biochem. Behav.* **30**, 303–308.
Heninger, C. & Gallager, D.W. (1988) *Neuropharmacology* **27**, 1073–1076.
Heninger, C., Saito, N., Tallman, J., Garrett, K., Vitek, M., Duman, R. & Gallager, D. (1990) *J. Mol. Neurosci.* **2**, 101–107.
Hernandez, T., Heninger, C., Wilson, M. & Gallager, D. (1989) *Eur. J. Pharmacol.* **170**, 145–155.
Hernandez, T., Rosen, J. & Gallager, D. (1990) *Brain Res.* **517**, 294–300.
Hunkeler, W., Mohler, H., Pieri, L., Polc, P., Bonetti, E., Cumin, R., Schaffner, R. & Haefly, W. (1981) *Nature* **290**, 514–516.
Johnston, G. & Skerritt, J. (1983) In *Actions and Interactions of GABA and Benzodiazepines.* (ed. Bowery, N.G.), pp 179–189. New York, Raven Press.
Klein, E., Uhde, T. & Post, R. (1986) *Am. J. Psychiatry* **143**, 235–236.
Krespan, B., Springfield, S.A., Haas, H. & Geller, H.M. (1984) *Brain Res.* **295**, 265–274.
Kunchandy, J. & Kulkarni, S.K. (1986) *Psychopharmacology* **90**, 198–202.
Lamb, R.J. & Griffiths, R.R. (1985) *Eur. J. Pharmacol.* **110**, 257–261.
Laurie, D.J. & Pratt, J.A. (1989) *Brain Res.* **504**, 101–111.
Levitan, E.S., Schofield, P.R., Burt, D.R., Rhee, L.M., Wisden, W., Kohler, M., Darlison, M.G., Barnard, E.A. & Seeburg, P.H. (1988) *Nature* **335**, 76–79.
Little, H., Nutt, D. & Taylor, S. (1984) *Br. J. Pharmacol.* **83**, 951–958.
Little, H., Dolin, S. & Halsey, M. (1986) *Life Sci.* **39**, 2059–2065.
Lolait, S., O'Carroll, A., Kusano, K. & Mahan, L. (1989a) *FEBS Lett.* **528**, 17–21.
Lolait, S., O'Carroll, A., Kusano, D., Muller, J., Brownstein, M. & Mahan, L. (1989b) *FEBS Lett.* **246**, 145–148.
Mamalaki, C., Stephenson, F.A. & Barnard, E.A. (1987) *EMBO J.* **6**, 561–565.
Marangos, P.J. & Crawley, J.N. (1982) *Neuropharmacology* **21**, 81–84.
Marks, J. (1985) In *The Benzodiazepines: Use, Overuse, Misuse, Abuse.* (ed. Marks, J.), pp 33–38. Lancaster, MPT Press Limited.
Marley, R.J. & Gallager, D.W. (1989) *Eur. J. Pharmacol.* **159**, 217–223.
Marley, R.J., Heninger, C., Hernandez, T.D. & Gallager, D.W. (1991) *Neuropharmacology* **30**, 245–251.
Martin, J., Kuwahara, A., Horii, I., Moreau, J., Jenck, F., Sepinwall, J. & Haefely, W. (1990) *Soc. Neurosci. Abstr.* **16**, 1104.

Massotti, M., Alleva, F., Balazs, T. & Guidotti, A. (1980) *Neuropharmacology* **19**, 951–956.
Mele, L., Sagratella, S. & Massotti, M. (1984) *Brain Res.* **323**, 93–102.
Miller, L.G., Greenblatt, D.J., Barnhill, J.G. & Shader, R.I. (1988) *J. Pharmacol. Exp. Ther.* **246**, 170–176.
Miller, L., Galpern, W., Greenblatt, D., Lumpkin, M. & Shader, R. (1990) *J. Pharmacol. Exp. Ther.* **254**, 33–38.
Mohler, H. & Okada, T. (1977) *Science* **198**, 845–851.
Mohler, H., Battersby, M.K. & Richards, J.G. (1980) *Proc. Natl Acad. Sci. USA* **77**, 1161–1670.
Moreau, J., Jenck, F., Pieri, L., Schoch, P., Martin, J. & Haefely, J. (1990) *Eur. J. Pharmacol.* **190**, 269–273.
Nutt, D. (1986) *Trends Pharm. Sci.* **8**, 457–460.
Nutt, D. & Costello, M. (1987) *Lancet*, August 22, 463.
Nutt, D. & Costello, M. (1988) *Life Sci.* **43**, 1045–1053.
Obata, T. & Yamamura, H.I. (1986) *Biochem. Biophys. Res. Commun.* **141**, 1–6.
Olsen, R.W. (1982) *Annu. Rev. Pharmacol. Toxicol.* **22**, 245–277.
Olsen, R.W. & Snowman, A.M. (1983) *J. Neurochem.* **41**, 1653–1663.
Olsen, R. & Tobin, A. (1990) *FASEB J.* **4**, 1469–1480.
Olsen, R. & Venter, J. (1986) In *Receptor Biochemistry and Methodology* (eds Olsen, R. & Venter, J.), pp 351. New York, Alan R. Liss.
Olsen, R.W., Wong, E.H.F., Stauber, G.B. & King, R.G. (1984) *Fed. Proc.* **443**, 2773–2778.
Overstreet, D.H. & Yamamura, H.I. (1979) *Life Sci.* **25**, 1865–1878.
Paul, S.M., Syapin, P.J., Pough, B.A., Moncada, V. & Skolnick, P. (1979) *Nature* **281**, 688–689.
Peters, J., Kirkness, E., Callachan, H., Lambert, J. & Turner, A. (1988) *Br. J. Pharmacol.* **94**, 1257–1269.
Petersen, E., Paschelke, G., Kehr, W., Nielsen, M. & Braestrup, C. (1982) *Eur. J. Pharmacol.* **82**, 217–221.
Polc, P. (1988) *Prog. Neurobiol.* **31**, 349–423.
Post, R.M. (1987) In *Psychopharmacology: The Third Generation of Progress* (ed. Meltzer, H.Y.), pp 567–576. New York, Raven Press.
Primus, R. & Gallager, D.W. (1991) Society Neuroscience Abstracts. (in press).
Pritchett, D., Luddens, H. & Seeburg, P. (1989a) *Science* **245**, 1389–1392.
Pritchett, D.B., Sontheimer, H., Shivers, B.D., Ymer, S., Kettenmann, H., Schofield, P.R. & Seeburg, P.H. (1989b) *Nature* **338**, 582–585.
Richards, J.G., Schoch, P., Haring, P., Takacs, B. & Mohler, H. (1987) *J. Neurosci.* **7**, 1866–1886.
Rickles, K., Schweizer, E., Csanalosi, I., Case, W.G. & Chung, H. (1988) *Arch. Gen. Psychiatry* **45**, 444–450.
Ries, R., Roy-Byrne, P., Ward, N., Neppe, V. & Cullison, S. (1989) *Am. J. Psychiatry* **146**, 536–537.
Rosenberg, H.C. & Chiu, T.H. (1981) *Eur. J. Pharmacol.* **70**, 453–460.
Sannerud, C., Cook, J. & Griffiths, R. (1989) *Eur. J. Pharmacol.* **167**, 333–343.
Savic, I., Widen, L. & Stone-Elander, S. (1991) *Lancet*, Jan. 19, **337**, 133–137.
Schiller, G.D. & Farb, D.H. (1986) *Ann. N.Y. Acad. Sci.* **463**, 221–223.
Schoch, P., Richards, J.G., Haring, P., Takacs, B., Stahli, C., Staehelin, T., Haefely, W. & Mohler, H. (1985) *Nature* **314**, 168–171.
Schofield, P. (1989) *Trends Pharm. Sci.* **10**, 470–475.

Schofield, P.R., Darllison, M.G., Barnard, E.A., Stephenson, F.A., Seeburg, P.H., Fujita, N., Burt, D.R. & Rodriguez, H. (1987) *Nature* **328**, 221–227.
Schweizer, E. & Rickels, K. (1986) *Am. J. Psychiatry* **143**, 1590–1592.
Sher, P.K., Study, R.E., Mazzetta, J., Barker, J.L. & Nelson, P.G. (1983) *Brain Res.* **268**, 171–176.
Shivers, B., Killisch, I., Sprengel, R., Sontheimer, H., Kohler, M., Schofield, P. & Seeburg, P. (1989) *Neuron* **3**, 327–337.
Siegel, R.E. (1988) *Neuron* **1**, 579–584.
Sieghart, W. (1989) *Trends Pharm. Sci.* **10**, 407–411.
Sigel, E., Baur, R., Trube, G., Mohler, H. & Malherbe, P. (1990) *Neuron* **5**, 703–711.
Squires, R., Casida, J., Richardson, M. & Saederup, E. (1983) *Mol. Pharmacol.* **23**, 326–336.
Squires, R. & Braestrup, C. (1977) *Nature* **166**, 732–734.
Stephens, D.N. & Schneider, H.H. (1985) *Psychopharmacology* **87**, 322–327.
Stephenson, F. (1988) *Biochem. J.* **249**, 21–32.
Sweetman, P.M. & Tallman, J.F. (1986) *Mol. Pharmacol.* **29**, 299–306.
Sweetman, P.M., Lloyd, J., Gallombardo, P., Malison, R.T., Gallager, D.W., Tallman, J.F. & Nestler, E.J. (1988) *J. Neurochem.* **51**, 1274–1284.
Tallman, J.F. & Gallager, D.W. (1985) *Ann. Rev. Neurosci.* **8**, 21–44.
Tallman, J.F., Thomas, J.W. & Gallager, D.W. (1978) *Nature* **274**, 383–385.
Tallman, J.F., Paul, S., Skolnick, P. & Gallager, D.W. (1980) *Science* **207**, 274–281.
Thomas, J.W. & Tallman, J.F. (1981) *J. Biol. Chem.* **156**, 9838–9842.
Thomsen, C., Pedersen, U.B. & Gallager, D.W. (1991) *Eur. J. Pharm.* In press.
Tietz, E.I. & Rosenberg, H.C. (1988) *Brain Res.* **438**, 41–51.
Verdoorn, T., Draguhn, A., Ymer, S., Seeburg, P. & Sakmann, B. (1990) *Neuron* **4**, 919–928.
Waterhouse, B.D., Moises, H.C., Hermes, H.H., Geller, H.M. & Woodward, D.J. (1984) *J. Pharmacol. Exp. Ther.* **228**, 257–267.
Wilson, M.A. & Gallager, D.W. (1987) *Eur. J. Pharmacol.* **136**, 333–343.
Wilson, M.A. & Gallager, D.W. (1988) *Brain Res.* **473**, 198–202.
Wilson, M.A. & Gallager, D.W. (1989) *J. Pharmacol. Exp. Ther.* **248**, 879–885.
Wisden, W., Morris, B., Darlison, M., Hunt, S. & Barnard, E. (1989) *Mol. Brain Res.* **5**, 305–310.
Woods, S. & Charney, D. (1988) In *Handbook of Anxiety Disorders* (eds Last, C. & Hersen, M.), pp 413–444. New York, Pergamon Press.
Ymer, S., Schofield, P., Draguhn, A., Werner, P., Kohler, M. & Seeburg, P. (1989) *EMBO J.* **8**, 1665–1670.
Yokoyama, N., Ritter, B. & Neubert, A.D. (1982) *J. Med. Chem.* **25**, 337–339.
Zharkovsky, A., Sayrin, A., Zharkovsky, T. & Cereska, K. (1989) *Acta Comm. Univ. Tartuensis.* **866**, 27–41.

CHAPTER 4

ETHANOL TOLERANCE AND PHYSICAL DEPENDENCE: THE ROLE OF CALCIUM CHANNELS AND OTHER POSSIBLE MECHANISMS

Hilary J. Little

Pharmacology Department, The Medical School, University Walk, Bristol, BS8 1TD, UK

Table of Contents

THE BIOLOGICAL BASES OF DRUG TOLERANCE AND DEPENDENCE
ISBN 0-12-564250-4

4.1 Introduction

There is considerable evidence to suggest that the important sites of action of ethanol are in the cell membrane, and much of this chapter will be concerned with the effects of ethanol on postsynaptic membrane function. Although ethanol has effects on neurotransmitter release (see Section 4.7), these are thought to be consequences of its membrane actions. Many of the effects discussed, including those on ion channels and on second messenger systems, are exerted at both pre- and postsynaptic sites.

I shall restrict the text to discussion of studies on the biochemical changes that occur during long-term intake of ethanol that might be responsible for ethanol tolerance and the withdrawal syndrome. I have not attempted to cover the extensive and valuable work on alcohol dependence in man. It should be borne in mind, however, that the biochemical changes described may be the cause of continued drinking in alcoholics. The first section of the chapter will concentrate on the possible role of calcium ions in ethanol dependence, in view of the many recent developments in this area.

In order to aid the interpretation of results described below, the blood concentrations of ethanol associated with certain behavioural effects are listed in Table 1. Blood concentrations of 5–10 mM are found in humans after

Table 1 Blood ethanol concentrations associated with the behavioural effects of ethanol. Reprinted with permission from Little (1991).

		Blood ethanol concentrations		
Species	Effects	(mM)	(mg/100 ml)	(% w/v)
Humans	Altered mood, impaired cognition	5.4	22	0.025
Humans	Increased risk of road traffic accidents	10.2	47	0.047
Humans	Impaired attention	11	50	0.05
Humans	Sedation, ataxia	20	91	0.09
Humans	Intoxication, ataxia	22	100	0.1
Rats	Sedation	22	100	0.1
Humans	Loss of conciousness	50	227	0.227
Rats	Hypothermia	40	184	0.184
Mice	Loss of righting reflex	65	300	0.3
Humans	Death	109	500	0.5
Mice	Sleep, hypothermia	122	562	0.562

ethanol doses that cause impaired behavioural responses such as loss of attention and inco-ordination, while 20 mM and above is associated with sedation, ataxia and confusion (Charness *et al.*, 1989). Between 50 and 100 mM causes considerable CNS depression, with loss of consciousness. Concentrations above about 100 mM may be fatal. In rodents, ataxic and anticonvulsant properties are seen after doses of 1–2 g/kg ethanol and sedative and hypnotic effects at 3–4 g/kg.

4.2 Effects of ethanol on neurotransmitter function and transmembrane signalling

4.2.1 The effects of ethanol on the neuronal membrane

The pharmacological properties of ethanol are said to be 'non-specific'. This does not mean that ethanol has the same effect at every site. The term is used in the pharmacological sense, indicating that ethanol does not act by binding to specific protein receptor sites. Because of the lack of such sites, it has been suggested that ethanol produces its effects through action on lipids rather than proteins. There is a considerable amount of evidence that ethanol can affect the lipids of cell membranes and this area of research has been summarized in the overview by Goldstein (1986).

The acute effect of ethanol is to increase lipid fluidity, that is, the amount of movement of the phospholipids in the membrane bilayer. Ethanol has this effect on neuronal membranes at concentrations of 10–20 mM (Chin and Goldstein, 1977a), but the changes are small, particularly when compared with those caused by alterations in temperature of a few degrees. The effects of ethanol, however, are not uniform throughout the membrane; the disordering was found to be greater when deeper ESR (electron spin resonance) probes were used than when measurements were made at the surface of the lipid bilayer (Goldstein and Chin, 1981). The changes were shown to be increased if gangliosides, normally removed during extraction, were included in the preparations (Harris *et al.*, 1984a).

Chronic ethanol treatment decreased the fluidizing effect of ethanol (Chin and Goldstein, 1977b) and decreased the fluidity of the membranes in the absence of ethanol (Lyon and Goldstein, 1982; Harris *et al.*, 1984b). Use of fluorescence polarization techniques has been found to demonstrate changes after chronic ethanol that were not apparent by ESR measurements (Harris *et al.*, 1984b). Tolerance to the fluidizing effects of ethanol was seen after chronic ethanol or chronic pentobarbitone treatment, but not after morphine administration (Johnson *et al.*, 1980). Taraschi *et al.* (1986) demonstrated transfer of the tolerance to the disordering effects of ethanol on multilamellar vesicles by addition of phosphatidylinositol from ethanol-fed rats and this transfer did not occur when other phospholipids, including phosphatidylserine, were used. The authors suggested that small changes in fatty acid composition might be responsible for the resistance to the action of the ethanol.

The capacity of membranes to bind ethanol, and other general anaesthetic compounds, was decreased by long-term ethanol administration (Rottenberg *et al.*, 1981). In some cases the membrane cholesterol content was found to be increased after chronic ethanol treatment (Chin *et al.*, 1978; Crews *et al.*, 1983), but in other studies where the chronic treatment schedule caused tolerance and dependence *in vivo*, no changes were found in the membrane cholesterol content (Lyon and Goldstein, 1983; La Droitte *et al.*, 1984). The ganglioside content of brain synaptic membrane was unaltered by a chronic treatment that caused dependence (Harris *et al.*, 1984b).

Littleton and John (1977) showed increased saturation of membrane phospholipid groups after 10 days ethanol inhalation. Harris *et al.* (1984b) found that this change occurred in the acyl groups of phosphatidylserine, but that chronic ethanol ingestion did not alter the acyl composition of other phospholipids. The amount of phosphatidylserine has been found to be increased after chronic ethanol treatment (Sun *et al.*, 1984). It appears that the changes in the lipid content of the membrane after long-term ethanol treatment are selective and may be confined to certain constituents. The membrane components affected, however, are important in neuronal transmission, and may be involved in the neuronal actions of ethanol.

The metabolism of brain phospholipids has more clearly been shown to be affected by long-term ethanol treatment. In 1980, Lee *et al.* measured phospholipid turnover in rat brain. An acute dose of ethanol, given *in vivo*, did not affect the incorporation of ^{32}P into phosphatidylcholine, phosphatidylinositol/phosphatidylserine or phosphatidylethanolamine. Increased incorporation of [^{3}H]glycerol into the three former compounds was found, but no tolerance developed to this effect after chronic ethanol treatment. Ethanol tolerance was found to be associated with an increase in ^{32}P incorporation into phosphatidylcholine, phosphatidylinositol/phosphatidylserine and phosphatidylethanolamine in microsomal membrane fractions and into phosphatidylinositol/phosphatidylserine in the synaptosomal fraction. During ethanol withdrawal, when a physical withdrawal syndrome was seen *in vivo*, there was a significant decrease in ^{32}P incorporation into microsomal phosphatidylinositol/phosphatidylserine.

There is therefore considerable evidence to show that ethanol can cause changes in the lipids of neuronal membranes. What is not so certain is whether these changes are the basis of the acute and chronic actions of ethanol and this has been the subject of some controversy. The theory of a lipid site of action for ethanol, however, should not be taken to mean that ethanol's action is mediated entirely through changes in the bilayer lipid. The primary action of ethanol may be on the lipid–protein interface surrounding the protein molecules within the membrane, but this site is very difficult to study. Small perturbations of this interface can cause considerable changes in the function of the membrane proteins. Effects on membrane transducer systems have been demonstrated (e.g. Rinon *et al.*, 1978; Loh and Law, 1980; Nelson and Delgardo-Escueta, 1986; Epaud and Lester, 1990). Changes at the lipid–protein interface could result in different changes at different sites, some membrane proteins being greatly affected and some to a lesser extent. Little is known as yet about the effects of such perturbations on ion channel function, but it is likely that some of the effects of ethanol described below are produced by this type of action.

4.2.2 Actions of ethanol on the polyphosphoinositide signalling system

Ethanol has been shown to have some effects on inositol lipid metabolism and these may play a role in ethanol dependence. An early paper (Allison and Cicero, 1980) reported that an acute dose of ethanol *in vivo* reduced myoinositol-1-phosphate levels in cerebral cortex by 60% within 30 min of injection. The change correlated with the ethanol blood concentrations, and normal values were reached 24 h later. Myoinositol concentrations were unaltered. The binding of [^{3}H]inositol has been found to be decreased by chronic ethanol treatment (Smith, 1987).

Comparison of the effects of acute and chronic ethanol on inositol phospholipid hydrolysis stimulated by various receptors was made by Gonzales *et al.* (1986) and Gonzales and Crews (1988). Inositide hydrolysis was measured by the release of [^{3}H]inositol phosphates from lithium-treated cerebrocortical slices incubated with [^{3}H]myoinositol. Only a high concentration of ethanol (500 mM) inhibited basal inositide hydrolysis and hydrolysis stimulated by KCl or glutamate. Noradrenaline-stimulated breakdown was more sensitive, as this was affected by 100 mM ethanol, while hydrolysis stimulated by carbachol or 5-HT was unaltered even by 500 mM. Some regional variations were seen, but KCl-stimulated breakdown was inhibited by ethanol in all brain areas studied. When rats were maintained on a liquid diet containing ethanol for 5 months, no changes were found in phosphatidylinositol hydrolysis, whether stimulated by muscarinic or noradrenergic agonists, KCl, glutamate or the calcium ionophore A23187. No tolerance was seen to the previously reported effect of *in vitro* ethanol on noradrenaline-stimulated hydrolysis. The authors pointed out that they measured only maximal responses to the agonists, not the ED_{50} values. Changes in the latter, such as that found by Hoffman *et al.* (1986) in the carbachol ED_{50} after chronic ethanol (see Section 4.5), would not have been detected.

Ethanol, added *in vitro* at 50 mM, decreased the activity of phospholipase A_2, the enzyme that catalyses the breakdown of membrane phospholipids (Hudspith *et al.*, 1985). Activity of the phospholipid base exchange enzymes, involved in the incorporation of serine into phospholipids in exchange for ethanolamine and choline, was also inhibited, to a lesser extent. Ethanol at 100 mM inhibited the basal activity of phospholipase C that transforms inositol phospholipids (phosphatidylinositol 4,5-biphosphate, PIP_2, and phosphatidyl inosotol, PI) into inositol triphosphate (IP_3) and diacylglycerol. The activity of all these enzymes was dependent on calcium and was increased by procedures that increased intracellular calcium.

Chronic ethanol treatment increased the turnover of membrane phospholipids, when measured before ethanol withdrawal (Hudspith *et al.*, 1985). The changes appeared to be presynaptic, rather than being a consequence of increased neurotransmitter release. Phospholipase A_2 activity was increased after the chronic treatment, as was the activity of the phospholipid base exchange enzymes. The breakdown of inositol phospholipids by phospholipase C was slightly greater after the ethanol administration, but the activity induced by depolarization using KCl, 40 mM, was more clearly increased following the chronic treatment.

Later work from this group showed that chronic ethanol administration increased the sensitivity of inositol phospholipid breakdown to the action of dihydropyridines (Hudspith *et al.*, 1987). Kendall and Nahorski (1985) had earlier demonstrated that dihydropyridine calcium channel antagonists, such as nifedipine, inhibited inositol phospholipid turnover and that this effect followed the same stereospecificity as the action of the dihydropyridines on voltage-dependent calcium channels. After the chronic ethanol treatment, the calcium channel activator Bay K 8644 was more effective in increasing depolarization induced inositol phosphate accumulation and this action was prevented by calcium channel antagonists. The stimulation of inositol phospholipid turnover by carbachol and noradrenaline was also increased. The increased effects of the dihydropyridines may be related to the changes in binding to these compounds found after chronic ethanol treatment. This aspect is discussed in detail below (see Section 4.3.4).

The results of Brennan and Littleton (1990) also suggested that protein kinase C was involved in the adaptations to chronic ethanol treatment. This was studied directly by Battaini *et al.* (1989), who showed that the addition of ethanol to the drinking water for 25 days decreased the number of binding sites for phorbol esters in rat cerebral cortex and hippocampus, but not in cerebellar or hypothalamic tissues. Phorbol esters are known to stimulate protein kinase C activity, in the same manner as diacylglycerol. Direct measurement of protein kinase activity, by the incorporation of ^{32}P into the protein histone type III S, showed decreases in activity in cytosolic and particulate fractions of hippocampus and cortex after the chronic ethanol treatment. Acute addition of ethanol *in vitro*, up to 500 mM, had no effect on the binding of phorbol esters or on the kinase activity.

4.2.3 Ethanol and adenyl cyclase

The effects of ethanol on cAMP levels have been contradictory. Although some changes have been reported, Redos *et al.* (1976) found no alterations after acute and/or chronic treatment *in vivo*. Shen *et al.* (1983) found decreases in cAMP on initial administrations of ethanol that continued during chronic treatment. On cessation of treatment, levels gradually returned to normal over the period of withdrawal hyperexcitability, but did not rise above control values. *In vitro*, however, ethanol increases adenyl cyclase activity, an effect that involves nucleotide-binding proteins (Luthin and Tabakoff, 1984). The effects were small at ethanol concentrations relevant to those found *in vivo* (50 mM), although regional variations were found (Hoffman *et al.*, 1987).

4.3 The involvement of calcium in ethanol dependence

4.3.1 The role of calcium channels in neuronal function

Calcium ions are involved in many neuronal functions, including postsynaptic responses and neurotransmitter release. Intracellular calcium ions interact with proteins such as calmodulin, and also act as second messengers. Calcium channels are divided into those operated by neurotransmitter–receptor interactions, and voltage-operated channels that increase their conductance on depolarization. Neurotransmitters that alter calcium conductance include noradrenaline, 5-HT and several peptides. In cultured cells of neuronal origin, Tsien and colleagues have demonstrated three subtypes of voltage-dependent channels (Nowycky *et al.*, 1985). The T subtype are activated at low voltages, but open only transiently. These have been suggested to be involved in bursting behaviour of neurones (Hernandez-Cruz and Pape, 1989). The L subtype is activated by strong depolarizations and the conductance change is long-lasting. Dihydropyridine compounds were found to be selective blocking agents for the L channels in the cultured cells, although the selectivity may not be as clear in normal mammalian neurones (see below). The N channels are also activated by strong depolarizations, but are of shorter duration. They are thought to be the subtype involved in neurotransmitter release from neurones (Hirning *et al.*, 1988). Omega-conotoxin was thought to block calcium channels of both the L and N subtypes in CNS tissue (Reynolds *et al.*, 1986) but recent work suggests selectivity for N-channels (Scroggs and Fox, 1991).

Calcium channels similar to those described in the cultured cells have been described in mammalian tissues, but the selectivity of the dihydropyridine calcium channel antagonists for the L subtype of channel in normal mammalian neurones is not apparent. Akaike *et al.* (1989) found that in hypothalamic cells, dihydropyridines affected channels that possessed the voltage dependence and inactivation characteristics of T channels as well as those with characteristics of the L type. Similar results were found by Takahashi *et al.* (1989) and Takahashi and Akaike (1990) in neurones acutely isolated from rat hippocampus. They identified the three types of channel, but all were blocked by a dihydropyridine antagonist, the greatest effect being on the T subtype. Whichever subtype is involved, the high-affinity binding sites for dihydropyridines found in the CNS are considered to represent voltage-sensitive calcium channels (Miller, 1987).

4.3.2 Effects of ethanol on calcium channels and related conductances

The acute action of ethanol is to decrease calcium conductance. This appears to be a selective effect; there is less blocking action on other types of current, at concentrations of ethanol that are achieved in the body during the behavioural effects (Pozos and Oakes, 1987). In contrast, the conductance of some channels, such as those permeable to chloride, and calcium-dependent potassium channels, may be increased by these relevant concentrations of ethanol (Celentano *et al.*, 1988; Carlen *et al.*, 1982). However, not all studies have demonstrated these effects (e.g. Siggins *et al.*, 1987). Evidence showing that ethanol decreased calcium currents and increased intracellular calcium was also obtained by Schwartz (1985) in Aplasia pacemaker neurones, but only one, very high, concentration of ethanol (880 mM, 4%) was used.

The majority of studies on the acute effect of ethanol on calcium uptake into neurones have shown that the calcium flux was decreased (Harris and Hood, 1980; Stokes and Harris, 1982). The fast and slow components of the uptake were measured by Leslie *et al.* (1983), using $^{45}Ca^{2+}$, who found that ethanol, 25–150 mM, decreased only the fast depolarization-dependent calcium uptake by rat brain synaptosomes. Similar results were reported by Harris *et al.* (1985) and Skattebol and Rabin (1987).

Tolerance has been found to the action of ethanol on calcium channels after chronic treatment. Friedman *et al.* (1980) reported that the action of ethanol was considerably reduced in tissues from mice treated with ethanol in a liquid diet for 10 days. In the absence of ethanol added to the medium, synaptosomes from animals receiving the chronic ethanol diet showed decreased calcium accumulation in both depolarizing and non-depolarizing conditions. The decrease in depolarization-dependent calcium uptake reported by Leslie *et al.* (1983) was lost after chronic ethanol treatment. In the latter two studies it was not stated whether or not the animals were withdrawn from the ethanol before tissue preparation. Wu *et al.* (1986) showed that calcium uptake into hippocampal P2 fraction was decreased by chronic ethanol treatment, when measured 18 h after withdrawal. In striatal slices, Lucchi *et al.* (1985) showed that chronic ethanol treatment decreased potassium-stimulated $^{45}Ca^{2+}$ uptake. However, Messing *et al.* (1986) found that cultured PC12 cells increased their uptake of $^{45}Ca^{2+}$ when grown in ethanol and that this resulted in tolerance to the inhibitory action of ethanol.

Durand and Carlen (1984a) reported that chronic ethanol treatment decreased calcium-dependent potassium currents in rat hippocampal slices, measured 3 weeks after ethanol withdrawal (Table 2). A later study from this group (Reynolds *et al.*, 1990) used a slightly different chronic ethanol treatment (lower doses, 3–8 g/kg per day instead of 10–15 g/kg per day, given for 15 rather than 20 weeks). In this case, the duration of the after-hyperpolarizations in hippocampal CA1 pyramidal cells, measured 16–24 h after the last dose of ethanol treatment, was found to be significantly increased compared with control values (Table 3). These potentials in dentate gyrus granule cells of the hippocampus were unchanged by the chronic treatment. No changes were found in GABA-mediated inhibitory synaptic potentials in either type of cell in this study. The pyramidal cells showed tolerance to the ethanol-induced potentiation of the after-hyperpolarizations after the chronic treatment; in fact, ethanol added to the bathing medium at 20 mM slightly decreased these potentials in these circumstances.

It is not certain how these electrophysiological changes are related to the behavioural effects of chronic ethanol treatment. The behavioural withdrawal syndrome in rats is seen a few hours after withdrawal from ethanol, with a peak around 8 h, depending on the method of ethanol administration. Whittington and Little (1990) demonstrated a pattern of changes in field potentials in mouse hippocampal slices, recorded extracellularly immediately on withdrawal from chronic ethanol treatment. The changes included decreased thresholds for elicitation of population spikes and increases in paired pulse potentiation. The individual changes followed different time-courses during the several hours of recording, suggesting that a complex series of alterations takes place in this tissue on withdrawal from ethanol. The dihydropyridine calcium channel antagonist PN 200-110 stereospecifically blocked all the signs of hyperexcitability in the hippocampal field potentials seen after the ethanol treatment (Figure 1; Whittington and Little, 1991a).

Table 2 Effects of long-term exposure to ethanol on intracellarly measured physiological parameters of CA1 pyramidal cells. Reproduced with permission from Durand and Carlen (1984a).

Measure	Control group	Ethanol group	*P* value
Resting potential (mV)	51.7 ± 2.22 (12)	52.5 ± 2.86 (12)	NS
Action potential (mV)	69.17 ± 2.21 (12)	72.5 ± 2.92 (12)	NS
IPSP (maximum) (mV)	5.54 ± 1.21 (11)	2.37 ± 0.61 (11)	NS
IPSP (maximum) (second)	0.44 ± 0.078 (11)	0.21 ± 0.06 (11)	<0.05
AHP (mV per spike)	1.72 ± 0.39 (9)	0.98 ± 0.29 (9)	NS
AHP (second per spike)	0.48 ± 0.14 (9)	0.16 ± 0.06 (9)	<0.05

Statistical analysis was done with a two-tailed t-test for all parameters except after-hyperpolarization (AHP) amplitude and duration, for which a two-tailed Mann-Whitney 'U' test was used because standard deviations for the two groups were significantly different by analysis of variance. Values are mean ± SEM (*n*). Slices were prepared 3 weeks after the end of a 23-week ethanol diet.

Table 3 Passive and synaptic membrane properties of hippocampal CA1 neurones from sucrose control and chronic ethanol-exposed rats. Reproduced with permission from Reynolds *et al.* (1990).

Measure	Control group	Ethanol group	*P* value
Resting potential (mV)	68 ± 1	67 ± 1	NS
Slope resistance (megohms)	46 ± 6	42 ± 4	NS
AHP (mV per spike)	0.54 ± 0.07	0.56 ± 0.07	NS
AHP (second per spike)	0.44 ± 0.04	0.64 ± 0.06	<0.05
EPSP (maximum) (mV/spike)	10.2 ± 0.7	10.4 ± 1.2	NS
IPSP (maximum) (mV/spike)	4.5 ± 0.6	4.8 ± 0.7	NS

EPSP–IPSP sequences just subthreshold for firing were generated by electrical stimulation of Schaffer collaterals. All values are mean ± SEM for eight control and eight chronic ethanol-exposed cells. Statistical analysis was performed using a t-test for unpaired data. Slices were prepared 16–24 h after the last p.o. dose of a 15-week ethanol treatment schedule.

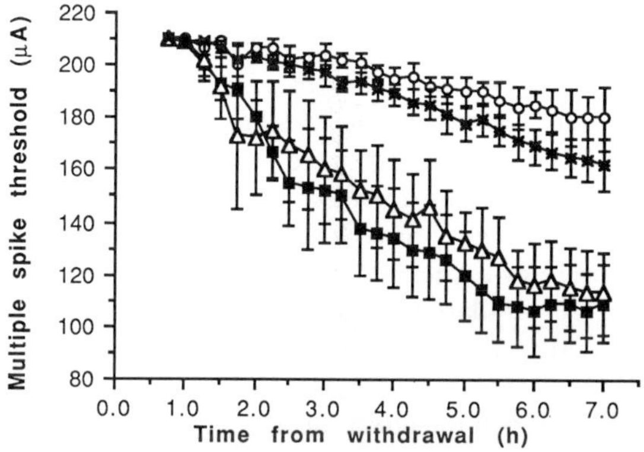

Figure 1 The effects of isomers of the calcium channel antagonist PN 200-110 on the hyperexcitability in hippocampal slices caused by withdrawal from chronic ethanol treatment. Mice were given ethanol in the drinking water for 12 weeks. Extracellular recordings were made from hippocampal slices prepared immediately on withdrawal from ethanol. PN 200-110 was added to the bathing medium at the beginning of recording. Values for the thresholds for elicitation of population spikes are the mean of five measurements ±SEM. Reproduced with permission from Whittington and Little (1991a).

This was a selective effect, as this compound did not alter the hyperexcitability in hippocampal slices from untreated mice produced by addition of the GABA antagonist bicuculline.

4.3.3 Changes in intracellular calcium concentrations with ethanol

The acute effect of ethanol appears to be to increase intracellular calcium concentrations, even though calcium influx is decreased. In the neurosecretory PC12 cell line, ethanol increased intracellular calcium concentrations when applied at 400 mM, but not at 100 mM (Rabe and Weight, 1988). Davidson *et al.* (1988) also found small increases in intracellular calcium when ethanol was added to synaptosomal preparations, but in this study ethanol was effective at lower concentrations, 50 mM and above. The increase occurred in both resting (5 mM K^+) and depolarized (55 mM K^+).

Measurements using the intracellular calcium-sensitive dye, Fura-2, showed that high concentrations of ethanol (350 mM and above) increased resting intracellular synaptosomal calcium concentrations in whole brain tissue (Daniell *et al.*, 1987; Daniell and Harris, 1988a,b). The increase in intracellular calcium was suggested to be due to calcium release from intracellular sites. The mechanism of this effect of ethanol was investigated by Daniell and Harris (1989), who showed that ethanol released calcium from intracellular stores in synaptosomes that were not sensitive to the calcium-releasing action of inositol 1,4,5-triphosphate (IP_3). The effects were seen when ethanol was added at comparatively low concentrations, 25–100 mM. The authors suggested that high concentrations of ethanol may have been required to show effects in the Fura-2 studies because Fura-2 chelates calcium, thus buffering small changes, and because Fura-2 accumulated in intracellular organelles, such as mitochondria, in which the calcium concentrations are higher than in the cytosol.

Daniell and Harris (1988b) studied the effects of chronic ethanol treatment on intracellular calcium concentrations in whole brain synaptosomes, using Fura-2. Ethanol, added *in vitro*, increased intracellular calcium. This effect was decreased by the chronic ethanol treatment. In the absence of ethanol, the intracellular calcium concentrations were not altered significantly after 7 days on a liquid diet containing ethanol, although the levels were somewhat lower than controls.

4.3.4 Ethanol and dihydropyridine-sensitive calcium channels

There has been much recent interest in the effects of chronic ethanol treatment on dihydropyridine-sensitive binding sites in the CNS. These sites are thought to represent voltage-sensitive calcium channels (see above). Although the exact role of these channels in normal neuronal function is not well understood, there is increasing evidence that they do have a role in controlling excitability and may be involved in epileptiform activity. Dihydropyridine calcium channel antagonists, such as nifedipine, have been used for many years for their effects on the cardiovascular system, but recently they have been shown to have actions on the CNS (Ramkumar and El-Fakahany, 1986; Raeburn and Gonzales, 1988). Pharmacological effects on the CNS include anticonvulsant (Hoffmeister *et al.*, 1982; Meyer *et al.*, 1986; De Sarro *et al.*, 1988; Larkin *et al.*, 1988) and some sedative actions (Hoffmeister *et al.*, 1982) and possible analgesic (Del Pozo *et al.*, 1987) and antidepressant effects (Czyrak *et al.*, 1989). They appear to have a selective action on drug-induced withdrawal syndromes, protecting against ethanol withdrawal (Little *et al.*, 1986), morphine withdrawal (Bongianni *et al.*, 1986; see Section 4.3.5.3) and nitrous oxide withdrawal (Dolin and Little, 1989a).

4.3.4.1 Acute interactions between ethanol and dihydropyridines

Calcium channel antagonists potentiated the acute pharmacological effects of ethanol *in vivo*, such as the ataxic action and the anaesthetic effects (Isaacson *et al.*, 1985; Dolin and Little, 1986; Pucilowski *et al.*, 1989). The calcium channel activator Bay K 8644 decreased the general anaesthetic action of ethanol (Dolin *et al.*, 1988b). The calcium channel antagonists possess some sedative properties, at high doses, so the interaction with ethanol may have been partly additive. However, dihydropyridines do not produce general anaesthesia, even at extremely high doses (Dolin and Little, 1986). The interaction could also have been due to effects of ethanol on the dihydropyridine receptor. Rius *et al.* (1987) found that ethanol, given acutely, increased the affinity of the dihydropyridine binding sites in rat brain. This effect was found when the binding was measured *in vivo*, even though ethanol had no effect on dihydropyridine binding measured *in vitro* (Greenberg and Cooper, 1984).

4.3.4.2 Changes in dihydropyridine-sensitive binding sites after chronic ethanol administration

The number of dihydropyridine binding sites in the CNS has been found to increase after chronic ethanol treatment (Dolin *et al.*, 1987; Dolin and Little, 1989b). Wu *et al.* (1987) found a temporal correlation between the increase in binding sites and the development of ethanol tolerance. Increases in binding occurred after various methods of administration of ethanol, including inhalation of ethanol by rats (10–20 g/kg per day) for 7 days, intraperitoneal injection of ethanol in rats at 2 g/kg, once daily, for 10 days, and administration of ethanol in the drinking fluid to mice (11–14 g/kg per day) for 12 weeks. All of these chronic treatment schedules caused tolerance to ethanol and a mild withdrawal syndrome (convulsive behaviour on handling), with the exception of the intraperitoneal schedule, which caused tolerance, but not withdrawal signs (Littleton *et al.*, 1990; Whittington and Little, 1988; Dolin and Little, 1989b). Wu *et al.* (1987) reported a correlation between the time-course of this increase in dihydropyridine binding site number and that of the development of ethanol tolerance.

An increase in dihydropyridine binding site number has also been found in studies on cultured cells when the cells were grown in media containing ethanol. Messing *et al.* (1986) found an increase of 92% in the B_{max} in cells of the cultured neural cell line PC12 grown in ethanol, 200 mM, for 6 days. Littleton's group have studied this increase in detail and shown that the change in dihydropyridine binding sites was prevented by the protein synthesis inhibitor cycloheximide, and by the mRNA synthesis inhibitor anisomycin (Table 4), suggesting that it was the result of synthesis of new channel protein and was under genetic regulation (Harper *et al.*, 1989). Marks *et al.* (1989a) demonstrated that the increase occurred in intact PC12 cells, in which the second messenger systems are functional.

Brennan and Littleton (1990) investigated the mechanism of the increase in dihydropyridine binding when cultured bovine chromaffin cells were grown

Table 4 Effect of growth in ethanol on binding sites for [^{3}H]DHP on membranes from bovine adrenal chromaffin cells. Reproduced with permission from Harper *et al.* (1989).

Treatment	Binding of [^{3}H]nitrendipine	
	B_{max} (fmol/mg protein)	K_D (nM)
Control	113 ± 18	0.40 ± 0.04
Ethanol	286 ± 24*	0.36 ± 0.11
Control + Cycloheximide	103 ± 25	0.68 ± 0.20
Ethanol + Cycloheximide	136 ± 12	0.20 ± 0.06
Control + Anisomycin	104 ± 17	0.52 ± 0.02
Ethanol + Anisomycin	100 ± 18	0.43 ± 0.02

Cells were prepared on four separate occasions, and on each occasion the binding studies were performed in duplicate on 3 separate days. Values given represent means ± standard errors of at least 12 determinations.
* $p < 0.01$ versus control.

in ethanol. Growth of the cells in pertussis toxin, which prevents the coupling of G proteins, mimicked the upregulation of binding sites. When the calcium concentration in the growth medium was increased, the upregulation due to ethanol was prevented. These results suggested that inhibition of membrane calcium flux, and a G protein, are involved in the response of dihydropyridine binding sites to chronic ethanol. Prolonged action of a phorbol ester causes inhibition of protein kinase and this was found to cause upregulation of dihydropyridine binding sites in these cells. The fact that this upregulation was not additive with that caused by ethanol suggested that protein kinase C is involved in the control of voltage- and dihydropyridine-sensitive calcium channels. These results were in agreement with those of Battaini *et al.* (1989), who found evidence that chronic ethanol treatment *in vivo* decreased protein kinase activity.

One report, by Lucchi *et al.* (1985), found a more complex pattern of changes in dihydropyridine binding. These workers studied striatal tissue and showed that calcium independent binding was increased, and calcium-dependent binding decreased, after administration of ethanol to rats at approximately 20 g/kg per day for 25 days. The difference between this and the above results may have been due either to the higher doses of ethanol given during the chronic treatment in the latter study, compared with those above, or to the brain region studied. A later communication from this laboratory (Bergamaschi *et al.*, 1987) found an increase in dihydropyridine binding B_{max} values in cerebral cortex on acute administration of ethanol and a decrease in B_{max} after chronic treatment.

Evidence for a causal relationship between increases in central dihydropyridine binding and the ethanol withdrawal syndrome was provided by the study of Brennan, Littleton and Crabbe (unpublished results) on binding changes in withdrawal-resistant and withdrawal-susceptible lines of mice. These strain lines have been selectively bred for many generations and show large differences in the severity of the ethanol withdrawal syndrome. The increase in dihydropyridine binding site number after chronic ethanol administration was greater in the withdrawal-susceptible line than in the withdrawal-resistant line.

Calcium channel binding in human tissues has not been found to be significantly increased in alcoholics (Marks *et al.*, 1989b; Kril *et al.*, 1989), although the former authors, studying small samples, found that the binding site number was increased by 26%. Neither paper included details of any pathological changes or cell loss. The latter authors found no change in benzodiazepine binding in the dependent population, suggesting that cell loss did not occur, but variable changes in benzodiazepine binding have been found experimentally after chronic ethanol treatment (see below). It has been shown that the characteristics of dihydropyridine binding are altered by postmortem delays (Quirion *et al.*, 1988); these authors cautioned against extrapolation from postmortem results on dihydropyridine binding to physiological conditions.

No experimental studies have yet reported the effects of chronic ethanol treatment on dihydropyridine binding measured *in vivo*. This is an important aspect, as dihydropyridine calcium channel antagonists bind preferentially to the inactivated form of the channel complex (Bean, 1984). Binding to homogenate preparations measures the interaction in a totally depolarized membrane, in which channels will be largely inactivated, and thus may not reflect the situation in the normal physiological state. This was clearly demonstrated by the results of Rius *et al.* (1987), who showed that a single dose (3 g/kg, i.p.) of ethanol, *in vivo*, caused a short-duration increase in the B_{max} for dihydropyridine binding, 40 min after ethanol administration, followed by an increase in affinity that peaked at 8 h, returning to normal by 36 h. Acute addition of ethanol *in vitro* has been shown by several authors not to affect dihydropyridine binding (Greenberg and Cooper, 1984; Harris *et al.*, 1985; Rius *et al.*, 1987).

The central dihydropyridine binding sites are thought to represent voltage-sensitive calcium channels. A change in their number is of interest only if it is accompanied by functional changes. That the increase in dihydropyridine binding is of functional importance was demonstrated by Dolin *et al.* (1987) and Littleton *et al.* (1988) using mammalian tissue. The *in vitro* effects of the

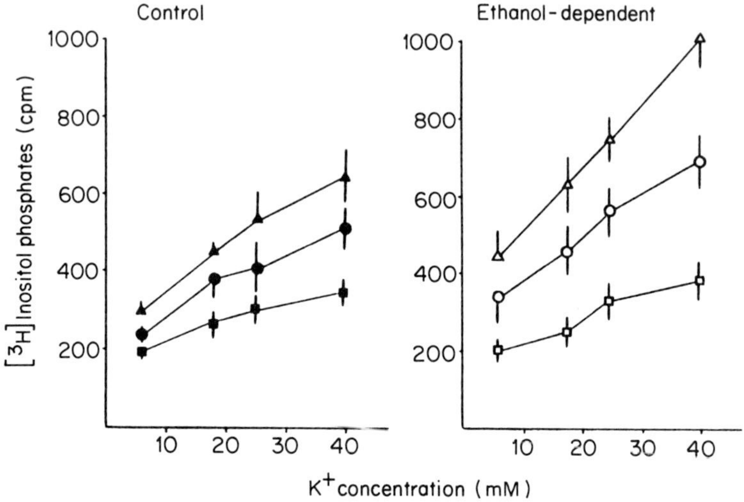

Figure 2 The effect of the Ca^{2+} channel activator BAYK8644 on depolarisation-induced accumulation of [^{3}H] inositol phosphates in cortical slices. Results show values from *control* animals (n = 5) on the left (filled symbols) and from *ethanol-dependent* animals (n = 5) on the right (open symbols). Error bars are S.E.M. ○, ● show the effect of increasing K^+ concentration (6 mM, 18 mM, 25 mM, 40 mM) on the accumulation of [^{3}H] inositol phosphates in the absence of BAYK8644. △, ▲ show the potentiating effect of BAYK8644, 5×10^{-7} M, on [^{3}H] inositol phosphate accumulation, whereas □, ■ show the inhibitory effect of BAYK8644 at 5×10^{-5} M. Reproduced with permission from Hudspith *et al.* (1987).

dihydropyridine calcium channel activator Bay K 8644 on neurotransmitter release and phosphatidylinositol turnover were increased in cortical tissue from rats treated chronically with ethanol by inhalation for 7 days (Figure 2). The increase in dihydropyridine binding sites appears, therefore, to reflect an increase in functional voltage-sensitive calcium channels. A similar conclusion was reached by Messing *et al.* (1986) in their study on cultured PC12 cells. They found that the increase in dihydropyridine binding was accompanied by an increase in calcium uptake by the cells, following the chronic ethanol treatment.

4.3.4.3 Can dihydropyridine compounds be used to modulate ethanol dependence?

Dihydropyridine calcium channel antagonists have been found to decrease the hyperexcitability that occurs during withdrawal from chronic ethanol treatment. This effect was seen when the compounds were given acutely, immediately on withdrawal, against a mild withdrawal syndrome, measured by convulsive behaviour and tremor on handling (Littleton and Little, 1987;

Littleton *et al.*, 1990) and against a severe withdrawal, following chronic treatment with higher doses of ethanol, measured by the incidence of spontaneous and audiogenic convulsions (Little *et al.*, 1986). A calcium channel blocking agent has been found to protect against the alcohol withdrawal syndrome in humans (Koppi *et al.*, 1987). The action of dihydropyridine antagonists in the above studies was a selective effect. These compounds have weak anticonvulsant actions against some other forms of convulsions, particularly those produced by pentylenetetrazol, but not against others, such as *N*-methyl-*d*-aspartate or electroshock seizures (Hoffmeister *et al.*, 1982; Dolin *et al.*, 1988a). We have repeatedly found that they have no protective action against bicuculline convulsions.

The dose of PN 200-110 effective against the ethanol withdrawal syndrome (Littleton *et al.*, 1990) was chosen to be the same as that shown by Supervilai and Karobath (1984) to be required to displace radiolabelled dihydropyridine from the CNS *in vivo*. We have measured the brain concentrations of nitrendipine and nimodipine, after the doses effective against the ethanol withdrawal syndrome, and found them to be in the low micromolar/high nanomolar range (Dolin *et al.*, 1988a; Dolin and Little, 1989b). This order of concentration is the same as that required to produce effects on brain tissues *in vitro* (see above).

It is now well established that the doses of the dihydropyridines required for CNS actions are higher than those needed to affect the cardiovascular system. This difference is not due to problems in entering the brain, as the compounds penetrate the CNS well. Higher concentrations of dihydropyridines are required to affect neuronal calcium channels than the corresponding channels in other tissues, although the binding affinities of neuronal and smooth muscle preparations, measured on homogenates, are of the same order of magnitude. This apparent discrepancy is probably due to the influence of membrane potential on the binding affinity (see above). The dihydropyridine calcium channel antagonists have a higher affinity for the inactivated state of the channel than for the open or closed states (Bean, 1984). At normal membrane potentials, in neuronal tissue, few of the channels would be activated, so few would be in the inactivated state. In homogenate preparations the tissues are totally depolarized, so binding affinities measured in this way do not reflect the affinity in the physiological situation. Studies on binding *in vivo*, such as that by Supervilai and Karobath (1984), provide a better indication of the affinities in functioning neurones.

The stereospecificity of the isomers of the dihydropyridine calcium channel antagonist, PN 200-110, in protecting against the ethanol withdrawal syndrome followed the same pattern as that on calcium channel conductance (Littleton *et al.*, 1990). The same stereoselectivity was seen when the effects of the isomers of PN 200-110 were studied on withdrawal hyperexcitability in isolated hippocampal slices (Whittington and Little, 1991a). This stereospecificity, and the correlation with the dose required to displace a radiolabelled dihydropyridine from binding sites in the CNS (Littleton *et al.*, 1990), showed that the effect was mediated by neuronal voltage-sensitive calcium channels, rather than being a non-specific action.

Nitrendipine, given acutely, was found to be ineffective in preventing the anxiogenic aspects of the ethanol withdrawal syndrome (File *et al.*, 1989). The dose used was the same as that which prevented the tremor and convulsions in other studies (Littleton *et al.*, 1990), so the results suggest that anxiety during ethanol withdrawal may be caused by different biochemical changes than the convulsive behaviour. The effects of chronic administration of nitrendipine (see below) on ethanol withdrawal-induced anxiogenic behaviour, however, have not yet been investigated.

Bay K 8644 is a dihydropyridine with calcium channel activating properties, that is, it increases the opening of the channels, thereby having the opposite effect to that of the antagonists. The (−) form possesses this action, but the (+) isomer is a calcium channel antagonist (Franckowiak *et al.*, 1985; O'Neill and Bolger, 1988). The racemic form of Bay K 8644 prevented the protective action of the calcium channel antagonists in ethanol withdrawal, but did not itself potentiate the withdrawal symdrome (Littleton and Little, 1987; Littleton *et al.*, 1990). The (−) isomer, however, increased the convulsive behaviour seen in mice on handling during ethanol withdrawal (unpublished results). This compound has convulsive effects when given alone (Bolger *et al.*, 1985), so this result needs to be compared with the action of the (−) isomer of Bay K 8644 in other convulsive states before conclusions can be drawn from these results.

4.3.4.4 Prevention of ethanol tolerance and withdrawal by dihydropyridines

The problem of a causal relationship between a biochemical change and a behavioural syndrome is, of course, almost impossible to solve, as the answer can never be fully proven. The fact that a biochemical change is produced by chronic ethanol treatment does not mean that such a change is the cause of the behavioural manifestations of dependence, such as tolerance and the withdrawal syndrome. If the biochemical change, however, can be prevented, and if such a manoeuvre also prevents the tolerance and withdrawal, then the evidence for causality is rather better.

Dihydropyridine calcium channel antagonists can prevent adaptations to chronic ethanol treatment if they are given chronically during the ethanol intake. Such administration prevented the development of alcohol tolerance in animal models of this condition (Wu *et al.*, 1987; Little and Dolin, 1987; Dolin and Little, 1989b). When nifedipine or nitrendipine was given

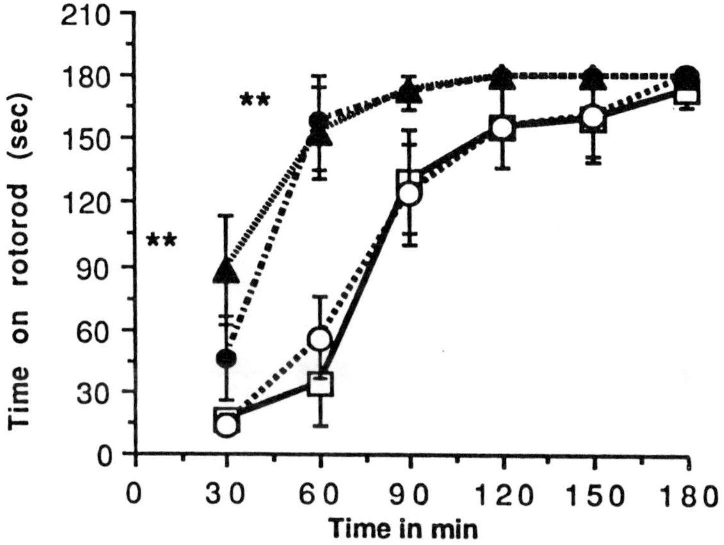

Figure 3 Time spent on the rotating rod after chronic ethanol treatment, with and without concurrent nitrendipine injections. All groups were given acute injections of ethanol, 2 g/kg, at the beginning of the testing period. Tolerance developed when ethanol was given alone, but not when nitrendipine was administered with the ethanol during the chronic treatment. Chronic treatment, once daily for 10 days, was: ▲, ethanol 1.5 g/kg; ○, ethanol 1.5 g/kg + nitrendipine 50 mg/kg; ●, ethanol 1.5 g/kg + nitrendipine 10 mg/kg; □, vehicles. Reproduced with permission from Dolin and Little (1989b).

continuously with the ethanol, significantly less tolerance developed to the ataxic action of ethanol than when rodents received the same amount of ethanol given alone (Figure 3). This effect was not due to alterations in central concentrations of ethanol. Residual dihydropyridine in the CNS at the time of testing could have produced this pattern of results, as, acutely, dihydropyridine calcium channel antagonists potentiate the behavioural effects of ethanol (Dolin and Little, 1986). To exclude this possibility, we measured the central nitrendipine concentrations. We found that, at the time the tolerance was measured, the concentrations were an order of magnitude lower than those that are necessary to have an acute effect on the actions of ethanol.

Chronic administration of a dihydropyridine calcium channel antagonist for 2 weeks or more also decreased the ethanol withdrawal syndrome, even though the dihydropyridine treatment was stopped 24 h or 48 h before the measurement of ethanol withdrawal severity (Figure 4) (Whittington and Little, 1988). Again, when we measured the central dihydropyridine

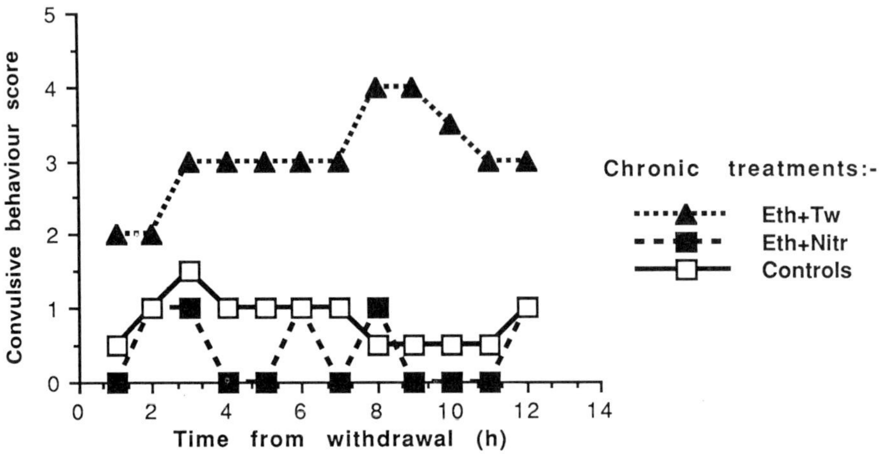

Figure 4 Median scores for convulsive behaviour after chronic ethanol (Eth) treatment, with and without concurrent nitrendipine (Nitr) injections. Signs of ethanol withdrawal syndrome were seen when ethanol was given alone, but not when nitrendipine was administered with the ethanol during the chronic treatment. Reproduced with permission from Whittington *et al.* (1991).

concentrations, they were found to be too low at the time of the ethanol withdrawal tests to have had an acute action on the withdrawal behaviour. The effect on withdrawal was not seen when only 2 days' dihydropyridine treatment was given. These results suggest that the chronic administration of a dihydropyridine calcium channel antagonist produced some form of adaptive response that prevented or reversed the adaptations to ethanol.

Evidence that the changes observed *in vivo* after these treatments were due to changes in neuronal excitability was obtained using hippocampal slices (Whittington and Little, 1990). Recordings were made from isolated slices, prepared after various chronic treatments. A clear pattern of hyperexcitability, including increased paired pulse potentiation and decreased thresholds for elicitation of field potentials, was found after chronic ethanol intake. When nitrendipine was given with the ethanol, the hyperexcitability in the slices was significantly decreased (Whittington and Little, 1991b).

The increase in the number of dihydropyridine-sensitive calcium channels caused by chronic ethanol treatment was also prevented by the concurrent dihydropyridine administration (Dolin *et al.*, 1988b; Dolin and Little, 1989b). This effect therefore may be due to an adaptive response to the long-term presence of the dihydropyridine. Panza *et al.* (1985) reported that chronic administration of a dihydropyridine calcium channel antagonist caused downregulation of dihydropyridine receptors in mouse brain. An effect such as this would counteract the upregulation caused by chronic ethanol administration (see Figure 5). Prevention of the increase in dihydropyridine binding caused by chronic ethanol treatment was also seen when bovine adrenal chromaffin cells were grown in ethanol plus a dihydropyridine (Harper *et al.*, 1989).

4.3.4.5 Do the effects of dihydropyridines represent a new development in the treatment of alcoholism?

This is the first time that a pharmacological treatment has been shown to prevent both the adaptive changes in the behavioural actions of ethanol (tolerance and the withdrawal syndrome) and a related biochemical change (the increase in number of dihydropyridine binding sites). Consistent results have been obtained from behavioural, receptor binding and electrophysiological studies on this effect (Wu *et al.*, 1987; Dolin *et al.*, 1987; Dolin and Little, 1989b; Whittington and Little, 1988, 1989a,b,c, 1991b; Whittington *et al.*, 1991). The evidence from all these types of study suggests that chronic administration of a dihydropyridine calcium channel antagonist with ethanol, during long-term ethanol intake, prevents the manifestations of ethanol dependence.

It will be of great interest if these results are found to be applicable to patients. Current pharmacological treatment of ethanol dependence is limited to symptomatic alleviation of the withdrawal syndrome, using benzodiazepines or similar compounds. The problems with these current 'substitution' treatments are several-fold. They have their own pharmacological actions, including sedation, and their own dependence liability (Finer, 1970; Busto *et al.*, 1983; Schuster and Humphries, 1981). They do not correct the underlying neuronal changes which are involved in alcohol dependence (Nutt *et al.*, 1989). Whilst they have a place in providing protection from the acute alcohol withdrawal syndrome, they do not appear to have any long-term corrective action. If dihydropyridine calcium channel antagonists could be given during drinking, to reverse the neuronal adaptation to ethanol, both the severity of the withdrawal and the tendency to relapse might be reduced.

At present we do not have compounds which are selective for neuronal dihydropyridine binding sites. This means that, in addition to the effects on the CNS described above, the dihydropyridine compounds also had cardiovascular actions. This would obviously be unsatisfactory in a therapeutic regime. If compounds selective for neurones could be synthesized, they might be of use in alcoholic patients. Our evidence suggests that the cardiovascular actions of the dihydropyridines were not involved in their effects on ethanol dependence. A further problem with the compounds studied so far is that,

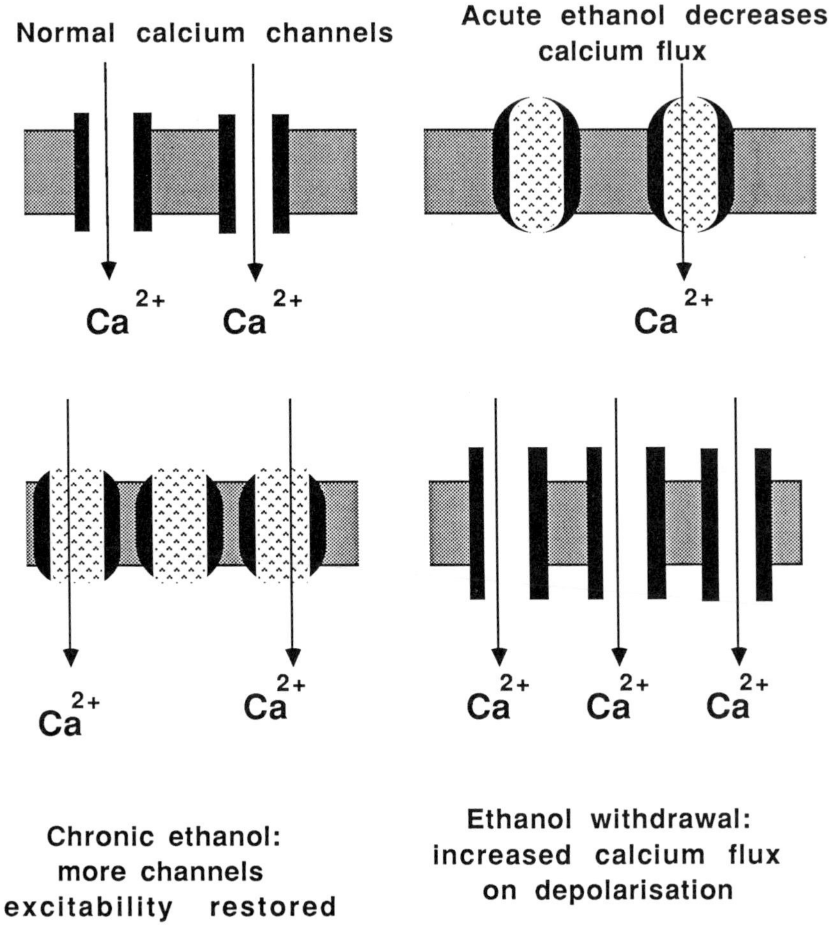

Figure 5 Schematic diagram of the theory put forward to explain the effects of dihydropyridine calcium antagonists on ethanol tolerance and withdrawal. The evidence so far for this theory is as follows: (i) Acute ethanol decreases calcium flux, not necessarily through dihydropyridine-sensitive channels. (ii) The number of dihydropyridine-sensitive calcium channels in the CNS is increased after chronic ethanol treatment. (iii) Concurrent chronic administration of dihydropyridine calcium channel antagonists prevents the upregulation of dihydropyridine binding, the development of ethanol tolerance and the behavioural and electrophysiological manifestations of the ethanol withdrawal syndrome. Reproduced with permission from Little (1991).

when given acutely in combination with ethanol, they potentiate its behavioural effects (Dolin and Little, 1986). Again, it may be possible to find selective compounds which have the required effects on ethanol dependence, without the acute interaction, as the two properties do not appear to occur exactly in parallel. This aspect is currently under investigation.

4.4 Excitatory amino acid transmission and ethanol dependence

Until recently, only a small amount of work had been done on the involvement of excitatory amino acid transmission in ethanol dependence. There is now considerable interest in this area, but it remains to be seen whether this is only a reflection of the current general interest in this area of research, or whether changes in excitatory amino acid transmission do play an important role in ethanol dependence. There are two main candidates for these neurotransmitter systems, glutamate and *N*-methyl-*d*-aspartate (NMDA), and the receptors have been divided into three subtypes (Watkins and Evans, 1981). These subtypes were named after the selective agonists NMDA, kainate and quisqualate, although the latter name has now been replaced by AMPA.

4.4.1 Effects of chronic ethanol treatment on excitatory amino acid receptor binding

Binding studies have suggested that long-term ethanol treatment increases excitatory amino acid binding in the CNS. Michaelis *et al.* (1978) showed that chronic ethanol administration increased the number of [^{3}H]glutamate binding sites in brain synaptosomal preparations. MK801 is a noncompetitive antagonist at the NMDA subtype of receptors. Grant *et al.* (1990) found a 17% increase in [^{3}H]MK801 binding in hippocampal tissue after a chronic ethanol treatment schedule that causes acute intoxication and spontaneous withdrawal signs.

4.4.2 Biochemical studies on chronic ethanol treatment and excitatory amino acid transmission

Chronic ethanol was found to increase potassium stimulated release of glutamate from hippocampal slices, when measured 36 hours into withdrawal (Keller *et al.*, 1983). In cerebrocortical slices, the increase in glutamate release on withdrawal was not significant, but a decrease in release from this tissue was found during the treatment. Glutamate release was unaffected by acute ethanol administration (4 g/kg) or addition of ethanol *in vitro* (56 mM).

A selective action of a high concentration of ethanol *in vitro* (100 mM) on the actions of quisqualate and kainate, with no effect on the actions of NMDA, glutamate or aspartate, was found by Teichberg *et al.* (1984), who measured $^{22}Na^{+}$ efflux from preloaded striatal slices. Recent work by Hoffman *et al.* (1989) showed that ethanol concentrations of 10–25 mM inhibited NMDA-stimulated calcium uptake in cultured cerebellar granule cells. Cyclic GMP accumulation stimulated by NMDA was also decreased by ethanol and the actions of kainate were less affected than those of NMDA. An earlier study (Riveros and Orrego, 1986) failed to find an effect of 100 mM ethanol on the glutamate-stimulated uptake of $^{45}Ca^{2+}$ into rat cerebrocortical slices.

4.4.3 Electrophysiological studies on ethanol and excitatory amino acid transmission

Acute effects of ethanol have been found in electrophysiological studies on excitatory acid transmission, but there has been little investigation so far of the effects of chronic ethanol. Gruol (1982) showed that low concentrations of ethanol (16 mM) decreased glutamate-evoked synaptic activity in cultured spinal cord neurones, but the direct responses to glutamate were little affected by ethanol concentrations up to 80 mM. Celentano *et al.* (1988) found no effect of acute ethanol (50 mM) on glutamate responses of cultured chick spinal cord neurones.

Selective blockade of NMDA responses has been seen at concentrations of ethanol that are relevant to the more subtle of ethanol's behavioural actions. The patch-clamp study of Lima-Landman and Albuquerque (1989) showed that very low concentrations of ethanol, 1.74–8.65 mM, increased the probability of NMDA-activated channel opening in cultured rat hippocampal cells, but did not affect channel open time, while concentrations of 86.5–174 mM decreased both the probability of channel opening and the mean open time. Lovinger *et al.* (1989) found an inhibitory action of ethanol on NMDA responses between 5 and 50 mM. Responses to kainate or quisqualate were affected only slightly by these concentrations.

Cerebellar Purkinje cells grown in a low concentration (19.5 mM) of ethanol showed reduced responsiveness to glutamate (Yool and Gruol, 1987). The blockade by chronic ethanol treatment of long-term potentiation (LTP) in hippocampal slices, reported by Durand and Carlen (1984b), may be related to its effects on NMDA responses, as NMDA has been shown to be involved in this form of synaptic plasticity (Collingridge *et al.*, 1983). Acute treatment with ethanol also decreased hippocampal LTP (Sinclair and Lo,

1986). It is difficult to reconcile the decrease in LTP after long-term ethanol administration (Durand and Carlen, 1984b) with the reported increase in NMDA receptor number after such treatment (Grant *et al.*, 1990), but the chronic schedule in the electrophysiological study lasted 9 months, while in the binding experiments treatment was for only 7 days. It is possible either that these treatment schedules may have resulted in different changes at NMDA sites or that changes at other sites may have caused the decrease in LTP.

4.4.4 Behavioural studies on ethanol and excitatory amino acid transmission

Freed and Michaelis (1978) showed that the glutamate antagonist glutamate diethyl ester decreased the seizure incidence during ethanol withdrawal, when given 5 h after removal of ethanol. They also found supersensitivity to the convulsant effects of kainic acid, but not to pentylenetetrazol, when these compounds were given during the chronic administration of ethanol.

Grant *et al.* (1990) reported that the overall severity of withdrawal was significantly reduced by the noncompetitive NMDA antagonist MK801 at 1 and 3 mg/kg i.p., given three times within 7 h, but limb tremor was unaffected. This protective effect of MK801 would be evidence for a role for NMDA receptors in the withdrawal syndrome only if MK801 were selective for convulsions initiated by changes at NMDA receptors. The evidence suggests that this is not the case. Kulkarni and Ticku (1989) showed that 1 mg/kg MK801, i.p., protected against the lethal, but not the convulsant, actions of picrotoxin. Tricklebank *et al.* (1989) reported that the intravenous ED_{50} values for MK801 for protection against NMDA convulsions, and against pentylentetrazol convulsions, were 0.22 mg/kg and 0.18 mg/kg, respectively. The effectiveness of MK801 in ethanol withdrawal does not therefore necessarily indicate that the withdrawal syndrome is initiated at NMDA receptors. Decreases in GABA transmission, for example, would result in convulsive behaviour that would be blocked by MK801.

Administration of NMDA to naive mice causes a convulsive syndrome that differs in many respects from the ethanol withdrawal syndrome. Although rodents show clonic convulsions and wild running, also seen during ethanol withdrawal, they demonstrate bizarre behaviour, violent tail movements and self-mutilation that are not caused by ethanol withdrawal. Grant *et al.* (1990) found an exacerbation of the withdrawal syndrome, measured by handling-induced seizures, when NMDA was given during ethanol withdrawal. The behavioural actions of MK801 were reduced during ethanol withdrawal, a result said to be consistent with an increase in NMDA binding sites.

4.5 Ethanol tolerance and dependence and the GABA–benzodiazepine receptor complex

Gamma-aminobutyric acid (GABA) is thought to be one of the main inhibitory transmitters in the CNS. The protein complex in which receptors for GABA are situated contains, in addition, several other receptor sites, that bind benzodiazepines, barbiturates and convulsant drugs such as picrotoxin. The benzodiazepine receptor is also the site at which benzodiazepine inverse agonists and antagonists act (Nutt *et al.*, 1982). The GABA receptor appears to exist in two forms, with low affinity and high affinity. The former is probably of greater physiological importance.

Ethanol has been reported to have acute effects on the GABA receptor ionophore complex, increasing the number of GABA receptors (Ticku, 1980), increasing benzodiazepine binding (Davis and Ticku, 1981) and decreasing binding at the picrotoxin site (Thyagarajan and Ticku, 1985; Sanna *et al.*, 1990). These effects may be of functional importance, as ethanol has been consistently found to potentiate the increase in chloride conductance caused by GABA agonists (e.g. Ticku *et al.*, 1986). However, electrophysiological studies on the action of ethanol on the effects of GABA or on GABA-mediated inhibition have not produced consistent results. Although some reports have found potentiating effects of ethanol (Davidoff, 1973; Nestoros, 1980; Wiesner *et al.*, 1987; Celentano *et al.*, 1988; Takada *et al.*, 1989), others have found no evidence for this (Gruol, 1982; Carlen *et al.*, 1982; Harris and Sinclair, 1984; Gage and Robertson, 1985; Mancillas *et al.*, 1986; Siggins *et al.*, 1987). Therefore, although it has become generally accepted that potentiation of GABA plays an important part in the behavioural effects of ethanol, the actual evidence is conflicting. The demonstration by Aguayo (1990) that ethanol potentiates the actions of GABA in some, but not all, neurones explains many of the earlier results.

4.5.1 The effects of chronic ethanol treatment on binding to the GABA receptor ionophore complex

Chronic ethanol treatment has been reported to decrease the number and affinity of GABA receptor sites. Ticku (1980) showed that there was a temporal correlation between the binding changes and the appearance of withdrawal behaviour in rats. Treatment with 11–17 g/kg per day ethanol, for 21 days, which caused a withdrawal syndrome, decreased the affinity of the low-affinity GABA binding site. This change was not seen after shorter treatment durations, which did not result in a withdrawal syndrome, and was found only over the period during which seizure activity was seen. Such decreases in GABA binding have been reported in several other papers (e.g. Ticku and Burch, 1980;

Linnoila *et al.*, 1981; Ticku *et al.*, 1983; Volicer and Biagioni, 1982), although Hunt and Dalton (1981) did not find changes.

Decreases in GABA binding could be responsible for tolerance to those actions of ethanol that are produced by potentiation of GABA transmission. However, Harris *et al.* (1983) found GABA binding to be increased in brain tissue from miniature swine after ethanol intake for 3 years. It is possible that species differences occur. Tran *et al.* (1981) found increased [^{3}H]muscimol binding in human alcoholics who were drinking up to the time of death. [^{3}H]Muscimol binds to the high-affinity GABA site, rather than to the low-affinity site. The low-affinity site is considered to be involved in the physiological effects of GABA and it is difficult to interpret the importance of changes in the high-affinity site.

Although some changes have been reported in benzodiazepine binding after chronic ethanol treatment, these have not been consistent. Benzodiazepine receptor binding was found to be decreased (Freund, 1980; Kochman *et al.*, 1981; Volicer and Biagioni, 1982) or unchanged (Karobath *et al.*, 1980; Hemmingsen *et al.*, 1982; Schoemaker *et al.*, 1983) by chronic ethanol treatment. It is possible that the reported changes are caused by the neuronal damage that occurs on very long-term ethanol treatment, as they appear to be seen after a longer duration of ethanol chronic treatment than is required to produce tolerance and dependence on ethanol (Freund, 1980; Rottenberg, 1985). Evidence for a possible selective interaction between benzodiazepine inverse agonists and ethanol was found by Mhatre *et al.* (1988), who showed that chronic ethanol administration selectively increased the binding of the inverse agonist Ro15-4513 in cerebral cortex and cerebellum. Binding to benzodiazepine agonists had been found to be unaltered by the same ethanol treatment schedule (Rastogi *et al.*, 1986).

The allosteric effect of GABA agonists in increasing benzodiazepine binding (Hemmingsen *et al.*, 1982) and binding to the picrotoxin, or 'TBPS', site (Thyagarajan and Ticku, 1985; Liljequist *et al.*, 1986) were reported to be unchanged after chronic ethanol administration, although Liljequist *et al.* (1989) found some evidence for alterations in the allosteric interactions between the components of the receptor complex, as diazepam stimulation of TBPS binding was slightly increased.

4.5.2 Chronic ethanol administration and chloride flux

Allan and Harris (1987) have shown that chronic ethanol treatment abolished the potentiation of muscimol-stimulated chloride uptake into microsacs (prepared from mouse cerebellar tissue) seen with low concentrations of ethanol, but no difference was seen in the chloride uptake in the absence of ethanol. Morrow *et al.* (1988) also demonstrated tolerance to the action of ethanol on chloride flux into synaptoneurosomes, after treatment with ethanol *in vivo* by inhalation for 14 days. In this study, the potentiation by ethanol of GABA agonist-stimulated chloride uptake was lost completely after the chronic treatment, but the direct action of ethanol on the chloride flux was unchanged. A correlation was found between the GABA agonist stimulation and the blood ethanol concentrations during the chronic treatment, and the changes disappeared 4 days after ethanol withdrawal, when ethanol tolerance and signs of physical dependence were no longer apparent.

4.5.3 Electrophysiological studies on the effects of chronic ethanol administration on GABA transmission

Durand and Carlen (1984a) found the amplitude and duration of inhibitory postsynaptic potentials (IPSPs) in hippocampal slices to be decreased 3 weeks after withdrawal from an ethanol liquid diet. Both GABA-mediated inhibition, and the after-hyperpolarization that is considered to be due to calcium-dependent potassium conductance, were decreased (Table 2). No overt withdrawal syndrome was seen after the chronic ethanol treatment used in this study. Such behaviour in rats would peak a few hours after withdrawal of ethanol. The persistence of the electrophysiological changes, therefore, suggests that they are unlikely to be the cause of the behavioural withdrawal signs, unless some compensatory adaptations take place to bring the withdrawal hyperexcitability to an end. Later experiments from the same group (Reynolds *et al.*, 1990) failed to show any change in IPSPs in hippocampal slices prepared 24 h after withdrawal from 15 weeks ethanol treatment (Table 3). These results therefore do not support the theory that decreases in GABA transmission are responsible for the ethanol withdrawal syndrome.

Takada *et al.* (1989) studied the effects of GABA by extracellular recordings on hippocampal slices prepared from rats 4 days after cessation of chronic ethanol treatment (2 g/kg, twice daily for 30 days). Inhibition by exogenous GABA of the population spikes (the simultaneous discharge of pyramidal cells) occurred to the same extent after this chronic treatment as in control slices. The potentiation of this effect by ethanol at concentrations above 70 mM, seen in control preparations, was, however, lost after the chronic treatment. Unfortunately, this study did not indicate how long tolerance lasted to the *in vivo* actions of ethanol after their chronic treatment schedule, so it is not clear whether the decreased effect of ethanol in potentiating the effects of GABA can be correlated with tolerance to its behavioural effects. The time-course of the change suggests that it is unlikely to be correlated with the withdrawal syndrome. Four days after cessation of treatment in rats, signs of withdrawal hyperexcitability would be unlikely. These results indicate that the chloride flux changes may be involved in ethanol tolerance, but the lack of change in the absence of added ethanol suggests that this site is unlikely to be the cause of the ethanol withdrawal syndrome.

We have demonstrated hyperexcitability in extracellular recordings from isolated hippocampal slices prepared immediately on withdrawal from chronic ethanol treatment (Whittington and Little, 1990). We suggested that several different mechanisms may underlie the withdrawal hyperexcitability, including a decrease in GABA-mediated inhibition. The signs of hyperexcitability were prevented by dihydropyridine calcium channel antagonists (Whittington and Little, 1989a,b). Extracellular recordings made using antidromic stimulation provided evidence of decreased inhibitory potentials in the CA1 area of the hippocampus after the ethanol treatment (Whittington and Little, 1989c).

4.5.4 Effects of chronic ethanol treatment on the behavioural effects of compounds acting at the GABA complex

Chronic ethanol treatment has been reported to decrease the behavioural effects of GABA agonists (Taberner and Unwin, 1981; Martz *et al.*, 1983), suggesting either downregulation of GABA receptors or alterations in coupling. Tolerance to the potentiation of ethanol hypnosis by muscimol, however, was not found by Mattucci-Schiavone and Ferko (1987) in rats that were tolerant to the action of ethanol.

Chronic ethanol treatment reduces the effects of benzodiazepines (Rosenberg *et al.*, 1983; Le *et al.*, 1986). Cross-tolerance between barbiturates and ethanol also occurs, although barbiturate treatment had more effect on the actions of ethanol than did ethanol treatment on the effects of barbiturates (Gougos *et al.*, 1986; Khanna *et al.*, 1988). Cross-dependence, defined by a demonstration that substitution of one drug completely prevents withdrawal after production of dependence on the other drug, has been demonstrated in mice between ethanol and chlordiazepoxide (Chan *et al.*, 1986).

Chronic administration of chlordiazepoxide with ethanol did not affect the degree of tolerance that developed to the ethanol, although the severity of the withdrawal syndrome was reduced, possibly because of the presence of metabolites of chlordiazepoxide (Chan *et al.*, 1982). In patients, cessation of long-term intake of alcohol plus a benzodiazepine resulted in a withdrawal syndrome with fewer autonomic disturbances than withdrawal from alcohol alone, but a higher incidence of neuropsychiatric symptoms (Benzer and Cushman, 1980).

The partial inverse benzodiazepine agonist Ro15-4513 increased seizure incidence during ethanol withdrawal (Lister and Karanian, 1987). Similarly, Mehta and Ticku (1988) showed that both Ro15-4513 and FG7142 caused seizures during ethanol withdrawal. This effect was blocked by the benzodiazepine receptor antagonist Ro15-1788 (Becker and Anton, 1988). The production of seizures by partial inverse agonists during ethanol withdrawal would be predicted from the intrinsic preconvulsant properties of these compounds.

The effects of GABA antagonists, or benzodiazepine inverse agonists, do not necessarily provide information on the origin of the ethanol withdrawal syndrome, as the effects of other convulsants that do not act by inhibiting GABA transmission are also increased during ethanol withdrawal. Seizure activity in the hippocampus due to physostigmine was increased during ethanol withdrawal (Gonzales, 1985). Increases in the convulsant effects of kainic acid, but not of pentylenetetrazol, were found when these compounds were given during the chronic administration of ethanol (Freed and Michaelis, 1978). The excitatory amino acid NMDA was reported to increase the severity of the withdrawal syndrome (Grant *et al.*, 1990). The calcium channel activator (−)-Bay K 8644 increased the severity of handling convulsions when given during ethanol withdrawal (Whittington and Little, unpublished results).

Although decreased GABA transmission results in seizures, the pattern of behaviour is not the same as that seen in ethanol withdrawal. In rodents, the main characteristics of ethanol withdrawal are tremor, hyperreactivity and convulsions (Goldstein and Pal, 1971). Blockade of GABA receptors, either directly with bicuculline or indirectly with a benzodiazepine inverse agonist or picrotoxin, does not cause tremor and does not produce the hyperreactivity characteristic of ethanol withdrawal. Wild running is seen in rats during ethanol withdrawal. This is not seen after postsynaptic blockade of GABA transmission, although it is produced by inhibitors of glutamic acid decarboxylase (Taberner, 1977). Wild running also occurs during the seizure activity produced by an audiogenic stimulus in genetically susceptible mice (Schelesinger *et al.*, 1965) and this type of pattern is also seen after systemic administration of the excitatory amino acid NMDA. Behaviourally, therefore, changes in GABA neurones could be responsible for part, but not all, of the ethanol withdrawal syndrome.

4.5.5 Treatment of ethanol withdrawal with GABA agonists and benzodiazepines

The GABA agonists muscimol and THIP, GABA itself, the GABA uptake blocking agent amino-oxyacetic acid, and sodium valproate (which increases GABA concentrations) have all been shown to decrease some signs of the ethanol withdrawal syndrome in experimental models (Goldstein, 1973, 1979; Cooper *et al.*, 1979; Frye *et al.*, 1983; Gonzales and Hettinger, 1984). Phenobarbitone also decreased tremor and convulsions. The $GABA_B$ agonist baclofen was not very effective (Tarika and Winger, 1980). Not all studies, however, have shown effects of this type of compound. Goldstein (1979) found that muscimol, over a range of doses, was ineffective against handling convulsions during withdrawal. Frye *et al.* (1983) found that GABA and GABA agonists provided no protection against tremor during ethanol withdrawal.

Benzodiazepines decrease the ethanol withdrawal syndrome and are widely used therapeutically for this purpose (Brown, 1982; Peachey and Naranjo, 1984). Not all signs of withdrawal, however, were prevented by these compounds. Okamoto *et al.* (1983) showed that tremor and bizarre behaviour in cats was not prevented by diazepam. Neither the protective effects of benzodiazepines in ethanol withdrawal, nor the actions of compounds that increase GABA transmission, are necessarily evidence that the ethanol withdrawal syndrome is due to decreases in GABA transmission. Benzodiazepines have anticonvulsant actions in syndromes that are not caused by deficits in GABA transmission. They are effective against seizures due to the excitatory amino acid NMDA (Moreau *et al.*, 1989), the cardiac glycoside digoxin (Kulkarni and Mehta, 1983) and the cholinergic agonist pilocarpine (Turski *et al.*, 1984). They had some action against strychnine and nicotine seizures (Sofia *et al.*, 1976). The doses of benzodiazepines effective in ethanol withdrawal were similar to those required to protect against these other types of seizures (e.g. diazepam 5–10 mg/kg, chlordiazepoxide 16 mg/kg) so it does not appear that there is any selectivity in this respect.

Although benzodiazepine agonists are drugs of choice in treating withdrawal in alcoholics, they do not prevent the dependence (Nutt *et al.*, 1989). It has also been reported that they prevent only part of the withdrawal syndrome (Aaronson *et al.*, 1982). There is evidence that treatment of alcoholics with benzodiazepines can result in abuse of these compounds in addition to alcohol (Schuster and Humfries, 1981; Finer, 1970; Busto *et al.*, 1983; Jaffe *et al.*, 1983). It has been suggested that an endogenous compound with properties of an inverse agonist at benzodiazepine receptors might be the cause of the ethanol withdrawal syndrome, but we have shown that the benzodiazepine receptor antagonist Ro15-1788 did not affect the ethanol withdrawal syndrome (Little *et al.*, 1983). This compound blocks the effects of benzodiazepine inverse agonists (Nutt *et al.*, 1982) so the involvement of an inverse agonist in ethanol withdrawal appears unlikely.

4.6 Changes in cholinergic transmission after ethanol treatment

The acute actions of ethanol on cholinergic transmission were described many years ago. The CNS concentration of acetylcholine was increased (Hunt and Dalton, 1976). Acetylcholine release appears to be more sensitive to the inhibitory actions of ethanol than other neurotransmitters (Carmichael and

Israel, 1975). Changes in cholinergic transmission have been reported after chronic ethanol treatment. Muscarinic receptor number in cortex and hippocampus (but not striatum) was increased (Tabakoff *et al.*, 1979). This change was seen at 0 h and 8 h into withdrawal, but not at 24 h, suggesting a possible involvement with the behavioural withdrawal syndrome. Nordberg and Wahlstrom (1982) found an increase in muscarinic receptors, in the striatum only, on the eighth day of withdrawal from a very long ethanol treatment. No change was found after one day of withdrawal. Withdrawal convulsions were seen at the time the receptor change was found, but the binding was increased only in those animals that did not have seizures. As with other transmitter systems, binding in human brain did not follow the pattern seen in the laboratory. Tran *et al.* (1981) showed that muscarinic binding was unaltered in postmortem brain samples from alcoholics.

The density of nicotinic receptors was decreased in the hippocampus but increased in the thalamus and hypothalamus by 5 months of ethanol drinking (Yoshida *et al.*, 1982). Ethanol added *in vitro* did not affect nicotinic binding except at very high concentrations (El-Fakahany *et al.*, 1983).

The relevance of the increase in muscarinic binding was not clear, as Smith (1983) showed that, although the binding was increased, the effects of carbachol on incorporation of ^{32}P into phosphatidylinositol or phosphatidic acid were unaltered after chronic ethanol treatment. The situation was further complicated by the results of Hoffman *et al.* (1986). They showed that although binding to the non-selective muscarinic ligand quinuclinylbenzilate was increased in both cortex and hippocampus after chronic ethanol intake, the stimulation of phosphatidylinositol 4,5-biphosphate by carbachol was increased in cortex but decreased in hippocampus. Use of the selective M_1 receptor ligand pirenzipine showed that M_1 binding was increased by the ethanol treatment in cortex but not in the hippocampus. The increase in muscarinic binding in cortex may therefore have functional consequences.

4.7 Monoamines and ethanol dependence

The evidence suggests that monoamine transmission can modulate ethanol dependence, but that changes in these systems may not be the initial cause of ethanol tolerance or the ethanol withdrawal.

4.7.1 Effects of acute ethanol treatment on monoamine transmission

Acute administration of ethanol has been reported to have a variety of effects on monoamines, depending on the system under study, the dose of ethanol, the species, and the time interval and route of administration. Changes in brain concentrations are not very informative about the synaptic effects of ethanol, but turnover studies are more useful. There was an increase in noradrenaline turnover after acute administration of ethanol (Hunt and Majchrowicz, 1974; Badawy *et al.*, 1983), followed by a decrease (Badawy *et al.*, 1983). Hunt and Majchrowicz (1974) found a decrease in dopamine turnover a few hours after a single dose of ethanol, but the turnover of this amine has also been found to increase, an effect suggested to be due to the formation of acetaldehyde from alcohol (Barbaccia *et al.*, 1982). The firing rate of dopaminergic neurones in the substantia nigra was raised by an acute dose of ethanol (4 g/kg) in unanaesthetized rats, but in anaesthetized animals only depressant actions of ethanol were seen (Mereu *et al.*, 1984).

A single injection of ethanol had little effect on 5-HT metabolism, although the concentrations of the metabolite 5-hydroxyindole acetic acid were transiently increased (Tabakoff and Boggan, 1974; Frankel *et al.*, 1974; Pohorecky *et al.*, 1978).

4.7.2 The effects of ethanol on monoamine release

The acute effects of ethanol on transmitter release have been found to vary with the transmitter studied, the brain region and the experimental conditions. In most cases the changes in transmitter release were attributed to alterations in calcium. The effects of ethanol on release therefore appear to be secondary to changes in calcium flux or concentrations, rather than to actions on other components of the release mechanism.

Daniell and Leslie (1986) found no effect of acute ethanol (25–200 mM) on noradrenaline release from several brain regions. Wu *et al.* (1986) found no change in 5-HT release from synaptosomal preparations of hippocampus and hypothalamus when ethanol was added up to 100 mM. Holman and Snape (1985) demonstrated an important point when they showed a difference between results obtained from measurement of the effects of ethanol added *in vitro* and injected *in vivo* on catecholamine release. Changes (increases in dopamine release) were seen only after *in vivo* administration of ethanol. The dose used, 3 g/kg, gave a maximal blood ethanol concentration of 78 mM.

Dopamine release in freely moving rats was measured by Di Chiara and Imperato (1986). They found that comparatively low doses (0.5 and 1 g/kg i.p.) selectively increased release from the nucleus accumbens, with little change in striatal release. The change in release followed a similar time-course to the behavioural effects of the ethanol and was suggested to be related to the reward properties of ethanol.

Lynch and Littleton (1983) showed that 50 mM ethanol reduced dopamine release from striatal slices evoked by potassium depolarization, while increasing that due to the calcium ionophore A23187, indicating that the effect on release was due to decreased entry of calcium into the terminal. Tolerance developed to these actions of chronic ethanol treatment, a change suggested to be due to increased sensitivity of the terminal to calcium entry. Harper *et al.* (1987) demonstrated inhibitory actions of ethanol (100 mM) on dopamine and noradrenaline release from control striatal slices. The acute effect on noradrenaline release was seen only when the intracellular concentration of calcium was increased. In preparations from ethanol-tolerant animals, release was increased by this concentration of ethanol, but was unchanged in the absence of this drug.

4.7.3 Changes in monoamine transmission after chronic ethanol treatment

Chronic ethanol administration was found to increase noradrenaline turnover and to decrease dopamine turnover, both during intoxication and during the withdrawal period (Hunt and Majchrowicz, 1974). A decrease in the sensitivity of dopamine receptors has been reported following long-term ethanol administration, 24 h, but not 8 h, after withdrawal (Hoffman and Tabakoff, 1977). The effect of dopamine antagonists in stimulating dopamine synthesis was decreased at both 8 h and 24 h, but returned to normal by 3 days into withdrawal. In contrast, Liljequist (1978), using a long ethanol treatment (5–9 months), found evidence for a supersensitivity of dopamine receptors that lasted 4 weeks after withdrawal. Subsensitivity to noradrenaline, measured by the cAMP response, was found in the cerebral cortex during chronic ethanol intake, followed by supersensitivity after 3 days of withdrawal (French *et al.*, 1975). Chronic ethanol treatment was found to decrease β-receptor number in some areas of the CNS and to lower the activation of adenyl cyclase by β-agonists, but the binding changes did not correlate with the functional alterations (Valverius *et al.*, 1989). β-Receptor numbers were increased in the later stages of ethanol withdrawal (Banerjee *et al.*, 1978; Kuriyama *et al.*, 1981) but significant changes were not found in α_1- or α_2-receptor numbers (Lynch *et al.*, 1983).

5-HT turnover appeared to be little altered by acute or chronic ethanol administration, apart from slight increases in 5-hydroxyindole acetic acid (Tabakoff and Boggan, 1974; Frankel *et al.*, 1974; Pohorecky *et al.*, 1978). Badawy *et al.* (1980) showed that chronic administration of glucose or sucrose increased 5-HT synthesis in rat brain. This is a very important result, as many chronic studies use such compounds, either to increase ethanol intake or to provide calories for control animals. This effect could mask, or alter, changes caused by ethanol.

4.7.4 Modification of ethanol tolerance by drugs acting on monoamine transmission

Changes in monoamine transmission can modulate ethanol tolerance. Frankel *et al.* (1975) reported that *p*-chlorophenylalanine, a 5-HT depletor, decreased tolerance to the ataxic action of ethanol, without altering its acute action. The 5-HT precursor 5-hydroxytryptophan had the opposite effect (Le *et al.*, 1979). The effect of 5-HT depletion on ethanol tolerance is thought to originate in the median raphe nucleus, which projects largely to the hippocampus, as lesions of this nucleus produced the effect (Le *et al.*, 1981a). Such lesions caused depletion of 5-HT in the hippocampus and cerebral cortex, but did not alter striatal 5-HT levels. This type of lesion has also been found to cause learning deficits. When lesions were placed in the dorsal or magnus nucleus of the raphe, tolerance to ethanol was unaltered.

Ritzmann and Tabakoff showed that 6-hydroxydopamine, a neurotoxin that acts on dopaminergic and noradrenergic terminals, prevented tolerance to ethanol, but not the ethanol withdrawal syndrome (Ritzmann and Tabakoff, 1976; Tabakoff and Ritzmann, 1977). The effect was seen only if the toxin was given before tolerance development, as there was no action on established tolerance. It was attributed to depletion of noradrenaline rather than dopamine, as co-administration of desipramine, a noradrenaline uptake blocking agent, prevented the effect. Le *et al.* (1981b) found that depletion of both noradrenaline and 5-HT prevented the development of ethanol tolerance, while depletion of noradrenaline or dopamine alone had no effect.

Tolerance to ethanol is increased by testing in surroundings in which the chronic treatment has been given (Le *et al.*, 1979). Such 'context-specific' tolerance may have a different physiological basis from tolerance that is not related to the surroundings. The study of Melchior and Tabakoff (1981) considered the importance of environmental cues in tolerance development. When tolerance to the hypnotic actions of ethanol was entirely dependent on the presence of a familiar environment, the depletion of noradrenaline decreased tolerance, but depletion of 5-HT increased the rate of tolerance development. The latter result was in contrast to previous reports (see above), but was complicated by the effects of the agent used, 5,7-dihydroxytryptamine, on the initial actions of ethanol. The increase in tolerance was suggested to be due to the increase in the initial action of ethanol caused by low doses of 5,7-dihydroxytryptamine. A later report (Melchior and Tabakoff, 1986) confirmed this suggestion and showed that 5,7-dihydroxytryptamine increased brain concentrations of ethanol.

In the above results, it was necessary to take into account the effects of the modulating agents on the initial actions of ethanol. It is difficult to interpret tolerance changes if there are alterations in the 'baseline' actions of ethanol. There have been other reports of such alterations after treatments that affect monoamine transmission. Induction of supersensitivity to dopamine by chronic administration of an antagonist, or by depletion, decreased the acute actions of ethanol, despite increased brain concentrations (Yanai and Feiggenbaum, 1983). Administration of an α_1-agonist (Menon and Kodama, 1985) or α_2-antagonists (Lister *et al.*, 1989) decreased the acute actions of ethanol. It is possible that changes in the acute actions of ethanol may be due to changes in acute tolerance, rather than in the initial actions of ethanol, although this clearly does not explain all the above results. Blockade of α_2-receptors (Edwards *et al.*, 1983) or lesions of the median raphe (Campanelli *et al.*, 1988) antagonized the phenomenon of acute tolerance to ethanol, without altering the initial actions.

4.7.5 Monoamine transmission and ethanol withdrawal

Some drugs that alter monoamine transmission have been found to affect ethanol withdrawal, but the results have not always been consistent. It should also be kept in mind, as explained previously (Section 4.5.5), that protective effects do not necessarily imply causal involvement of the particular transmitter system affected. Some selectivity of action needs to be shown before such conclusions are drawn. The α_2-agonist clonidine has been reported to decrease the ethanol withdrawal syndrome (Bjorkquist, 1975; Wilkins *et al.*, 1983), but one report found an increase in severity (Blum *et al.*, 1983) and another no effect (Hemmingsen *et al.*, 1984). The differences in these results could have been due to differences in the dosage of clonidine, as this compound may have both pre- and postsynaptic actions (Nutt and Glue, 1986).

4.8 Neuroactive peptides and ethanol dependence

There is now considerable evidence that ethanol tolerance can be modulated by certain peptides that have neuronal actions. Interest in the effects of such peptides on drug tolerance originated in the demonstration by de Weid (1965) that lysine-vasopressin restored deficits in learning and memory produced by hypophysectomy. Krivoy *et al.* (1974) extended these ideas to opiate dependence and found that intracerebral vasopressin increased morphine tolerance. Later work showed that an analogue, desglycinamide-arginine-vasopressin, that lacked the endocrine properties of vasopressin, was effective. Hoffman *et al.* (1978) studied the effects of a similar analogue, arginine-vasopressin, on ethanol tolerance and found that it prolonged the duration of tolerance after the cessation of ethanol treatment. The responses of naive animals to ethanol were unaffected. Although an early study by Kalant's group suggested that a vasopressin analogue inhibited development of ethanol tolerance, this was not confirmed by these authors subsequently (Le *et al.*, 1982) and it is generally aggreed that tolerance development is unaffected.

These results were confirmed and extended by Rigter and Crabbe (1980), who considered the effect not to be on the learned component of tolerance, i.e. that due to practice in the test while under the influence of ethanol, as it was seen when ethanol was given by inhalation, when there is little learning component to the tolerance. This group also showed that desglycinamide-arginine-vasopressin increased ethanol withdrawal seizures (Rigter *et al.*, 1980). This was a selective effect as the compound did not affect seizures caused by the convulsant pentylenetetrazol. Administration of 6-hydroxy-dopamine prevented the effect of arginine-vasopressin (Hoffman *et al.*, 1983).

The action of desglycinamide-arginine-vasopressin in prolonging ethanol tolerance was prevented by electrolytic lesion of the median raphe, but not the dorsal raphe or raphe magnus (Le *et al.*, 1982). Selective destruction of the fibres of 5-HT neurones innervating the hippocampus also prevented the effect of desglycinamide-arginine-vasopressin, suggesting an important role for the hippocampus in ethanol tolerance (Speisky and Kalant, 1985). Lesions of the pathways from the raphe nuclei to the septum did not alter the effect of the peptide on ethanol tolerance. The vasopressin analogue did not affect 5-HT synthesis in hippocampal or septal tissue, suggesting that the interaction might occur at a postsynaptic site (Speisky and Kalant, 1987).

4.9 Drinking and dependence

This chapter has described the effects of ethanol on various transmitter and signalling systems, and the actions of various compounds on ethanol tolerance and the withdrawal syndrome. I have tried to evaluate the evidence to see how much we know about the mechanism(s) of ethanol dependence. However, perhaps the most important question from a clinical point of view is what makes someone drink. The factors that initiate drinking in alcoholics are probably not the same as those that maintain continued drinking or that cause relapses after abstinence. The former involve on the one hand social and psychological reasons, the neurophysiological bases of which are as yet little understood, and on the other hand the acute pharmacological actions of ethanol. Ethanol has both reinforcing and aversive effects, but just which of its many actions on neurotransmitter systems are responsible for these is not clear.

Many of the models used in the laboratory to investigate this aspect of ethanol dependence determine the preference of animals for ethanol. There are many ways in which this can be measured, from the simple choice between drinking bottles containing water or dilute ethanol to complex schedule-induction techniques. Self-administration of ethanol can also be measured using indwelling cannulae, as with other compounds with addition liability. The remainder of this chapter will briefly describe various pharmacological and physiological manipulations of ethanol preference.

It is noticeable that the drugs that have so far been shown to decrease ethanol preference are not the same as those that prevent the ethanol withdrawal syndrome or those that act on systems that are supposed to mediate the pharmacological effects of ethanol. This suggests two possibilities. The known effects of ethanol on transmitter and signalling systems that are thought to mediate the more obvious behavioural actions of ethanol may not be involved in the reinforcing effect of ethanol on first administration. In addition, the adaptations of ethanol that occur on long-term intake may not be related to continued drinking in alcoholics. The latter appears unlikely. It is more probable that we simply do not yet know sufficient about the adaptations to chronic ethanol to be able either to understand the physiological basis of craving and relapses or to manipulate this by pharmacological means.

One of the problems in this area is that there is no good rodent model in which long-term ethanol drinking leads to an increased preference for alcohol. In the ethanol-preferring C57 strain of mice, for example, chronic ethanol intake reduced the preference for ethanol solutions over water (Unwin and Taberner, 1982). The schedule-induction methods can produce ethanol polydipsia by intermittent food delivery, but the increased ethanol intake in these studies is not necessarily due to the adaptations to prolonged high ethanol brain concentrations, as solutions of other compounds also produce polydipsia, and it is very much affected by environmental conditions (Tang *et al.*, 1982).

Drugs that affect 5-HT transmission appear to alter ethanol preference in animal studies. Compounds that increase 5-HT transmission have been shown to decrease the amount of ethanol drunk in a free-choice situation (Myers and Martin, 1973). Both the precursor of 5-HT and 5-HT uptake blockers have this effect. The latter type of compound has been tested in patients, and found to have some effect in decreasing drinking (Naranjo *et al.*, 1986). Little is known of the mechanism of this effect. It may be related to the effect of 5-HT inhibitors in decreasing food intake (Gill and Amit, 1987) or to the effects on the renin–angiotensin system, described below (Grupp *et al.*, 1988a). Lesions of the raphe nucleus decreased ethanol preference (Rodriguez-Echandia and Foscolo, 1988).

Some rodent studies have suggested that benzodiazepines may decrease ethanol intake (Chan *et al.*, 1983a,b), but others did not show any effect

(Beaman *et al.*, 1984; Daoust *et al.*, 1987a). There is little evidence in patients that they have any beneficial effect in preventing relapses after abstinence. It is possible that the effects in the animal studies were due to potentiation of the pharmacological actions of ethanol. GABA agonists acting at the $GABA_A$ site and the GABA antagonist bicuculline did not alter ethanol preference (Boismare *et al.*, 1984; Daoust *et al.*, 1987a). A possible role for $GABA_B$ receptors, however, was suggested by the effects of the agonist baclofen in decreasing ethanol intake in a free-choice situation (Daoust *et al.*, 1987a). A novel compound, calcium bis-acetylhomotaurine, has also been shown to decrease ethanol choice (Daoust *et al.*, 1987b; Le Magnen *et al.*, 1987a). This drug has been suggested to act at $GABA_B$ receptors or on noradrenergic transmission, but its mechanism of action is unclear. It did not alter the pharmacological effects or toxicity of ethanol (Le Magnen *et al.*, 1987b).

The changes reported in cholinergic receptors after chronic ethanol treatment (see Section 4.6) may be related to subsequent ethanol intake. Wahlstrom and Nordberg (1988) demonstrated a correlation in rats between striatal muscarinic binding and voluntary ethanol intake after long-term drinking. Administration of amphetamine or nicotine has been shown to increase ethanol intake (Potthoff and Ellison, 1982). This effect appears to be mediated through noradrenergic transmission (Levy and Ellison, 1985). Despite the involvement of dopamine transmission in reward mechanisms, compounds affecting this system do not appear to have much effect on ethanol intake. Dopamine uptake inhibitors did not alter ethanol preference (Daoust *et al.*, 1986), but dopamine antagonists lowered the intake in ethanol-preferring rats (Fadda *et al.*, 1987).

Recently, angiotensin II has been shown to cause a reduction in ethanol preference (Grupp *et al.*, 1988b). This was not due to changes in fluid intake or pharmacokinetics. Inhibitors of angiotensin converting enzyme, such as captopril and enalapril, also reduced ethanol drinking (Spinosa *et al.*, 1988). Vasopressin, which prolongs ethanol tolerance (see Section 4.8), was found to decrease ethanol polydipsia in the Brattleboro rat, which shows diabetes insipidus due to vasopressin deficiency (Myers *et al.*, 1983a). However, it did not alter ethanol choice in other models (Myers *et al.*, 1983a) and it was considered that the effect was secondary to the polydipsic state rather than to an action on ethanol preference (Rigter and Crabbe, 1985). Other peptides have been found to modulate ethanol preference, including bombesin (Kulkosky *et al.*, 1987) and cholecystokinin (Kulkosky and Glazner, 1988).

Opioid transmission has been suggested to be involved in the reinforcing effects of ethanol. The antagonist naloxone was found to decrease the acquisition of ethanol preference by a conditioning forced ethanol exposure (Sandi *et al.*, 1988). Naltrexone decreased voluntary selection of alcohol in monkeys selected for established excess drinking (Myers *et al.*, 1986). Opioid mechanisms have been invoked to explain the actions of tetrahydroisoquinoline and β-carboline compounds that cause large increases in ethanol drinking. This area has been recently reviewed by Myers (1989). It has been suggested that these compounds are formed in the CNS after ethanol administration.

The involvement of calcium in ethanol choice has received little attention so far. Wu *et al.* (1987) showed that rats with higher preference for ethanol showed greater potassium-evoked calcium uptake in synaptosomal preparations. If a good model of increased ethanol drinking induced by chronic treatment were available it would be of interest to determine the effects of the chronic calcium channel antagonist treatments that prevent ethanol tolerance and withdrawal (see Section 4.3.4).

Certain areas of the CNS may be involved in voluntary drinking. Neurochemical lesions of the hippocampus were found to decrease ethanol choice in a self-selection test (Myers *et al.*, 1983b). Hypothalamic stimulation has been found to cause large increases in the choice of ethanol solutions over water (Amit *et al.*, 1970). This has been suggested to be due to changes in energy balance (Atrens *et al.*, 1983). Stressful stimuli that activated the hypothalamic-pituitary-adrenocortical axis caused increased ethanol choice after the stress and this was abolished by hypophysectomy (Nash and Maickel, 1988). Lesions of the hippocampus produced by kainic acid did not affect the ethanol self-selection (Swartzwelder and Myers, 1983). Area postrema lesions increased ethanol intake, but did not affect the aversive effect of ethanol (Stewart *et al.*, 1988), while amygdaloid lesions decreased conditioned taste aversion to ethanol (Kolakowska *et al.*, 1985).

4.10 Conclusions

The above description of the effects of ethanol on neurotransmission is not exhaustive, but I have tried to select those areas that appeared from the evidence to be the most important. The various systems have been described separately, but this should not be taken to indicate that they are alternative explanations. The systems all interact and all may be involved in dependence on ethanol.

I have spent some time on the role of calcium because considerable data have now been obtained implicating this messenger in both the acute actions of ethanol and in physical dependence. Recent results suggest that manipulation of voltage-sensitive calcium channels can modulate the adaptations to ethanol in a way that has not previously been possible. Ethanol has long been suggested to act on GABA transmission, but the evidence is more conflicting than is normally realized. I have tried to re-examine critically the older data and to challenge some of the assumptions behind the conclusions. Excitatory amino acid transmission is a field in which there is much current interest, and in which ethanol has been shown to cause changes. Perhaps the most exciting of these are the effects of very low concentrations of ethanol in the patch-clamp studies. It would be of great interest if this electrophysiological approach were applied to other transmitter systems. The actions of the peptides, such as vasopressin analogues, in modulating ethanol tolerance show that drug tolerance and learning may be closely related.

Acknowledgement

H.J.L. is a Wellcome Trust Senior Lecturer.

References

Aaronson, L.M., Hinman, D.J. & Okamoto, M. (1982) *J. Pharmacol. Exp. Ther.* **221**, 319–325.

Aguayo, L.G. (1990) *Eur. J. Pharmacol.* **187**, 127–130.

Akaike, N., Kostyuk, P. G. & Osipchuk, Y.V. (1989) *J. Physiol.* **412**, 181–195.

Allan, A.M. & Harris, R.A. (1987) *Pharmacol. Biochem. Behav.* **27**, 665–670.

Allison, J.H. & Cicero, T. (1980) *J. Pharmacol. Exp. Ther.* **213**, 24–27.

Amit, Z., Stern, M.H. & Wise, R.A. (1970) *Psychopharmacology* **17**, 367–377.

Atrens, D.M., Marfaing-Jallat, P. & LeMagnen, J. (1983) *Pharmacol. Biochem. Behav.* **19**, 571–575.

Badawy, A.A.-B., Punjani, N.F. & Evans, M. (1980) *Subst. Alcohol Actions Misuse* **1**, 507.

Badawy, A.A.-B., Williams, D.L. & Evans, M. (1983) *Pharmacol. Biochem. Behav.* **18** (Suppl. 1), 389.

Banerjee, S.P., Sharma, V.K. & Khanna, J.M. (1978) *Nature* **276**, 407–409.

Barbaccia, M.L., Bosio, A., Lucci, L., Spano, P.F. and Trabucci, M. (1982) *Life Sci.* **30**, 2163–2170.

Battaini, F., Del Vasco, R., Govoni, S. & Trabucci, M. (1989) *Alcohol* **6**, 169–172.

Beaman, C.M., Hunter, G.A., Dunn, L.L. & Reid, L.D. (1984) *Alcohol* **1**, 39–42.

Bean, B.P. (1984) *Proc. Natl Acad. Sci. USA* **81**, 6388–6392.

Becker, H.C. & Anton, R.F. (1988) *Pharmacol. Biochem. Behav.* **32**, 163–167.

Benzer, D. & Cushman, P. (1980) *Alcoholism: Clin. Exp. Res.* **4**, 243–247.

Bergamaschi, A., Govoni, S. & Trabucchi, M. (1987) *Pharmacol. Res. Commun.* **19**, 975–976.

Bjorkquist, S.E. (1975) *Acta Psychiatr. Scand.* **52**, 256–263.

Blum, K., Briggs, A.H. & DeLallo, L. (1983) *Subst. Alcohol Actions Misuse* **4**, 59–63.

Boismare, F., Daoust, M., Moore, N., Saligaut, C., Lhuintre, J.P., Chretien, P. and Durlach, J. (1984) *Pharmacol. Biochem. Behav.* **21**, 787–789.

Bolger, G.T., Weissman, P. & Skolnick, P. (1985) *Naunyn-Schmeideberg's Arch. Pharmacol.* **328**, 373–377.

Bongianni, F., Carla, V., Moroni, F. & Pellegrini-Giampietro, D.E. (1986) *Br. J. Pharmacol.* **88**, 561–567.

Brenna, C.H. & Littleton, J.M. (1990) *Neuropharmacology* **29**, 689–693.

Brown, C.G. (1982) *Ann. Emerg. Med.* **11**, 276–280.

Busto, V., Simpkins, J., Sellers, E.M., Sisson, B. & Segal, R. (1983) *Br. J. Addict.* **78**, 429–435.
Campanelli, C., Le, A.D. & Kalant, H. (1988) *Psychopharmacology* **96**, 454–457.
Carlen, P.L., Gurevich, N. & Durand, D. (1982) *Science* **215**, 306–309.
Carmichael, F.J. & Israel, Y. (1975) *J. Pharmacol. Exp. Ther.* **193**, 824–834.
Celentano, J.J., Gibbs, T.T. & Farb, D.H. (1988) *Brain Res.* **455**, 377–380.
Chan, A.W.K., Schanley, D.L., Leong, F.W. & Casbeer, D. (1982) *Pharmacol. Biochem. Behav.* **17**, 1239–1244.
Chan, A.W.K., Leong, F.W. & Schanley, D.L. (1983a) *Pharmacol. Biochem. Behav.* **18**, 797–802.
Chan, A.W.K., Schanley, D.L. & Leong, F.W. (1983b) *Pharmacol. Biochem. Behav.* **19**, 275–280.
Chan, A.W.K., Langan, M.C., Leong, F.W., Penetrante, M.L., Schanley, D.L. & Aldrich-Castanik, L. (1986) *Alcohol* **3**, 309–316.
Charness, M.E., Simon, R.P. & Greenburg, D.A. (1989) *N. Engl. J. Med.* **321**, 442–454.
Chin, J.H. & Goldstein, D.B. (1977a) *Mol. Pharmacol.* **13**, 435–441.
Chin, J.H. & Goldstein, D.B. (1977b) *Science* **196**, 684–685.
Chin, J.H., Parsons, L.M. & Goldstein, D.B. (1978) *Biochim. Biophys. Acta* **513**, 358–363.
Collingridge, G.L., Kehl, S.J. & McLennan, A. (1983) *J. Physiol.* **334**, 33–46.
Cooper, B.R., Ferris, R.M. & White, H.L. (1979) *J. Pharmacol. Exp. Ther.* **209**, 396–403.
Crews, F.T., Majchrowicz, E. and Meeks, R. (1983) *Psychopharmacology* **81**, 208–213.
Czyrak, A., Mogilnicka, E. & Maj, J. (1989) *Europharmacology* **28**, 229–233.
Daniell, L.C. & Harris, R.A. (1988a) *J. Pharmacol. Exp. Ther.* **245**, 1–7.
Daniell, L.C. & Harris, R.A. (1988b) *Alcoholism* **12**, 179–183.
Daniell, L.C. & Harris, R.A. (1989) *J. Pharmacol. Exp. Ther.* **250**, 875–881.
Daniell, L.C. & Leslie, S.W. (1986) *Brain Res.* **377**, 18–28.
Daniell, L.C., Brass, E.P. & Harris, R.A. (1987) *Mol. Pharmacol.* **32**, 831–837.
Daoust, M., Moore, N., Saligaut, C., Lhuintre, J.P., Chretien, P. & Boismare, F. (1986) *Alcohol* **3**, 15–17.
Daoust, M., Saligaut, C., Lhuitre, J.P., Moore, N., Flipo, J.L. & Boismare, F. (1987a) *Alcohol* **4**, 469–472.
Daoust, M., Lhaintre, J.P., Saligaut, C., Moore, N., Flipo, J.L. & Boismare, F. (1987b) *Alcohol* Suppl. 1, 319–322.
Davidoff, R.A. (1973) *Arch. Neurol.* **28**, 60–63.
Davidson, M., Wilce, P. & Shanley, B. (1988) *Neurosci. Lett.* **89**, 165–169.
Davis, W.C. & Ticku, M.K. (1981) *Mol. Pharmacol.* **20**, 287–295.
Del Pozo, E., Caro, G. & Baeyens, J.M. (1987) *Eur. J. Pharmacol.* **137**, 155–160.
De Sarro, D.B., Meldrum, B.S. & Nistico, G. (1988) *Br. J. Pharmacol.* **93**, 247–256.
De Weid, D. (1965). *Nature* **232**, 58–59.
Di Chiara, G. & Imperato, A. (1986) *Symposia in Neuroscience.* Fidia Research Series, vol. 3, pp 89–96. Springer-Verlag, Berlin, Heidelberg, New York and Tokyo.
Dolin, S.J. (1988) The effects of calcium antagonists on sedative drug action in rodents: anaesthesia, physical dependence and tolerance. PhD Thesis, University of London.
Dolin, S.J. & Little, H.J. (1986) *Br. J. Pharmacol.* **88**, 909–914.
Dolin, S.J. & Little, H.J. (1988) *Br. J. Pharmacol.* **93**, 7P.
Dolin, S.J. & Little, H.J. (1989a) *Anaesthesiology* **70**, 91–97.
Dolin, S.J. & Little, H.J. (1989b) *J. Pharmacol. Exp. Ther.* **250**, 985–991.
Dolin, S.J., Little, H.J., Hudspith, M., Pagonis, C. & Littleton, J. (1987) *Neuropharmacology* **26**, 275–279.

Dolin, S.J., Hunter, A.B., Halsey, M.J. & Little, H.J. (1988a) *Eur. J. Pharmacol.* **152**, 19–27.
Dolin, S.J., Patch, T., Siarey, R.J., Whittington, M.A. & Little, H.J. (1988b) *Br. J. Pharmacol.* **95**, 877P.
Durand, D. & Carlen, P.L. (1984a) *Science* **224**, 1359–1361.
Durand, D. & Carlen, P.L. (1984b) *Brain Res.* **308**, 325–332.
Edwards, F., Schabinsky, V.V., Jackson, D.M., Starmer, G.A. & Jenkins, O. (1983) *Psychopharmacology* **79**, 246–250.
El-Fakahany, E.F., Miller, E.R., Abbassy, M.A., Eldefrawi, A.T. & Eldefrawi, M.E. (1983) *J. Pharmacol. Exp. Ther.* **224**, 289–296.
Epaud, R.M. & Lester, D.S. (1990) *Trends Pharmacol. Sci.* **11**, 317–320.
Fadda, F., Franch, F., Mosca, E., Meloni, R. & Gessa, G.L. (1987) *Alcohol Drug Res.* **7**, 285–290.
File, S.E., Baldwin, H.A. & Hitchcott, P.K. (1989) *Psychopharmacology* **98**, 262–264.
Finer, M.J. (1970) *J. A. M. A.* **213**, 1342.
Franckowiak, G., Bechem, M., Schramm, M. & Thomas, G. (1985) *Eur. J. Pharmacol.* **114**, 223–226.
Frankel, D., Khanna, J.M., LeBlanc, A.E. & Kalant, H. (1974) *Psychopharmacology* **44**, 247–252.
Freed, W.J. & Michaelis, E.J. (1978) *Pharmacol. Biochem. Behav.* **8**, 509–514.
French, S.W., Palmer, D.S., Narod, M.E., Reid, P.E. & Ramey, C.W. (1975) *J. Pharmacol. Exp. Ther.* **194**, 319–326.
Freund, G. (1980) *Life Sci.* **27**, 987–992.
Friedman, M.B., Erickson, C.K. & Leslie, S.W. (1980) *Biochem. Pharmacol.* **29**, 1903.
Frye, G.D., McGowan, J. & Breese, G.R. (1983) *J. Pharmacol. Exp. Ther.* **226**, 720–726.
Gage, P.W. & Robertson, B. (1985) *Br. J. Pharmacol.* **85**, 675–681.
Gill, K. & Amit, Z. (1987) *Alcoholism* **11**, 444–449.
Goldstein, D.B. (1973) *J. Pharmacol. Exp. Ther.* **186**, 1–9.
Goldstein, D.B. (1979) *J. Pharmacol. Exp. Ther.* **208**, 223–227.
Goldstein, D.B. (1986) *Recent Dev. Alcohol.* **4**, 231–240.
Goldstein, D.B. & Chin, J.H. (1981) *Alcoholism: Clin. Exp. Res.* **5**, 256–258.
Goldstein, D.B. & Pal, W. (1971) *Science* **172**, 288–290.
Gonzales, L.P. (1985) *Brain Res.* **335**, 384–388.
Gonzales, L.P. & Hettinger, M.K. (1984) *Brain Res.* **298**, 163–166.
Gonzales, R.A. & Crews, F.T. (1988) *Alcoholism* **12**, 94–98.
Gonzales, L.P., Theiss, C. & Crews, F.T. (1986) *J. Pharmacol. Exp. Ther.* **237**, 92–98.
Gougos, A., Khanna, J.M., Le, A.D. & Kalant, H. (1986) *Pharmacol. Biochem. Behav.* **24**, 801–807.
Grant, K.A., Valverius, P., Hudspith, M. & Tabakoff, B. (1990) *Eur. J. Pharmacol.* **176**, 289–296.
Greenberg, D.A. & Cooper, E.C. (1984) *Alcoholism: Clin. Exp. Res.* **8**, 568–571.
Gruol, D.L. (1982) *Brain Res.* **243**, 25–33.
Grupp, L.A., Perlanski, E. & Stewart, R.B. (1988a) *Pharmacol. Biochem. Behav.* **30**, 823–827.
Grupp, L.A., Perlanski, E. & Stewart, R.B. (1988b) *Pharmacol. Biochem. Behav.* **31**, 813–916.
Harper, J.C., Pagonis, C. & Littleton, J.M. (1987) *Alcohol Alcoholism* Suppl., 725–729.
Harper, J.C., Brenna, C.H. & Littleton, J.M. (1989) *Neuropharmacology* **28**, 1299–1302.
Harris, D.P. & Sinclair, J.G. (1984) *Gen. Pharmacol.* **15**, 449–454.
Harris, R.A. & Hood, W.F. (1980) *J. Pharmacol. Exp. Ther.* **213**, 562–568.

Harris, R.A., Fenner, D., Feller, D., Sieckman, G., Lloyd, S., Mitchell, M., Dexter, J.D., Tumbleson, M.E. & Bylund, D.B. (1983) *Pharmacol. Biochem. Behav.* **18**, 363–367.
Harris, R.A., Groh, G.I., Baxter, D.M. & Hitzemann, R.J. (1984a) *Mol. Pharmacol.* **25**, 410–417.
Harris, R.A., Baxter, D.M., Mitchell, M.A. & Hitzemann, R.J. (1984b) *Mol. Pharmacol.* **25**, 401–409.
Harris, R.A., Jones, S.B., Bruno, P. & Bylund, D.B. (1985) *Biochem. Pharmacol.* **34**, 2187–2191.
Hemmingsen, R., Braestrup, C., Nielsen, M. & Barry, D.I. (1982) *Acta Psychiatr. Scand.* **65**, 120–126.
Hemmingsen, R., Clemmesen, L. & Barry, D.I. (1984) *J. Stud. Alcohol* **45**, 310–315.
Hernandez-Cruz, A. & Pape, H.C. (1989) *J. Neurophysiol.* **61**, 1270–1283.
Hirning, L.D., Fox, A.P., McCleskey, E.W., Olivera, R.M., Thayer, S.A., Miller, R.J. & Tsien, R.W. (1988) *Science* **239**, 57–61.
Hoffman, P.L. & Tabakoff, B. (1977) *Nature* **268**, 551.
Hoffman, P.L., Ritzmann, R.F., Walter, R. & Tabakoff, B. (1978) *Nature* **276**, 614–616.
Hoffman, P.L., Melchior, C.L. & Tabakoff, B. (1983) *Life Sci.* **32**, 1065–1071.
Hoffman, P.L., Moses, F., Luthin, G.R. & Tabakoff, B. (1986) *Mol. Pharmacol.* **30**, 13–18.
Hoffman, P.L., Saito, T. & Tabakoff, B. (1987) *Ann. N. Y. Acad. Sci.* **492**, 396–397.
Hoffman, P.L., Rabe, C.S., Moses, F. & Tabakoff, B. (1989) *J. Neurochem.* **52**, 1937–1940.
Hoffmeister, F., Benz, U., Heise, A., Karuse, H.P. & Neuser, V. (1982) *Arzneim.-Forsch.* **32**, 347–360.
Holman, R.B. & Snape, B.M. (1985) *J. Neurochem.* **44**, 357–363.
Hudspith, M., John, G.R., Nhamburo, P.T. & Littleton, J.M. (1985) *Alcohol* **2**, 133–138.
Hudspith, M.J., Brennan, C.H., Charles, S. & Littleton, J.M. (1987) *Ann. N. Y. Acad. Sci.* **492**, 156–170.
Hunt, W.A. & Dalton, T.K. (1976) *Brain Res.* **109**, 628–631.
Hunt, W.A. & Dalton, T.K. (1981) *Pharmacol. Biochem. Behav.* **14**, 733–739.
Hunt, W.A. & Majchrowicz, E. (1974) *J. Neurochem.* **23**, 549–552.
Isaacson, R.L., Molina, J.C., Draski, L.J. & Johnston, J.E. (1985) *Life Sci.* **36**, 2195–2199.
Jaffe, J.H., Domenic, A.C., Nies, A., Dixon, R.B. & Monroe, L.L. (1983) *Clin. Pharmacol. Ther.* **34**, 623–630.
Johnson, D.A., Lee, N.M, Cooke, R. & Loh, H. (1980) *Mol. Pharmacol.* **17**, 52–55.
Karobath, M., Rogers, J. & Bloom, F.E. (1980) *Neuropharmacology* **19**, 125–128.
Keller, E., Cummins, J.T. & Von Hungen, K. (1983) *Subst. Alcohol Actions Misuse* **4**, 383–392.
Kendall, D.A. & Nahorski, S.R. (1985) *Eur. J. Pharmacol.* **115**, 31–36.
Khanna, J.M., Le, A.D., Gougos, A. & Kalant, H. (1988) *Pharmacol. Biochem. Behav.* **31**, 179–186.
Kochman, R.L., Hirsch, J.D. & Clay, G.A. (1981) *Res. Commun. Subst. Abuse* **2**, 135–144.
Kolakowska, L., Laure-Achagiotis, C. & Le-Magnen, J. (1985) *Pharmacol. Biochem. Behav.* **23**, 333–338.
Koppi, S., Eberhardt, G., Haller, R. & Konig, P. (1987) *Neuropsychobiology* **17**, 49–52.
Kril, J.J., Gundlach, A.L., Sodd, P.R., Johnston, G.A.R. & Harper, C.G. (1989) *Ann. Neurol.* **26**, 395–397.
Krivoy, W.A., Zimmermann, E. & Lande, S. (1974) *Proc. Natl Acad. Sci. USA* **71**, 1852–1856.

Kulkarni, S.K. & Mehta, A.K. (1983) *Psycopharmacology* **79**, 287–289.
Kulkarni, S.K. & Ticku, M.K. (1989) *Life Sci.* **44**, 1317–1323.
Kulkosky, P.J. & Glazner, G.W. (1988) *Alcoholism* **12**, 277–281.
Kulkosky, P.J., Sanchez, M.R., Chui, N. & Glazner, G.W. (1987) *Neuropharmacology* **26**, 1211–1216.
Kuriyama, K., Muramatsu, M., Aiso, M. & Ueno, E. (1981) *Neuropharmacology* **20**, 659–666.
Lace, J.W., Schneider, C.W. & Hartline, R.A. (1986) *Pharmacol. Biochem. Behav.* **24**, 1137–1140.
La Droitte, P., Lamboeuf, Y. & de Saint-Blanquat, G. (1984) *Biochem. Pharmacol.* **33**, 615–624.
Larkin, J.G., Butler, E. & Brodie, M.J. (1988) *Br. Med. J.* **296**, 530–531.
Le, A.D., Kalant, H. & Khanna, J.M. (1979) *Psychopharmacology* **61**, 125–129.
Le, A.D., Khanna, J.M., Kalant, H. & Le Blanc, A.E. (1981a) *J. Pharmacol. Exp. Ther.* **218**, 525–529.
Le, A.D., Khanna, J.M., Kalant, H. & Le Blanc, A.E. (1981b) *Psychopharmacology* **75**, 231–235.
Le, A.D., Lalant, H. & Khanna, J.M. (1982) *Eur. J. Pharmacol.* **80**, 337–345.
Le, A.D., Khanna, J.M., Kalant, H. & Grossi, F. (1986) *Pharmacol. Biochem. Behav.* **24**, 93–98.
Le Magnen, J., Tran, G., Durlach, J. & Martin, C. (1987a) *Alcohol* **4**, 99–102.
Le Magnen, J., Tran, G. & Durlach, J. (1987b) *Alcohol* **4**, 103–108.
Leslie, S.W., Barl, E., Chandler, J. & Farrar, R.P. (1983) *J. Pharmacol. Exp. Ther.* **225**, 571–575.
Levy, A.D. & Ellison, G. (1985) *Psycopharmacology* **86**, 233–236.
Liljequist, S. (1978) *Acta Pharmacol. Toxicol.* **43**, 19–28.
Liljequist, S., Culp, S. & Tabakoff, B. (1986) *Life Sci.* **38**, 1931–1939.
Liljequist, S., Culp, S. & Tabakoff, B. (1989) *Pharm. Toxicol.* **65**, 362–367.
Lima-Landman, M.T. & Albuquerque, E.X. (1989) *FEBS Lett.* **247**, 61–67.
Linnoila, M., Stowell, L., Marangos, P.J. & Thurman, R.G. (1981) *Acta Pharmacol. Toxicol.* **49**, 407–411.
Lister, R.G. & Karanian, J.W. (1987) *Alcohol* **4**, 409–411.
Lister, R.G., Durcan, M.J., Nutt, D.J. & Linnoila, M. (1989) *Life Sci.* **44**, 111–119.
Little, H.J. (1991) *Prog. Neurobiol.* **36**, 171–194.
Little, H.J. & Dolin, S.J. (1987) *Br. J. Pharmacol.* **92**, 606P.
Little, H.J., Taylor, S.C., Nutt, D.J. & Cowen, P.J. (1983) *Eur. J. Pharmacol.* **107**, 375–377.
Little, H.J., Dolin, S.J. & Halsey, M.J. (1986) *Life Sci.* **39**, 2059–2065.
Littleton, J.M. & John, G.R. (1977) *J. Pharm. Pharmacol.* **29**, 579–580.
Littleton, J.M. & Little, H.J. (1987) *Br. J. Pharmacol.* **92**, 663P.
Littleton, J., Harper, J., Hudspith, M., Pagonis, Dolin, S.J. & Little, H.J. (1988) In *The Psychopharmacology of Addiction* (ed. Lader, M.), pp 61–72. New York, Tokyo, Oxford University Press.
Littleton, J.M., Little, H.J. & Whittington, M.A. (1990) *Psychopharmacology* **100**, 387–392.
Loh, H.H. & Law, P.Y. (1980) *Annu. Rev. Pharmacol.* **20**, 201–234.
Lovinger, D.M., White, G. & Weight, F.F. (1989) *Science* **243**, 1721–1724.
Lucchi, L., Govoni, S., Battaini, F., Pasinetti, G. & Trabucci, M. (1985) *Brain Res.* **332**, 376–379.
Luthin, G.R. & Tabakoff, B. (1984) *J. Pharmacol. Exp. Ther.* **228**, 579–587.
Lynch, M.A. & Littleton, J.M. (1983) *Nature* **303**, 175.
Lynch, M., Littleton, J., McKernan, R.M., Durcan, M.J., McMillan, T. &

Campbell, I.C. (1983) *Brain Res.* **288**, 145–149.
Lyon, R. & Goldstein, D.B. (1983) *Mol. Pharmacol.* **23**, 86–91.
Mancillas, J.R., Siggins, G.R. & Bloom, F.E. (1986) *Science* **231**, 161–163.
Marks, S.S., Watson, D.L., Carpenter, C.L., Messing, R.O. & Greenberg, D.A. (1989a) *J. Neurochem.* **53**, 168–172.
Marks, S.S., Watson, D.L., Carpenter, C.L., Messing, R.O. & Greenberg, D.A. (1989b) *Brain Res.* **478**, 196–198.
Martz, A., Deitrich, R.A. & Harris, R.A. (1983) *Eur. J. Pharmacol.* **89**, 53–62.
Mattucci-Schiavone, L. & Ferko, A.P. (1987) *Pharmacol. Biochem. Behav.* **27**, 745–748.
Mehta, A.K. & Ticku, M.K. (1988) *J. Pharmacol. Exp. Ther.* **246**, 558–564.
Melchior, C.L. & Tabakoff, B. (1981) *J. Pharmacol. Exp. Ther.* **219**, 175–180.
Melchior, C.L. & Tabakoff, B. (1986) *Pharmacol. Biochem. Behav.* **24**, 955–961.
Menon, M.K. & Kodama, C.K. (1985) *Neuropharmacology* **24**, 927–939.
Mereu, G., Fadda, F. & Gessa, G.L. (1984) *Brain Res.* **292**, 63–69.
Messing, R.O., Carpenter, C.L., Diamond, I. & Greenberg, D.A. (1986) *Proc. Natl Acad. Sci. USA* **83**, 6213–6215.
Meyer, F.B., Tally, P.W., Anderson, R.E., Sundt, Jr, T.M., Yaksh, T.L. & Sharbrough, F.W. (1986) *Brain Res.* **384**, 180–183.
Meyer, F.B., Anderson, R.E. & Sundt, T.M. (1986) *Mayo Clinic. Proc.* **61**, 239.
Mhatre, M., Mehta, A.K. & Ticku, M.K. (1988) *Eur. J. Pharmacol.* **153**, 141–145.
Michaelis, E.K., Mulvaney, M.J. & Freed, W.J. (1978) *Biochem. Pharmacol.* **27**, 1685–1691.
Miller, R.J. (1987) *Science* **235**, 46–52.
Moreau, J.L., Pieri, L. & Prud'hon, B. (1989) *Br. J. Pharmacol.* **98**, 1050–1054.
Morrow, A.L., Suzdak, P.D., Karanian, J.W. & Paul, S.M. (1988) *J. Pharmacol. Exp. Ther.* **246**, 158–164.
Myers, R.D. (1989) *Experientia* **45**, 436–443.
Myers, R.D. & Martin, G.E. (1973) *Ann. N. Y. Acad. Sci.* **215**, 135–144.
Myers, R.D., Critcher, E.C. & Cornwell, N.N. (1983a) *Peptides* **4**, 359–366.
Myers, R.D., Swartzwelder, H.S. & Holahan, W. (1983b) *Brain Res. Bull.* **10**, 333–338.
Myers, R.D., Borg, S. & Mossberg, R. (1986) *Alcohol* **3**, 383–388.
Naranjo, C.A., Sellers, E.M. & Lawrin, M.O. (1986) *J. Clin. Psychiatry* **47**, 16–22.
Nash, J.F. & Maickel, R.P. (1988) *Prog. Neuropsychopharmacol. Biol. Psychiatry* **12**, 653–671.
Nelson, L. & Delgardo-Escueta, A.V. (1986) *Brain Res.* **386**, 32–40.
Nestoros, J.N. (1980) *Life Sci.* **26**, 519–523.
Nordberg, A. & Wahlstrom, G. (1982) *Life Sci.* **31**, 277–287.
Nowycky, M.C., Fox, A. & Tsien, R.W. (1985) *Nature* **316**, 440–443.
Nutt, D. & Glue, P. (1986) *Br. J. Addict.* **81**, 327–338.
Nutt, D.J., Cowen, P.J., Batts, C.C., Grahame-Smith, D.G. & Green, A.R. (1982) *Psychopharmacologia* **76**, 84–87.
Nutt, D.J., Adinoff, B. & Linnolia, M. (1989) *Recent Dev. Alcohol.* **7**, 283–313.
Okamoto, M., Aaronson, L. & Hinman, D. (1983) *J. Pharmacol. Exp. Ther.* **225**, 589–594.
O'Neill, S.K. & Bolger, G.T. (1988) *Brain Res. Bull.* **21**, 865–872.
Panza, G., Grebb, J.A., Sanna, E., Wright, A.G. & Hanbauer, L. (1985) *Neuropharmacology* **24**, 1113–1117.
Peachey, J.E. & Naranjo, C.A. (1984) *Drugs* **27**, 171–182.
Pohorecky, L.A., Newman, B., Sun, J. & Bailey, W.H. (1978) *J. Pharmacol. Exp. Ther.* **204**, 424–432.

Potthoff, A.D. & Ellison, G. (1982) *Psychopharmacology* **77**, 242–245.
Pozos, R.S. & Oakes, S.G. (1987) *Recent Dev. Alcohol.* **5**, 327–345.
Pucilowski, O., Krascik, P., Trzaskowska, E. & Kostowski, W. (1989) *Alcohol* **6**, 165–168.
Quirion, R., Lal, S., Olivier, A., Robitaille, Y., Vassavan Nair, N.P., Ford, R.M. & Stratford, J.G. (1988) *Ann. N. Y. Acad. Sci.* **522**, 203–206.
Rabe, C.S. & Weight, F.F. (1988) *J. Pharmacol. Exp. Ther.* **244**, 417–422.
Raeburn, D. & Gonzales, R.A. (1988) *T.I.P.S.* **9**, 117–118.
Ramkumar, V. & El-Fakahany, E.E. (1986) *Trends Pharmacol. Sci.* **7**, 171–172.
Rastogi, S.K., Thyagarajan, R., Clothier, J. & Ticku, M.K. (1986) *Neuropharmacology* **25**, 1179–1184.
Redos, J., Hunt, W.A. & Catravas, G. (1976) *Life Sci.* **18**, 989.
Reynolds, I.J., Wagner, J.A., Snyder, S.A., Thayer, S.A., Olivera, B.B. & Miller, R.J. (1986) *Proc. Natl Acad. Sci. USA* **83**, 8804–8807.
Reynolds, J.N., Wu, P.H., Khanna, J.M. & Carlen, P.L. (1990) *J. Pharmacol. Exp. Ther.* **252**, 265–271.
Rigter, H. & Crabbe, J. (1980) In *Pharmacology of Alcohol* (ed. Sandler, M.), pp 179–189. New York, Raven Press.
Rigter, H. & Crabbe, J.C. (1985) *Peptides* **6**, 669–676.
Rigter, H., Rijk, H. & Crabbe, J.C. (1980) *Eur. J. Pharmacol.* **64**, 53–68.
Rinon, G., Hanski, E., Braun, S. & Levitski, A. (1978) *Nature* **276**, 394–396.
Ritzmann, R.F. & Tabakoff, B. (1976) *Nature* **263**, 418–420.
Rius, R.A., Bergamaschi, S., DiFonso, F., Govoni, S., Trabucci, M. & Rossi, F. (1987) *Brain Res.* **402**, 359–361.
Riveros, N. & Orrego, F. (1986) *Neuroscience* **17**, 541–546.
Rodriguez-Echandia, E.L. & Foscolo, M.R. (1988) *Drug Alcohol Depend.* **21**, 141–146.
Rosenberg, H., Smith, S. & Chiu, T.H. (1983) *Life Sci.* **32**, 279–285.
Rottenberg, H. (1985) *Alcohol* **2**, 203–207.
Rottenberg, H., Waring, A. & Rubin, E. (1981) *Science* **213**, 583–585.
Sandi, C., Borrelli, J. & Guaza, C. (1988) *Pharmacol. Biochem. Behav.* **29**, 39–43.
Sanna, E., Concas, A., Serra, M. & Biggio, G. (1990) *J. Neurochem.* **54**, 696–698.
Schelesinger, K., Boggan, W.G. & Freedman, D.X. (1965) *Life Sci.* **4**, 2345–2351.
Schoemaker, H., Smith, T.L. & Yamamura, H.I. (1983) *Brain Res.* **258**, 347–350.
Schuster, C.L. & Humphries, R.H. (1981) *Conn. Med.* **45**, 11–13.
Schwartz, M.H. (1985) *Brain Res.* **332**, 337–353.
Scroggs, R.S. and Fox, A.P. (1991) *J. Neurosci.* **11**, 1334–1346.
Shen, A., Jacobyansky, A., Pathman, D. & Thurman, R.G. (1983) *Eur. J. Pharmacol.* **89**, 103–110.
Siggins, G.R., Pittman, Q.J. & French, E.D. (1987) *Brain Res.* **414**, 22–34.
Sinclair, J.G. & Lo, G.F. (1986) *Gen. Pharmacol.* **17**, 231–233.
Skattebol, A. & Rabin, R.A. (1987) *Biochem. Pharmacol.* **36**, 2227–2229.
Smith, T.L. (1983) *Neuropharmacology* **22**, 661–663.
Smith, T.L. (1987) *Life Sci.* **41**, 2863–2868.
Sofia, R.D., Solomon, T.A. & Barry III, H. (1976) *Eur. J. Pharmacol.* **35**, 7–16.
Speisky, M.B. & Kalant, H. (1985) *Brain Res.* **326**, 281–290.
Speisky, M.B. & Kalant, H. (1987) *Alcohol Alcoholism* Suppl. 1, 455–459.
Spinosa, G., Perlanski, E., Leenen, F.H., Stewart, R.B. & Grupp, L.A. (1988) *Alcoholism* **12**, 65–70.
Stewart, R.B., Perlanski, E. & Grupp, L.A. (1988) *Alcoholism* **12**, 698–704.
Stokes, J.A. & Harris, R.A. (1982) *Mol. Pharmacol.* **22**, 99.

Sun, G.Y., Huant, H.M., Lee, D.Z. & Sun, A.Y. (1984) *Life Sci.* **35**, 2127–2133.
Supervilai, P. & Karobath, M. (1984) *J. Neural Transmission* **60**, 149–167.
Swartzwelder, H.S. & Myers, R.D. (1983) *Neurosci. Lett.* **36**, 99–104.
Tabakoff, B. & Boggan, W.D. (1974) *J. Neurochem.* **22**, 759–764.
Tabakoff, B. & Ritzmann, R.F. (1977) *J. Pharmacol. Exp. Ther.* **203**, 319–331.
Tabakoff, B., Munoz-Marcus, M. & Fields, J.A. (1979) *Life Sci.* **25**, 2173–2180.
Taberner, P.V. (1977) *J. Pharm. Pharmacol.* **29**, 256.
Taberner, P.V. & Unwin, J.W. (1981) *Br. J. Pharmacol.*, **74**, 276P.
Takada, R., Saito, K., Matsura, H. & Inoki, R. (1989) *Alcohol* **6**, 115–119.
Takahashi, K. & Akaike, N. (1990) *Br. J. Pharmacol.* **100**, 705–710.
Takahashi, K., Wakamori, M. & Akaike, N. (1989) *Neurosci. Lett.* **104**, 229–234.
Tang, M., Brown, C. & Falk, J.L. (1982) *Pharmacol. Biochem. Behav.* **16**, 155–158.
Taraschi, T.F., Ellingson, J.S., Zimmerman, R. & Rubin, E. (1986) *Proc. Natl Acad. Sci. USA* **83**, 9398–9402.
Tarika, J.S. & Winger, G. (1980) *Psychopharmacology* **70**, 201–208.
Teichberg, V.I., Tal, N., Goldberg, D. & Luini, A. (1984) *Brain Res.* **291**, 285–292.
Thyagarajan, R. & Ticku, M.K. (1985) *Brain Res. Bull.* **15**, 343–345.
Ticku, M.K. (1980) *Br. J. Pharmacol.* **70**, 403–410.
Ticku, M.K. & Burch, T. (1980) *J. Neurochem.* **34**, 417–423.
Ticku, M.K., Burch, T.P. & Davis, W.C. (1983) *Pharmacol. Biochem. Behav.* **18**, 15–18.
Ticku, M.K., Lowrimore, P. & Lehoullier, P. (1986) *Brain Res. Bull.* **17**, 123–126.
Tran, V.T., Snyder, S.H., Major, L.F. & Hawley, R.J. (1981) *Ann. Neurol.* **9**, 289–292.
Tricklebank, M.D., Singh, L., Oles, R.J., Preston, C. & Iversen, S.D. (1989) *Eur. J. Pharmacol.* **167**, 127–135.
Turski, W.A., Cavalheiro, E.A., Bortolotto, Z.A., Mello, L.M., Schwartz, M. & Turski, L. (1984) *Brain Res.* **321**, 237–253.
Unwin, J.W. & Taberner, P.V. (1982) *Psychopharmacology* **78**, 361–364.
Valverius, P., Hoffman, P.L. & Tabakoff, B. (1989) *J. Neurochem.* **52**, 492–497.
Volicer, L. & Biagioni, T.M. (1982) *Neuropharmacology* **21**, 283–286.
Volicer, L., Morin, R. & Gold, B.I. (1977) *J. Stud. Alcohol.* **38**, 11–13.
Wahlstrom, G. & Nordberg, A. (1988) *Brain Res.* **474**, 189–191.
Watkins, J.C. & Evans, R.H. (1981) *Annu. Rev. Pharmacol. Toxicol.* **21**, 165–204.
Whittington, M.A. & Little, H.J. (1988) *Br. J. Pharmacol.* **94**, 885P.
Whittington, M.A. & Little, H.J. (1989a) *Br. J. Pharmacol.* **98**, 923P.
Whittington, M.A. & Little, H.J. (1989b) *Br. J. Pharmacol.* **96**, 137P.
Whittington, M.A. & Little, H.J. (1989c) *Br. J. Pharmacol.* **97**, 435P.
Whittington, M.A. & Little, H.J. (1990) *Brain Res.* **523**, 237–244.
Whittington, M.A. & Little, H.J. (1991a) *Br. J. Pharmacol.* **103**, 1313–1320.
Whittington, M.A. & Little, H.J. (1991b) *Br. J. Pharmacol.* **103**, 1677–1684.
Whittington, M.A., Siarey, R.J., Patch, T.L., Butterworth, A.R., Dolin, S.J. & Little, H.J. (1991) *Br. J. Pharmacol.* **103**, 1669–1676.
Wiesner, J.B., Henriksen, S.J. & Bloom, F.E. (1987) *Neurosci. Lett.* **79**, 169–173.
Wilkins, A.J., Jenkins, W.J. & Steiner, J.A. (1983) *Psychopharmacology* **81**, 78–80.
Wu, P.H., Naranjo, C.A. & Fan, T. (1986) *Neurochem. Res.* **11**, 801–812.
Wu, P.H., Fan, T. & Narajo, C.A. (1987) *Pharmacol. Biochem. Behav.* **27**, 355–357.
Yanai, J. & Feiggenbaum, J.J. (1983) *Res. Commun. Subst. Abuse* **4**, 263–266.
Yool, A.J. & Gruol, D.L. (1987) *Brain Res.* **420**, 205–219.
Yoshida, K., Engel, J. & Liljequist, S. (1982) *Naunyn-Schmiedeberg's Arch.* **321**, 74–76.

CHAPTER 5

THE NEUROCHEMICAL MECHANISMS UNDERLYING NICOTINE TOLERANCE AND DEPENDENCE

David J.K. Balfour

Department of Pharmacology and Clinical Pharmacology, University Medical School, Ninewells Hospital, Dundee DD1 9SY, UK

Table of Contents

5.1 Introduction

It is now generally accepted that a majority of people who smoke tobacco do so in order to experience the psychopharmacological properties of the nicotine present in the smoke and that a significant proportion of habitual smokers become dependent upon nicotine (Balfour, 1984b). This conclusion is supported by the fact that nicotine, given in the form of Nicorette chewing gum or as a skin patch, is reported to alleviate the symptoms associated with

THE BIOLOGICAL BASES OF DRUG TOLERANCE AND DEPENDENCE
ISBN 0-12-564250-4

smoking withdrawal (Fagerstrom, 1988; Abelin *et al.*, 1989). The behavioural responses to nicotine are complex in nature and appear to be influenced by a number of factors, including the dose, the test environment used for the measurements and the duration of the experimental trial (Clarke, 1987). Nevertheless, the predominant effect of chronic nicotine in most animals is psychostimulation and it is clear that there are many similarities between the responses to chronic nicotine and those seen in animals given other psychostimulants such as amphetamine. As a result it has been suggested that the mechanisms which underlie the development of nicotine dependence may be the same as those that mediate amphetamine dependence (Wise and Bozarth, 1987) although it is important to remember that the psychopharmacological properties of nicotine are by no means identical to those of amphetamine (for review see Balfour, 1984b). In addition it is clear that many people become regular smokers without apparently developing a strong dependence upon nicotine and are able to quit the habit without much difficulty (Balfour, 1984b; Gilbert, 1979; Chapter 2). Thus, any hypothesis proposed to explain the role of nicotine in the tobacco-smoking habit must take account of this fact. This review will focus on the evidence which supports the hypothesis that nicotine exerts effects on pathways in the limbic system which control emotional responses to aversive environmental stimuli and that exposure to such stimuli enhances the development of nicotine dependence.

5.2 Behavioural and endocrinological consequences of chronic nicotine administration

5.2.1 Locomotor activity

In experimental animals the acute administration of moderate or high degrees of nicotine often results in suppression of spontaneous locomotor activity (Morrison and Stephenson, 1972; Stolerman *et al.*, 1973) although if a long trial is used a stimulation of activity may be observed towards the end of the trial (Clarke and Kumar, 1983). In contrast, if animals are pretreated with a number of injections of nicotine prior to the test day, they seem to become tolerant to the depressant effects of the drug and locomotor stimulation becomes the predominant response observed (Morrison and Stephenson, 1972; Stolerman *et al.*, 1973). In nicotine-tolerant rats locomotor activity is increased in a dose-dependent way up to a subcutaneous dose of 0.4 mg/kg. If a higher dose (0.8 mg/kg s.c.) is used, the animals do not appear to become fully tolerant and the activity observed during the first 60 min after the injection, although often higher than that observed for saline-treated controls, is lower than that recorded for rats treated chronically with 0.2 or 0.4 mg/kg (Clarke and Kumar, 1983). In some reviews (Gilbert, 1979) the suppressant effect of nicotine on locomotor activity has been equated to a 'sedative' action of the drug. While this conclusion cannot be totally excluded, it seems more likely that the decrease in activity observed in rats treated acutely with moderate doses of nicotine or chronically with higher doses is associated with the mechanisms which evoke ataxia and prostration in these animals rather than a sedative action similar to that seen in animals given a 'conventional' sedative drug. There is no evidence that experimental animals become tolerant to the stimulant action of nicotine (Clarke, 1987).

5.2.2 Models of nicotine dependence

Addictive drugs are thought to exert two effects which contribute to the maintenance of drug-taking behaviour. Firstly they are said to be 'rewarding' to take and many addicted individuals appear to develop a 'craving' to re-experience this potent reinforcing property of the drug. Wise and Bozarth (1987) have proposed that for most drugs of dependence, including particularly amphetamine and cocaine, this effect is so potent that it alone accounts for the desire to maintain the drug-taking behaviour. Secondly, however, there is evidence that the withdrawal of many, if not all, drugs of dependence can be associated with an unpleasant abstinence syndrome which addicts seek to avoid by maintaining their intake of drug. In the case of drugs, such as the opiates or the barbiturates, which cause physical dependence, the abstinence syndrome can be severe and even life-threatening and the use of drugs to ameliorate the symptoms has a clear place in the treatment of withdrawal. There is no evidence, however, that nicotine evokes a withdrawal effect of this type, and nicotine dependence appears to be predominantly psychological in nature (Balfour, 1984b, 1990a). Nevertheless, many habitual smokers experience significant and unpleasant withdrawal effects when they first stop smoking which can be ameliorated by giving nicotine in another form (Fagerstrom, 1988; West, 1988). Experimental studies designed to investigate the mechanisms which mediate the development of nicotine dependence have, therefore, examined both the ability of nicotine to act as a rewarding stimulus and the effects of nicotine withdrawal.

The putative rewarding properties of nicotine have been examined, primarily, using two paradigms—self-administration and conditioned place preference. When compared with many other drugs of dependence, nicotine is found to be a relatively weak substrate in drug self-administration schedules and its effects in this type of experiment appear to be influenced to a significant degree by the conditions of the experiment (Balfour, 1984b; Clarke, 1987). For example, Lang *et al.* (1977) reported that nicotine self-administration could be demonstrated in rats providing the animals were maintained at a reduced body weight. They also found that nicotine self-administration was enhanced if the injections were paired with food delivery. A subsequent study from the same group found that it was not necessary to pair food delivery with the nicotine injections in order to demonstrate nicotine self-administration although reduced body weight did seem to be important (Smith and Lang, 1980). A more recent study by Cox *et al.* (1984) suggested that neither reduced body weight nor schedule reinforcement was essential for the demonstration of nicotine self-administration in rats although pressing rates for nicotine were always fairly slow when compared with those reported for rats trained to self-administer amphetamine or cocaine and the increased rates observed for the rats pressing for nicotine could be explained, in part, by the stimulant effects of the nicotine *per se*. Nicotine self-administration has also been demonstrated in squirrel monkeys (Goldberg *et al.*, 1981) using a schedule in which a visual stimulus was occasionally paired with a nicotine injection. In another study, Hutchinson and Emley (1985) showed that, whereas non-stressed squirrel monkeys preferentially drank nicotine-free water, this preference was reversed if they were exposed to a stressful stimulus (tail shocks).

In a conditioned place preference study, drug administration is paired with a specific and distinguishable environment. If the drug is rewarding, when the animals are subsequently given a choice, they will opt to spend most time in the environment which was paired with the drug. Fudala *et al.* (1985) reported that the rewarding properties of nicotine could be demonstrated using this technique providing the nicotine injection was paired with the less-preferred compartment of the apparatus. The study reported by Clarke and Fibiger (1987), using a more standard procedure in which the initial preference was not used as a factor in the experimental design, failed to confirm the ability of nicotine to act as a reward in a place preference paradigm. More recently Iwamoto (1990), using a conditioned place preference paradigm in which the nicotine was given intracerebroventricularly, has reported that a place preference for nicotine can be demonstrated which is independent of the animal's initial preference for one of the compartments of the apparatus. It may be, therefore, that place preference studies with systemic nicotine may be compromised by aversive properties of the drug which are mediated peripherally.

It is consistently reported that tobacco smoke can exert a 'tranquillizing' effect and that the craving to smoke can be enhanced by exposure to aversive environments (Gilbert, 1979; Pomerleau and Pomerleau, 1987). A number of investigators, therefore, have sought to examine the putative anxiolytic properties of nicotine. Early studies failed to find any convincing evidence that nicotine did exert anxiolytic activity (Morrison, 1969; Morrison and Stephenson, 1970). More recently, however, Costall *et al.* (1989) have shown that nicotine does exert anxiolytic-like activity in mice tested in a two-compartment apparatus in which one compartment is made more aversive than the other. In contrast, Balfour *et al.* (1986b) failed to demonstrate anxiolytic-like activity in the elevated X-maze test for anxiety, a paradigm which is clearly able to detect the anxiolytic activity of the benzodiazepine anxiolytics (Pellow *et al.*, 1985). A subsequent study examined the possibility that the anxiolytic properties of nicotine were only revealed following a longer period of treatment with the drug. The results of these experiments (Table 1) did appear to suggest that chronic nicotine was anxiolytic. Analysis of covariance, however, showed that the increase in open runway entries was not independent of the increase in enclosed runway entries and, therefore, that the increased proportion of total activity occurring in the open runways OE:TA ratio could not be taken as unequivocal evidence for an anxiolytic response to chronic nicotine (Pellow *et al.*, 1985). Thus, if nicotine does, indeed, exert anxiolytic activity it seems reasonable to suggest that the neural systems which underlie the effect differ from those which mediate the responses to the benzodiazepines.

There appear to be no reliable reports that the withdrawal of nicotine from animals treated chronically with the drug has any effects on spontaneous activity *per se*. Benwell and Balfour (1979), however, showed that the withdrawal of nicotine from unstressed rats resulted in a modest but significant

Table 1 The effects of chronic nicotine and its withdrawal on the behavioural and plasma corticosterone responses to the elevated X-maze test for anxiety.

Drug treatment				
Chronic	Test day	Total activity	Responses (OE:TA ratio)	PC (μg/100 ml)
Saline	Saline	18 ± 2	0.23 ± 0.08	18 ± 2
Nicotine	Nicotine	$38 \pm 5^*$	0.38 ± 0.03	24 ± 4
Nicotine	Saline	18 ± 3	0.23 ± 0.08	24 ± 4

The responses were measured using male Sprague-Dawley rats pretreated with daily subcutaneous injections of saline or nicotine (0.4 mg/kg) for 19 days prior to the test day (chronic treatment). The treatment on the test day was given 5 min before the animals were placed in the maze for 20 min. Plasma corticosterone (PC) was measured using blood samples collected at the end of the trial. The total activity was calculated by summing the total entries into all four arms of the maze; the OE:TA ratio was calculated by dividing the number of entries made into the open runways by the total activity. Significantly different when compared with rats treated on the test day with saline: $^*P < 0.01$.

increase in the plasma corticosterone concentration. These data are consistent with the hypothesis that nicotine withdrawal is mildly anxiogenic in rats although other explanations for the effect were also proposed. Nevertheless, the drug discrimination study of Harris *et al.* (1986) also suggested that nicotine withdrawal was anxiogenic to the extent that it generalized to an anxiogenic stimulus (pentylenetetrazol) and that it could be attenuated by the prior administration of diazepam. The generalization, however, was not impressive and, as a result, the authors concluded that nicotine withdrawal was only weakly anxiogenic. Costall *et al.* (1989), using their two-compartment model of anxiety, were able to demonstrate that the withdrawal of nicotine from mice following a period of chronic treatment evoked changes in behaviour which were characteristic of an anxiogenic drug. In contrast, studies in our laboratory (Balfour, 1991a) have failed to demonstrate an anxiogenic response to nicotine withdrawal in the rat using the elevated X-maze test for anxiety (Table 1). At this time it is not possible to provide a clear explanation for this discrepancy although it is, perhaps, worth noting that the tests described by some groups are not specific for nicotine withdrawal (Costall *et al.*, 1990; Emmett-Oglesby *et al.*, 1990). Similar behavioural responses were observed following the withdrawal of addictive drugs with totally different mechanisms of action and it is possible, therefore, that the tests may detect the novelty of the no-drug state rather than being a specific measure of nicotine withdrawal. If this is the case then it is, perhaps, also likely that the changes in plasma corticosterone reported by Benwell and Balfour (1979) may also be a measure of drug withdrawal which is not a true indicator of dependence.

Operant conditioning schedules have also revealed behavioural changes which occur as a consequence of nicotine withdrawal. For example, Carroll *et al.* (1989) have reported that if nicotine is withdrawn from rats trained to lick for a sweetened glucose solution, the response is markedly suppressed. It was reinstated immediately the nicotine injections were restarted. In another study Corrigal *et al.* (1989) showed that rats can become tolerant to the suppressant effects of high nicotine doses (2 mg/kg per day s.c.) on lever-press responding for food. When, after a 50-day treatment schedule, the nicotine was withdrawn, responding for the food reward was initially depressed, although after 3 days it had returned to control levels. In both cases the authors suggested that the behavioural deficits could be a measure of nicotine abstinence although in neither study was there evidence that the effects were sustained for many days or that the effects were not the result of state-dependent learning upon nicotine. In a much earlier study, Morrison (1974) reported that the withdrawal of nicotine from rats trained on a shock avoidance schedule under the influence of the drug caused disruption of avoidance performance to the extent that it became significantly worse than that observed for saline-treated controls. In addition she reported that the disruption was significantly less marked if the schedule was made less stressful by the introduction of a warning signal prior to the delivery of each shock or a feedback signal after each successful lever-pressing response. She concluded that, since the acute administration of nicotine to rats trained with saline had no effect on avoidance performance, the effects of nicotine withdrawal could not be attributed to state-dependent learning and that the behavioural deficit, therefore, reflected the development of nicotine dependence. In addition she suggested that the dependence appeared to develop more readily in more stressful test environments. These conclusions, however, must remain speculative until confirmed by other studies although recent experiments in this laboratory have confirmed the development of the behavioural deficit following nicotine withdrawal (Balfour, 1990b) and shown that it persists for at least 5 days (Balfour, unpublished observations).

5.3 Neurochemical mechanisms

5.3.1 Studies on the role of central nicotinic receptors

In vitro radioligand binding studies have shown that $[^3H](-)$-nicotine binds reversibly, stereoselectively and with high affinity to membranes prepared from mammalian brain (Reavill *et al.*, 1988; Romano and Goldstein, 1980). The nicotine binding site also has high affinity for acetylcholine (ACh) and for other componds which act as agonists at the nicotinic cholinoreceptor located on autonomic ganglia but little or no affinity for agonists at non-cholinergic receptors (Martino-Barrows and Kellar, 1987; Clarke *et al.*, 1985b; Romano and Goldstein, 1980; Benwell and Balfour, 1985). Thus, it is widely assumed that the binding site represents the ACh recognition site on a central nicotinic receptor (Clarke *et al.*, 1985b; Wonnacott, 1987). This receptor appears to mediate a number of the behavioural responses to nicotine, including, particularly, its ability to act as a locomotor stimulant (Clarke and Kumar, 1983) and a cue in drug discrimination paradigms (Reavill *et al.*, 1988; Stolerman, 1988), to the extent that the potency of many, although not all, nicotonic agonists in these behavioural tests appears to correlate well with their affinity for the receptor (Reavill and Stolerman, 1990; Reavill *et al.*, 1990). In addition, both the locomotor stimulant response to nicotine and its ability to act as a discriminative cue can be attenuated by the systemic administration of pempidine or mecamylamine, non-quaternary compounds which block the nicotinic receptors found on autonomic ganglia but which also penetrate into the central nervous system (Clarke and Kumar, 1983; Stolerman, 1988; Romano *et al.*, 1981). In contrast the systemic administration of quaternary antagonists which do not readily cross the blood–brain barrier has little or no effect on the responses to nicotine. Although these observations provide clear support for the hypothesis that the responses are mediated by a central nicotinic receptor with characteristics similar to those of the receptor on autonomic ganglia, they do not correlate with the ability of the antagonists to displace [^{3}H](−)-nicotine in *in vitro* binding assays using membranes prepared from brain tissue. Indeed, when assayed *in vitro*, the central nervous system (CNS) nicotinic receptor is found to have little or no affinity for almost all nicotinic antagonists (Benwell and Balfour, 1985; Romano and Goldstein, 1980), the only exception being dihydro-β-erythroidine, whose affinity for the binding site is still approximately 50 times lower than that for (−)-nicotine (Reavill *et al.*, 1988; Wonnacott, 1987).

The reason for the marked discrepancy between the effects of nicotinic antagonists such as mecamylamine on the behavioural responses to nicotine thought to be mediated by the central nicotinic receptor with high affinity for nicotine and their apparent lack of affinity for the receptors *in vitro* remains to be established with certainty. One relatively simple explanation, proposed by Wonnacott (1987) and Reavill *et al.* (1988), is that these antagonists act noncompetitively at another site on the receptor complex. There is evidence that the nicotinic receptor in the CNS is an allosteric protein which appears to undergo a fairly rapid desensitization if it is exposed to agonist for a period of time (Wonnacott, 1987). Recently, Takayama *et al.* (1989) have suggested that radioligand binding studies using tritiated agonist as the ligand essentially measure binding to the desensitized form of the receptor, a conformation of the receptor complex which has a particularly high affinity for agonist. In their studies, in which they used [^{3}H]methylcarbamylcholine as the ligand, they found that mecamylamine did reduce agonist binding to the receptor, but that, in agreement with the hypothesis proposed by Wonnacott (1987) and by Reavill *et al.* (1988), the antagonist appeared to exert its effects allosterically rather than by competing for the agonist recognition site.

Studies with experimental animals have shown that the chronic administration of nicotine can result in an increase in the density of nicotinic receptors in the brain (Marks *et al.*, 1983; Nordberg *et al.*, 1985; Schwartz and Kellar, 1983). Studies with human tissue taken at postmortem also suggest that tobacco smoking is associated with an increase in the density of the receptors (Table 2). The mechanism which mediates the upregulation of the receptors remains to be clarified although the data currently available appear most consistent with the conclusion that the effect probably reflects an adaptation to the prolonged or repeated desensitization of the receptor complex by nicotine (Wonnacott, 1987). In the animal studies, upregulation of the receptors has been observed following both the chronic infusion of nicotine (Marks *et al.*, 1983) and the repetitive subcutaneous administration of the drug, often at

Table 2 Effects of tobacco smoking on the density of nicotinic receptors in human brain.

Brain region	Receptor density (fmol/mg protein)	
	Non-smokers	Smokers
Hippocampal formation	71 ± 8	144 ± 25**
Hippocampal neocortex	144 ± 13	310 ± 39**
Gyrus rectus	68 ± 6	98 ± 8*
Cerebellar cortex	84 ± 7	140 ± 17**
Median raphe nuclei	75 ± 10	112 ± 10**
Medulla oblongata	48 ± 6	50 ± 5

The density of nicotinic receptors was measured in membrane fractions prepared from postmortem brain tissue taken from 18 non-smokers (7 male and 11 female) and 12 smokers (6 male and 6 female) using $[^3H](-)$-nicotine as the radioligand. The results are expressed as means ± SEM. Significantly different when compared with the data for non-smokers: * $P < 0.05$; ** $P < 0.01$. The data are derived from the study reported by Benwell *et al.* (1988).

relatively high doses (Marks *et al.*, 1986a; Schwartz and Kellar, 1983, 1985). In contrast, the chronic administration of a centrally acting inhibitor of acetylcholinesterase activity has been shown to cause a decrease in the receptor density (Costa and Murphy, 1983; Schwartz and Kellar, 1985), which implies that prolonged exposure to the putative natural agonist for the receptor evokes down- rather than upregulation of the receptor. However, a recent study by De Sarno and Giacobini (1989) has shown that the repeated intracerebroventricular administration of the short-acting cholinesterase inhibitor physostigmine, over a period of 21 days, evokes an increase in the receptor density similar to that found in animals given chronic nicotine. These authors concluded that, for ACh at least, desensitization of the receptor complex was a response to repetitive rather than prolonged exposure to agonist and they suggested that desensitization occurred when 'activated' agonist–receptor complex was exposed to a further dose of agonist. Interestingly, although the plasma nicotine level of habitual smokers tends to increase steadily during the day, substantial peaks of plasma nicotine are superimposed on the basal levels following each cigarette and, possibly, following the inhalation of each puff of cigarette smoke (Russell, 1988). Thus, it seems likely that the brains of habitual smokers are exposed to nicotine in a way which, according to De Sarno and Giacobini (1989), is most likely to cause receptor desensitization and, thus, upregulation. It is, perhaps, not surprising, therefore, that the increases in receptor density evoked by smoking tobacco appear to be amongst the highest reported (Benwell *et al.*, 1988).

The molecular mechanism underlying the change in receptor density evoked by chronic nicotine administration remains to be established with certainty. Since it is likely that the receptor is an allosteric protein and that the radioligand studies used to measure the receptor density defect, primarily, a conformation of the receptor with high affinity for agonist, it is possible that the apparent increase in receptor density reflects an increased prevalence of this conformation of the receptor. Indeed, Romanelli *et al.* (1988) have suggested that this is the case. This view, however, has not been accepted by others who believe that the increased binding of [^{3}H](−)-nicotine or [^{3}H]ACh to brain membranes prepared from chronically treated rats reflects an increase in the synthesis of receptor protein (Wonnacott, 1987).

It is clearly tempting to suggest that the effects of chronic nicotine on the density of nicotinic receptors in the brain may be related to the development of tolerance to and/or dependence upon the drug. Both Marks *et al.* (1983) and Ksir *et al.* (1985) have drawn attention to the fact that the development of tolerance to the depressant effects of nicotine on locomotor behaviour correlates reasonably closely with the increase in receptor density. The data reported in a more recent paper by Ksir *et al.* (1987) suggest that locomotor simulation to nicotine is only observed if the doses given are high enough to evoke an increase in receptor density, results which, the authors claimed, imply a possible causative relationship. Other studies (Benwell and Balfour, 1985; Marks *et al.*, 1986a; Collins *et al.*, 1988), however, suggest that the development of tolerance to the depressant effects of nicotine on locomotor activity and the enhanced locomotor stimulant responses observed in animals treated chronically with the drug are unlikely to be associated with changes in the density of the receptors. Indeed, it would be surprising if this was the case since there is evidence that tolerance to the depressant effects of the drug persists for many weeks (Stolerman *et al.*, 1973) whereas the receptor density returns to control levels within 21 days of cessation of treatment (Schwartz and Kellar, 1985).

Another attractive possibility is that the increased density of receptors mediates the effects of nicotine withdrawal although, to date, this hypothesis has been the subject of very little direct investigation. If it is the case, then it is important to establish if the withdrawal effects are associated with increased responses to ACh mediated by an increased density of 'active' nicotinic receptors or diminished responses to the transmitter caused by a proliferation of inactive or desensitized receptors. One of the few studies to address this problem is that described by Lapchak *et al.* (1989). It showed that the release of ACh from slices of frontal cortex or hippocampus evoked by the addition of the nicotinic agonist methylcarbamylcholine was abolished if the slices were prepared from rats pretreated with nicotine using a treatment regime which caused upregulation of nicotinic receptors. If treatment was terminated 4 days prior to the preparation of the slices, there was a partial recovery of the responses to methylcarbamylcholine but no evidence of sensitization of the responses to the agonist. Thus, the data provide clear support for the hypothesis that the chronic treatment had caused desensitization of the receptors located on the cholinergic terminals of the frontal cortex and hippocampus, but they failed to provide any support for the hypothesis that nicotine withdrawal is associated with the expression of enhanced nicotinic responses.

Radioligand binding studies suggest that, in addition to the receptors labelled with [^{3}H](−)-nicotine, there is another population of nicotinic receptors present on brain membranes which have high affinity for α-bungarotoxin but little affinity for nicotine (Wonnacott, 1987). The distribution of these sites within mammalian brain differs considerably from that of the sites labelled by nicotine or ACh and there is little doubt that they represent a totally different population of binding sites (Marks and Collins, 1982; Marks *et al.*, 1986b; Clarke *et al.*, 1985b). There is little evidence that they mediate many, if any, of the behavioural responses observed following the administration of low or moderate doses of nicotine although it is possible that they may be implicated in the seizure activity which can occur following the administration of high doses of nicotine (Collins *et al.*, 1986; Miner *et al.*, 1984). There is, nevertheless, evidence that, in mice, chronic infusions of nicotine, albeit at a relatively high dose, can cause an increase in [^{125}I]α-bungarotoxin binding to brain membranes (Marks *et al.*, 1983, 1986a). In rats, however, treatment with a chronic nicotine injection schedule which increases the density of [^{3}H](−)-binding sites failed to increase [^{125}I]α-bungarotoxin binding (Marks *et al.*, 1986b).

5.3.2 Studies on the role of specific neurotransmitter systems in the responses to chronic nicotine

The receptors discussed in the previous section are clearly located on neuronal membranes and, thus, their stimulation could be expected to result in changes in neurotransmitter secretion which, ultimately, produce the psychopharmacological responses to nicotine. The effects of nicotine on neurotransmitter secretion in the brain are complex and by no means fully understood. Nevertheless, in some cases, it has proved possible to relate some of the psychophysiological and behavioural properties of the drug to its effects on specific neural pathways. Thus, for example, there is evidence that the reported ability of the drug to improve cognitive processes may be associated with the increase in ACh secretion evoked by nicotine administration (Wesnes and Warburton, 1983, 1984). Edwards and Warburton (1984) have expressed the view that this response is mediated primarily by the effects of the drug in the reticular formation. However, there is evidence for the presence of presynaptic nicotinic receptors on the membranes of cholinergic terminals in the hippocampus and cerebral cortex and that the density of these receptors declines sharply as the cholinergic fibres which innervate these areas of the brain degenerate in Alzheimer's disease (Flynn and Mash, 1986; Kellar *et al.*, 1987; London *et al.*, 1989; Perry *et al.*, 1987; Whitehouse *et al.*, 1986). Since stimulation of these receptors results in increased ACh secretion (Rowell and Winkler, 1984) it is clearly possible that they also may be implicated in the mechanisms which mediate the putative nootropic properties of nicotine.

There is also clear evidence that nicotine influences the secretion of monoamines in mammalian brain (Balfour, 1984a) and it is studies on these systems which have contributed most significantly to our understanding of the mechanisms which mediate the development of tolerance and, particularly, dependence upon nicotine. The remainder of this chapter will, therefore, focus on the effects of nicotine on brain monoamine systems.

5.3.2.1 Noradrenaline

Early studies, reviewed in detail by Balfour (1984a), indicated that the systemic administration of nicotine increased the turnover of noradrenaline in a number of areas of the brain although, in many cases, the responses were observed following the injection of rather high doses of the drug which did not even approximate to the dose a smoker might receive by inhaling the smoke from a cigarette. Subsequent studies, using more modern measures of noradrenaline turnover, have provided further support for the conclusion that the acute administration of moderately high doses (0.8 or 1 mg/kg) of the drug increases noradrenaline turnover in mammalian brain (e.g, Amano *et al.*, 1989; Kubo *et al.*, 1989; Mitchell *et al.*, 1989). It is widely assumed that the increased turnover reflects an increase in noradrenaline release, although Mitchell *et al.* (1990) are the only group who have used a more direct measure, *in vivo* microdialysis, to show that the increase in noradrenaline turnover in the hippocampus evoked by nicotine administration is associated with increased levels of the monoamine in the extracellular fluid.

The mechanism by which nicotine exerts its effect on brain noradrenaline systems remains to be established. *In vitro* studies suggest that nicotine can evoke the secretion of noradrenaline from superfused brain slices (Hall and Turner, 1972; Westfall, 1974) and synaptosomes (Balfour, 1973; Yoshida *et al.*, 1980) by stimulating presynaptic nicotinic receptors located on the nerve terminal membranes although, with the possible exception of the hypothalamus, the concentrations of nicotine required were high and probably of little pharmacological significance. It is, therefore, perhaps more likely that the effects of the drug on noradrenergic systems are caused by stimulation of the nicotinic receptors located on the somatic membrane of these cells (Egan and North, 1986; Engberg and Svensson, 1980; Svensson and Engberg, 1982). It is important to remember, however, that the noradrenergic neurones of the locus coeruleus also fire in response to novel or anxiogenic stimuli (Mason and Fibiger, 1979; Nakamura *et al.*, 1989) and, therefore, an increase in the firing rate of locus coeruleus neurones in response to acute nicotine does not, in itself, prove that the drug has exerted a direct effect on the neurones. Indeed, the data reported by Engberg (1989) suggest that the increased rate of firing of these neurones is an indirect response to the effects of acute nicotine on the peripheral nervous system which results in the release of excitatory amino acids from fibres which innervate the locus coeruleus. In this context, therefore, it is interesting to note that there is some evidence that the ganglionic antagonists such as mecamylamine and pempidine which, in the past, have been used to show that the effects of nicotine on monoamine secretion are mediated by a putative nicotinic receptor, also appear to act as non-competitive antagonists of the *N*-methyl-D-aspartate (NMDA) glutamatergic receptor and have been shown to antagonize the increase in noradrenaline secretion from superfused hippocampal slices evoked by the addition of NMDA (Snell and Johnson, 1989). Thus, the fact that responses to nicotine are antagonized by mecamylamine cannot now be taken as unequivocal evidence that they mediated by a nicotinic receptor.

The effects of chronic nicotine treatment on noradrenaline turnover remain controversial. Kirch *et al.* (1987) reported that infusions of nicotine, delivered continuously from subcutaneous minipumps, caused a significant decrease in the concentrations of noradrenaline in the frontal cortex. In contrast the study reported by Mitchell *et al.* (1989) showed that the chronic administration of nicotine in the form of daily subcutaneous injections enhanced the increase in noradrenaline turnover observed in the hippocampus. This effect was sustained for at least 7 days following withdrawal of the drug from rats which had been treated with nicotine for 28 days. The authors concluded that these data were consistent with the hypothesis that chronic pretreatment with nicotine sensitized the noradrenergic pathway which innervates the hippocampus to a subsequent challenge with the drug. A subsequent microdialysis study (Mitchell *et al.*, 1990) has shown that the increase in extracellular noradrenaline levels in the hippocampus evoked by the administration of nicotine is also enhanced by pretreatment with the drug. Interestingly, although their procedure measured total catecholamine turnover and, therefore, their data for the frontal cortex reflected the biosynthesis of both noradrenaline and dopamine, Mitchell *et al.* (1989) found no significant effect of nicotine on catecholamine turnover in this region of the brain. It is clear from the studies outlined above that the route of nicotine administration probably contributes significantly to the changes in brain noradrenaline systems which result from chronic treatment. It seems reasonable to suggest that the effects reported by Mitchell *et al.* (1989, 1990) probably reflect repeated stimulation of the noradrenegic fibres which innervate the hippocampus whereas the changes reported by Kirch *et al.* (1987) may well be the consequence of prolonged receptor desensitization. Kirch *et al.* (1987) argued that the procedure they used would mimic more closely the pattern of nicotine absorption experienced by an habitual smoker than the daily injection schedule used by Mitchell *et al.* (1989, 1990). This may well be the case to the extent that plasma nicotine levels will be maintained in a way which is similar, but not identical, to that found in regular smokers (Russell *et al.*, 1976). To date no attempts have been made to correlate the changes in noradrenaline turnover in either frontal cortex or hippocampus with the behavioural responses to chronic nicotine although Mitchell *et al.* (1990) have suggested that the effects in hippocampus may be implicated in the development of behavioural tolerance to the drug. As a result the significance of the results in relation to the tobacco-smoking habit must remain a matter of speculation.

5.3.2.2 Dopamine turnover and release

The effects of nicotine, particularly when it is given chronically, are similar in many respects to those of *d*-amphetamine. Since there is clear evidence that a majority of the psychopharmacological responses to amphetamine are related to its ability to stimulate dopamine secretion in the brain (e.g. Kelly *et al.*, 1975), it is, perhaps, not surprising that a number of laboratories have examined the effects of nicotine on these systems and found consistent evidence that the drug also stimulates dopamine turnover in rat brain. For example, Andersson *et al.* (1981) reported that both the systemic and intraventricular administration of nicotine increased the turnover of dopamine in a number of brain nuclei. If relatively high doses of the drug are given the increase in dopamine turnover appears to occur in most, if not all, of the dopamine pathways of the brain (Amano *et al.*, 1989; Haikala and Ahtee, 1988). However, if rats are treated with lower doses of the drug which yield plasma levels closer to those found in the plasma of human subjects who have smoked a cigarette (Pratt *et al.*, 1983) nicotine is reported to act preferentially on the mesolimbic system. This has been shown using both *ex vivo* measures of dopamine turnover (Clarke *et al.*, 1988; Grenhoff and Svensson, 1988; Mitchell *et al.*, 1989) and the technique of *in vivo* microdialysis in freely moving rats (Imperato *et al.*, 1986). The administration of nicotine to rats in the form of intermittent doses of tobacco smoke has also been shown to result in a preferential increase in dopamine utilization in mesolimbic areas of the brain (Fuxe *et al.*, 1986). The effects of nicotine on these systems appear to be mediated by a central nicotinic receptor to the extent that they are blocked by systemic injections of mecamylamine but not by the quaternary antagonists hexamethonium or chlorisondamine. In addition, Clarke *et al.* (1988) found that the effects of nicotine on dopamine turnover in the nucleus accumbens and olfactory tubercle were stereoselective, the biologically active (−)-enantiomer with high affinity for the central nicotinic receptors being significantly more active than the (+)-enantiomer. Further support for this conclusion comes from the study of Clarke and Pert (1985) which used a lesioning technique to show that nicotinic receptors with high affinity for nicotine were present on both the nerve terminal membrane and cell bodies of dopamine-secreting cells.

Studies using *in vitro* perfused brain slice or synaptosome preparations have shown that nicotine can stimulate release of dopamine from dopaminergic nerve terminals of striatum (Giorguieff-Chesselet *et al.*, 1979; Rapier *et al.*, 1988; Sakurai *et al.*, 1982; Westfall *et al.*, 1983) and nucleus accumbens (Rowell *et al.*, 1987). The response to nicotine is stereoselective, the (−)-enantiomer being approximately 100 times more potent than the (+)-enantiomer (Rapier *et al.*, 1988) and is attenuated, but not abolished, by the inclusion of ganglionic nicotinic antagonists in the superfusion medium (Rowell *et al.*, 1987; Westfall *et al.*, 1983). In a more recent study, Mifsud *et al.* (1989) used a microdialysis probe to investigate the effects of nicotine, administered directly into the nucleus accumbens of the rat, on the release of endogenous dopamine. These studies showed that the local application of nicotine into this region of the brain evoked the release of dopamine by a mechanism which could be antagonized by systemic injections of mecamylamine. These data, taken together, provide support for the conclusion that nicotine can stimulate the secretion of dopamine by stimulating presynaptic nicotinic receptors located on the nerve terminal membrane. However, there is no convincing evidence that the terminals in the nucleus accumbens are more sensitive to nicotine than the terminals in the striatum. Stimulation of the nicotinic receptors on the cell bodies results in excitation of the dopamine-secreting cells in both the substantia nigra (Clarke *et al.*, 1985a) and ventral tegmental area (Calabresi *et al.*, 1989). However, the mesolimbic neurones which originate in the ventral tegmental area are stimulated preferentially following the systemic administration of nicotine (Mereu *et al.*, 1987). It seems likely, therefore, that the preferential increase in mesolimbic dopamine secretion evoked by systemic nicotine is associated with increased firing of mesolimbic dopamine neurones rather than a preferential effect on the terminals in the nucleus accumbens.

The effects of chronic nicotine on brain dopamine systems seem to depend to a large extent on the dose of drug used and the route of administration. In studies in which rats were given daily injections of nicotine both Mitchell *et al.* (1989) using an *ex vivo* measure of dopamine turnover and Damsma *et al.* (1989) using *in vivo* microdialysis found that chronic administration of the drug resulted in the development of neither tolerance nor sensitization of the response. However, Lapin *et al.* (1989), using the dopamine/metabolite ratio as a measure of dopamine turnover, found that repeated daily injections of nicotine resulted in decreased dopamine turnover in the nucleus accumbens. This group have also reported that the same dosing schedule increases the density of dopamine receptors in the nucleus accumbens (Reilly *et al.*, 1987), results which provide additional support for the hypothesis that the treatment schedule decreases dopamine secretion in this region of the brain. In contrast, recent *in vivo* microdialysis studies in our laboratory have shown that rats pretreated with daily injections of nicotine (0.1 or 0.4 mg/kg) for 5 days prior to the test day exhibit an enhanced response to the drug (Figure 1). The reason for the discrepancy between the results reported from the different laboratories remains unclear although one factor which may merit further investigation is the nature of the test environment used for the studies.

In contrast to the effects of repeated daily injections of nicotine, constant infusion of the drug from subcutaneous osmotic minipumps is reported to decrease dopamine turnover in the striatum (Kirch *et al.*, 1987) and to increase the sensitivity of postsynaptic dopamine receptors in this region of the brain (Fung and Lau, 1988, 1989). In the nucleus accumbens, however, chronic exposure to nicotine infusions has been shown to potentiate the increase in dopamine biosynthesis and release evoked by challenging slices, prepared from this area of the brain, with amphetamine or nicotine, data which support the hypothesis that the treatment schedule results in enhanced neurotransmission at these synapses (Fung, 1989).

5.3.2.3 The role of dopamine in behavioural responses to nicotine

Studies designed to investigate the extent to which the discriminative properties of nicotine generalize to other drugs have revealed that, if a relatively high dose of the drug is used during training, the nicotine cue partially generalizes to amphetamine, data which suggest that the effects of nicotine on brain dopamine systems contribute to, but do no fully account for, mechanisms which mediate the responses (Stolerman *et al.*, 1984). There is more substantial evidence, however, that the changes in dopamine secretion do mediate the increases in locomotor activity observed in animals treated chronically with the drug. Thus, Clarke *et al.* (1988) reported that selective lesions of

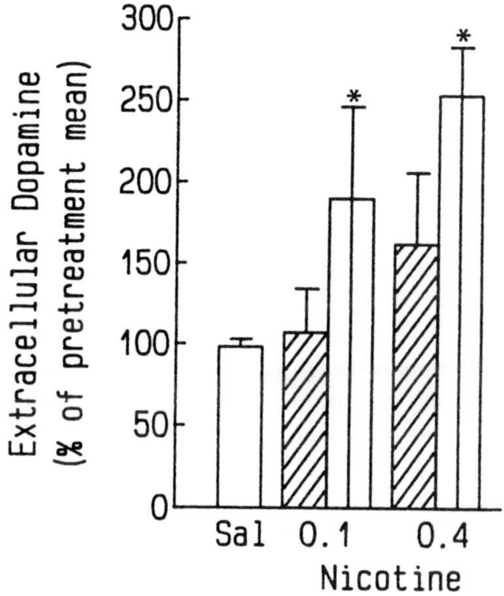

Figure 1 The effects of acute and subchronic nicotine on the extracellular levels of dopamine in the nucleus accumbens. The effects of nicotine on the extracellular dopamine (DA) levels in nucleus accumbens of conscious freely moving rats were studied in rats pretreated with daily injections of saline (hatched bars) or 0.1 or 0.4 mg/kg nicotine (striped bars) for 5 days prior to the test day using *in vivo* microdialysis. Control responses were measured in rats which were both pretreated and tested with saline (open bar). The measurements were made during the period 20–40 min after the injections when the peak increases in extracellular DA evoked by nicotine were observed. The data are the means ± SEM of 6–8 observations and are expressed as a percentage of the mean DA levels in the three dialysate samples collected prior to the injections of nicotine or saline. * Significantly different from saline-treated controls: $P < 0.05$. (The author is grateful to Dr M.E.M. Benwell for permission to publish these data.)

the mesolimbic dopamine system evoked by the bilateral injection of 6-hydroxydopamine into the nucleus accumbens blocked the locomotor response to the drug. A more recent study by Reavill and Stolerman (1990) has also shown that the administration of nicotine or cytisine directly into the ventral tegmental area evokes an increase in locomotor activity similar to that observed in rats treated systemically with the drug. Infusions of these drugs into the nucleus accumbens, striatum, dorsal hippocampus or the motor thalamus had no effects on ambulatory or repeated movements. These results, therefore, provide clear support for the hypothesis that, as appears to be the case for *d*-amphetamine and cocaine (Kelly *et al.*, 1975; Swerdlow *et al.*, 1986), the locomotor stimulant properties of nicotine are mediated by its ability to stimulate dopamine secretion in the mesolimbic system although, unlike the responses to the other psychostimulants, the effects of nicotine reflect an action on the cell bodies rather than an effect in the terminal field. Preliminary studies in this laboratory (Benwell and Balfour, 1990) suggest that the enhanced locomotor responses to nicotine observed in animals treated chronically with the drug may be related to an enhancement of the increase in extracellular dopamine levels in the nucleus accumbens evoked by nicotine although further experiments are necessary to establish this relationship with any certainty.

There is now a considerable body of evidence to support the hypothesis that the mesolimbic dopamine system forms an important component of the 'reward pathways' of the brain and that drugs which enhance neurotransmission within the system are perceived as rewarding by both humans and experimental animals (Wise and Bozarth, 1981, 1987; Wise, 1990). As a result, experimental animals can be trained to self-administer many of the drugs which either evoke the secretion of dopamine at synapses in the mesolimbic system or potentiate its effects in the synaptic cleft. Since, as has been outlined above, this system also appears to mediate the psychostimulant properties of many of the drugs, Wise and Bozarth (1987) have proposed their 'psychomotor stimulant theory of addiction' in which they suggest that the rewarding properties of a wide range of addictive agents, including particularly the classical psychostimulants such as the amphetamines, cocaine, the opiates and ethanol, are mediated by their ability to stimulate dopamine secretion in the mesolimbic system and that, providing the drugs are given at the correct dose, all can also evoke psychostimulation. This hypothesis is supported by the data reported by Di Chiara and Imperato (1988) who, using the *in vivo* microdialysis technique, showed that all these drugs preferentially increase extracellular dopamine concentrations in the mesolimbic system of freely moving rats. In explaining their hypothesis, Wise and Bozarth (1987) argued that the effects of *d*-amphetamine and cocaine on the mesolimbic dopamine system evoked such a powerful reward that this response, in itself, was sufficient to explain the craving for the drugs and that any abstinence effects which might occur following drug withdrawal probably contribute little to the maintenance of drug-taking behaviour. Both Wise and Bozarth and Di Chiara and Imperato included nicotine amongst the drugs which conformed to the hypothesis and, indeed, there is evidence that the rewarding properties of the drug are attenuated by lesions of the mesolimbic dopamine system (Singer *et al.*, 1982). However, when compared with the effects of *d*-amphetamine and cocaine, the increase in dopamine secretion evoked by nicotine is relatively modest (Di Chiara and Imperato, 1988; Benwell and Balfour, in preparation) and nicotine is a relatively weak substrate in drug self-administration schedules (Balfour, 1984b; Clarke, 1987).

An earlier section of this chapter on models of nicotine dependence has already drawn attention to the fact that nicotine appears to exert a 'tranquillizing' effect and that a number of groups have reported that self-administration of the drug is enhanced by exposure to stressful environments. Exposure to stress itself increases dopamine secretion in the mesolimbic system although, in many cases, the effects of stress appear to be greater in the mesocortical system (Abercombie *et al.*, 1989; Imperato *et al.*, 1990). However, there is evidence that repeated exposure to an aversive environment results in sensitization of the mesolimbic system to the extent that animals subsequently challenged with *d*-amphetamine exhibit an exaggerated locomotor response to the drug (Herman *et al.*, 1984). The ability of antidepressant drugs to attenuate the behavioural consequence of exposure to an unavoidable stress is also reported to depend upon an increase in dopamine secretion in the mesolimbic system and there is evidence that chronic treatment with these drugs is associated with sensitization of neurotransmission at mesolimbic dopamine synapses (Cervo and Samanin, 1988; Maj *et al.*, 1987). These data, taken together, appear consistent with the hypothesis that increased dopamine secretion in the mesolimbic and mesocortical system may form part of the mechanism by which animals and, presumably, man cope with aversive environments. If this is the case, then it seems reasonable to suggest that the effects of nicotine on the mesolimbic dopamine system may contribute to its reported ability to attenuate some of the behavioural responses to stress (Costall *et al.*, 1989; Vale and Balfour, 1989). In this context it is interesting to note that a recent study in this laboratory (Balfour, 1990b) has shown that *d*-amphetamine, like nicotine, enhances acquisition of a stressful shock avoidance task and that withdrawal of the drug also results in a marked disruption of the avoidance performance (Figure 2). These experiments also showed that the administration of *d*-amphetamine attenuated the disruption of avoidance performance evoked by the withdrawal of nicotine from rats trained with nicotine. The results suggest that, in this paradigm at least, enhanced dopamine secretion may improve the ability of the rats to 'cope' with the aversive test schedule. The data also suggest that exposure to stressful environments may enhance the addictive properties of psychostimulant drugs, including nicotine, because animals become dependent upon the increased levels of synaptic dopamine, evoked by psychostimulant administration, in order to attenuate the disruptive effects of the aversive environmental stimuli on behavioural performance (Balfour, 1991b).

5.3.2.4 5-Hydroxytryptamine

To date there is little evidence that nicotine exerts direct effects on the secretion of 5-HT in mammalian brain. Nevertheless, studies in a number of laboratories have shown that the administration of nicotine to experimental rats alters the

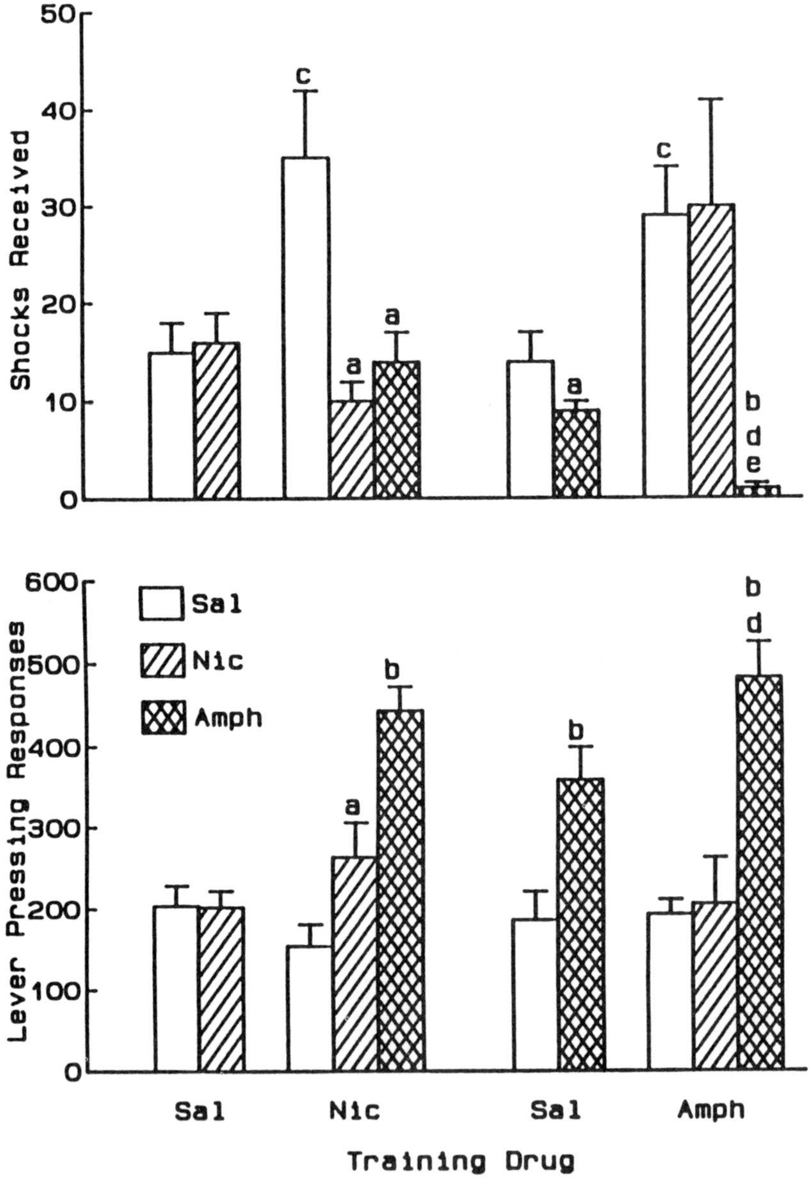

Figure 2 The effects of nicotine and *d*-amphetamine on shock avoidance behaviour in the rat. Rats were trained on an unsignalled shock avoidance schedule using the protocol described by Morrison (1974). The rats were given subcutaneous injections of saline (Sal) or 0.4 mg/kg nicotine (Nic) 3 min, or saline (Sal) or 0.5 mg/kg *d*-amphetamine (Amp) 30 min prior to each training session, a separate saline-treated

concentration and turnover of 5-HT in discrete areas of the brain. For example, Rosecrans (1971a) reported that acute injections of nicotine lowered the concentration and turnover of 5-HT in the forebrain of female rats which had been selected for their high levels of spontaneous activity. In contrast, in rats which exhibit low levels of activity, nicotine decreases 5-HT turnover in the midbrain and hindbrain. Similar, although less marked, changes are also observed in the brains of male rats (Rosecrans, 1971b). Repeated daily injections of nicotine result in a consistent and regionally selective reduction in the concentration of 5-HT in the hippocampus (Benwell and Balfour, 1979). Other results from our laboratory suggest that the reduction in hippocampal 5-HT evoked by chronic nicotine reflects a decrease in the turnover of the amine since the concentration of 5-hydroxyindole acetic acid (5-HIAA) in the hippocampus is also reduced by chronic administration of the drug. In addition, subsequent studies (Benwell and Balfour, 1982b) showed that 5-HT biosynthesis in synaptosomes prepared from the hippocampus of rats treated acutely or chronically with nicotine was reduced when compared with controls and that chronic administration resulted in a reduction in the number of tryptophan carrier sites present on the membranes of hippocampal synaptosomes. In each case the effects were regionally selective for the hippocampus, results which clearly suggest that nicotine exerts a selective effect on the 5-HTergic pathways which innervate this structure. However, the recent study reported by Mitchell *et al.* (1989) failed to find any evidence for an effect of nicotine on 5-HT turnover in the hippocampus. The reason for the discrepancy between the data from the two laboratories remains unclear although results reported from this laboratory have shown that it is important to ensure that the rats are not stressed by the handling procedures associated with administration of the drug since the reduction in hippocampal 5-HT evoked by nicotine is not apparent if the drug is given to stressed rats (Balfour *et al.*, 1975; Benwell and Balfour, 1982a).

The results outlined above suggest that rats do not become tolerant to the effects of nicotine on hippocampal 5-HT. The dosing regime used in these studies (single daily injections), however, was not designed to resemble the

---

◀

control group being used for the study with *d*-amphetamine. Once trained to criterion, the avoidance behaviour of the rats was tested at weekly intervals after injections of saline (open columns), 0.4 mg/kg nicotine (hatched columns) or 0.5 mg/kg *d*-amphetamine (cross-hatched columns). Significantly different from rats tested after saline: a, $P < 0.05$; b, $P < 0.01$. Significantly different from rats trained and tested after saline: c, $P < 0.05$; d, $P < 0.01$. Significantly different from rats trained with saline but tested after *d*-amphetamine: e, $P < 0.01$. Reproduced from Balfour (1991a) with the permission of the publisher.

dosing schedule experienced by habitual smokers who may smoke many cigarettes in a day. It is interesting to observe, therefore, that a recent postmortem study in this laboratory (Benwell *et al.*, 1990) has shown that the concentrations of 5-HT and 5-HIAA in human hippocampus are also reduced if the tissue is taken from subjects who had been habitual smokers (Figure 3). The effect was regionally selective to the extent that tobacco

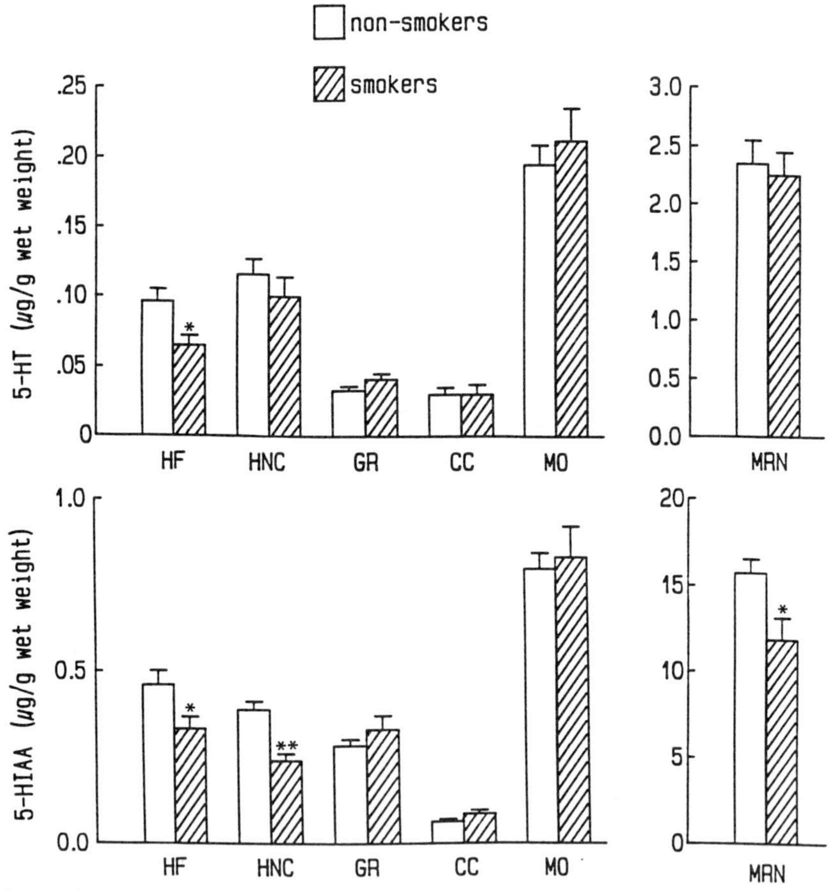

Figure 3 The effects of smoking on the 5-HT and 5-HIAA concentrations in human brain. The concentrations of 5-HT and 5-HIAA were measured in the hippocampal formation (HF), hippocampal neocortex (HNC), gyrus rectus (GR), cerebellar cortex (CC), medulla oblongata (MO) and median raphe nuclei (MRN) of tissue taken from subjects who had been tobacco smokers (hatched columns; $N = 8$) and from age-matched controls (open columns; $N = 12$). Significantly different from non-smokers: $*P < 0.05$; $**P < 0.01$. Reproduced from Benwell *et al.* (1990) with the permission of the publisher.

smoking had no significant effects on the concentrations of 5-HT or 5-HIAA in an area of the cerebral cortex (gyrus rectus), the cerebellum or the medulla oblongata. There was, however, a modest but statistically significant reduction in the concentration of 5-HIAA in the median raphe nuclei, the area of the brain which provides the major 5-HTergic innervation to the hippocampus. Tobacco smoking was also associated with a regionally selective increase in the density of 5-HT_{1A} receptors in the hippocampus (Figure 4). The changes in 5-HT and 5-HIAA are very similar to those found in unstressed rats treated with nicotine and, therefore, it seems reasonable to suggest that they are mediated by the nicotine present in the smoke that these subjects had inhaled. If this is the case the data imply that the repetitive inhalation of nicotine in tobacco smoke evokes the same effects on hippocampal 5-HT systems as those seen in experimental animals treated with nicotine injections and that, as far as 5-HT systems are concerned, the studies with experimental animals may have some relevance to the role of nicotine in the tobacco-smoking habit. In addition, the data, when taken together, appear to provide further evidence for the hypothesis that nicotine decreases 5-HT release and turnover in the hippocampus.

The possible psychopharmacological significance of the changes in hippocampal 5-HT evoked by nicotine administration remains to be established FitzGerald *et al.* (1985) used an automated tunnel maze to investigate the behavioural responses to nicotine in animals which had been pretreated with *p*-chlorophenylalanine (pCPA) to inhibit the biosynthesis of 5-HT. In these studies pCPA attenuated the increase in locomotor activity evoked by administration of the drug but had no effect on the activity of the saline-treated controls. Surprisingly, however, this group also found that pretreatment with 5-hydroxytryptophan, at doses which should have increased 5-HT formation in the brain, also reduced the locomotor response to nicotine. In a subsequent study using the elevated X-maze test of anxiety, Balfour *et al.* (1986a) employed the neurotoxin 5,7-dihydroxytryptamine to evoke selective lesions in the principal 5-HTergic fibres which innervate the hippocampus. The lesions had no effect on the enhanced locomotor activity seen in rats treated subchronically with nicotine prior to the test day and they did not influence the locomotor activity of the saline-treated control rats. Thus, it seems unlikely that changes in 5-HT secretion in the hippocampus are involved in the locomotor responses to the drug. In this study, however, the lesions did evoke a statistically significant, although modest, reduction in the proportion of activity occurring in the open runways of the maze, data which suggest that reduced 5-HT secretion in the hippocampus could be associated with the expression of anxiogenic-like behaviour in this test. Interestingly File *et al.* (1987) have reported that increased avoidance of the open runways of the maze correlates with decreased 5-HT secretion in the hippocampus measured 24 hours earlier

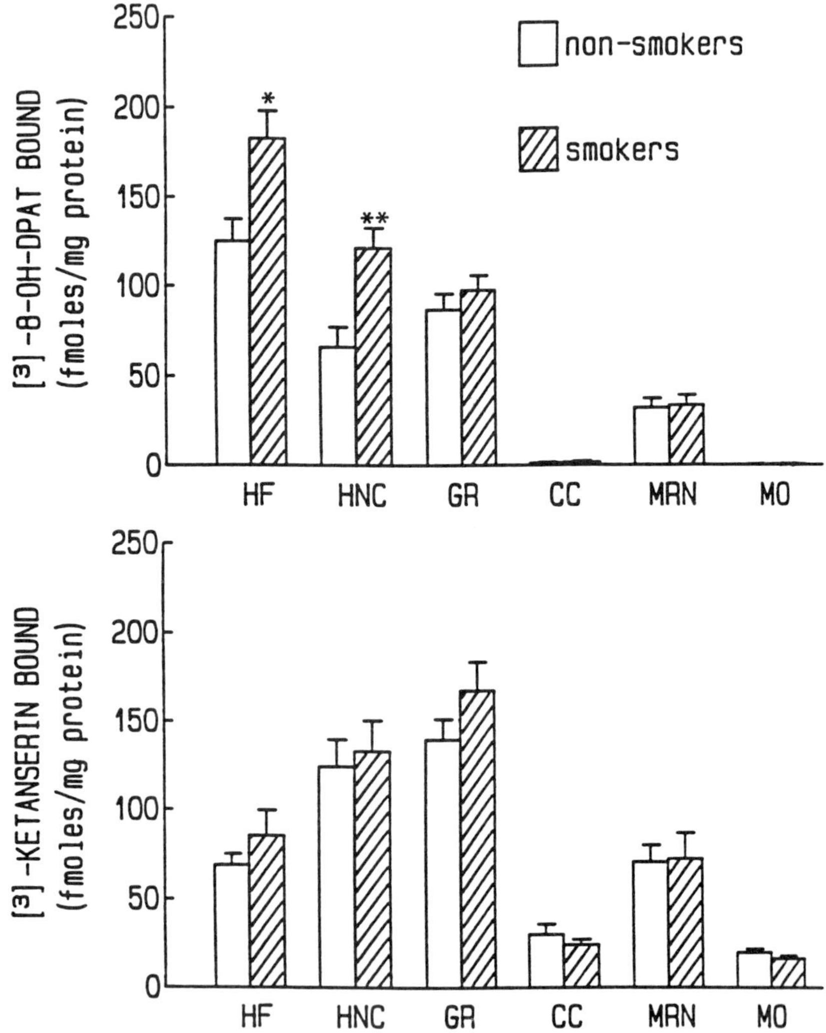

Figure 4 The effects of smoking on 5-HT_{1A} and 5-HT_2 receptor binding to human brain. Radioligand binding, using [^{3}H]8-hydroxy-2-(di-propylamino)-tetralin ([^{3}H]8-OH-DPAT) to label 5-HT_{1A} receptors and [^{3}H]ketanserin to label 5-HT_2 receptors, was measured in membranes prepared from the hippocampal formation (HF), hippocampal neocortex (HNC), gyrus rectus (GR), cerebellar cortex (CC), median raphe nuclei (MRN) and medulla oblongata (MO) of tissue taken from subjects who had been tobacco smokers (hatched columns; $N = 8$) and age-matched non-smokers (open columns; $N = 12$). Significantly different from non-smokers: $*P < 0.05$; $**P < 0.01$. Reproduced from Benwell *et al.* (1990) with the permission of the publisher.

using *in vivo* microdialysis. However, in another study, Balfour *et al.* (1986b) showed that nicotine appeared to reduce 5-HT turnover in the hippocampus of rats tested in the X-maze but to have no effect on avoidance of the open runways. Thus, when taken together, these data seem to provide little evidence for the hypothesis that the effects of nicotine on hippocampal 5-HT are associated with the expression of behavioural responses which are characteristic of anxiolytic or anxiogenic drugs.

Studies completed some years ago in our laboratory showed that if the plasma corticosterone level was reduced either by inhibiting corticosterone biosynthesis with metyrapone (Balfour *et al.*, 1975) or by inhibiting adrenocorticotrophic hormone (ACTH) secretion with betamethasone (Balfour and Benwell, 1979) the concentration and turnover of 5-HT in the hippocampus is decreased in a regionally selective way which appears to resemble the effects of nicotine. These results led Benwell and Balfour (1979) to suggest that the increase in plasma corticosterone seen following the withdrawal of nicotine from unstressed rats might be associated with its effect on hippocampal 5-HT. Subsequent studies have shown that if rats are repeatedly exposed to an aversive elevated open platform, the plasma corticosterone response habituates so that after approximately 20 sessions, the response is significantly lower than that found for rats tested acutely on the apparatus (Benwell and Balfour, 1982a; Copland and Balfour, 1987). Habituation of the response is associated with the development of a significant positive correlation between the plasma corticosterone concentration and the concentration of 5-HT in the hippocampus. The administration of nicotine prior to each session on the platform significantly attenuates the reduction in the plasma corticosterone response to the stress of the platform and results in the development of a significant but negative correlation between plasma corticosterone and the hippocampal 5-HT (Benwell and Balfour, 1982a). If rats which had been treated with nicotine prior to each session on the platform were tested after the injection of saline, the plasma corticosterone levels remained elevated but the correlation with hippocampal 5-HT was lost. These results provide some evidence for the hypothesis that nicotine interacts with the process by which animals habituate to an aversive environment and that this interaction may contribute to the development of nicotine dependence (Balfour, 1984b; Benwell and Balfour, 1982a). However, in the repeatedly stressed rats, plasma corticosterone did not correlate with the concentration of 5-HIAA in the hippocampus and, indeed, there is no direct evidence that habituation to the open platform stress is associated with changes in 5-HT release or turnover in this area of the brain. The data seem more consistent with the possibility that the treatments cause a change in the amount of 5-HT available for release, although it must be emphasized that this is a very speculative conclusion which requires further study.

Studies designed to examine the possible role of brain 5-HTergic systems in the mechanism of action of anxiolytic drugs have tended to focus on the pathways which originate in the dorsal raphe since there is reasonably good evidence that a number of different anxiolytic drugs inhibit the 5-HT-secreting cells in these nuclei (Costall *et al.*, 1988; Higgins *et al.*, 1988). Although it has not yet been established with certainty, the data currently available appear more consistent with the possibility that chronic nicotine acts predominantly on the pathways which emanate from the median, rather than the dorsal, raphe, a conclusion which is consistent with the fact that the drug exerts neither anxiolytic nor anxiogenic effects in most tests of anxiety (Balfour, 1991a, b). If this is the case, then it is tempting to suggest that nicotine may act preferentially on the 5-HTergic pathways involved in controlling mood and which form the primary site of action of a number of antidepressent drugs. The evidence for this at the present time is almost entirely circumstantial. Nevertheless, it is interesting to note that nicotine appears to interact with habituation to a form of unavoidable stress similar to that employed in many paradigms used to detect the putative antidepressant activity of drugs (Benwell and Balfour, 1982a; Willner, 1990). In addition, recent studies suggest that the effects of antidepressant drugs on the behavioural responses to aversive environments may depend upon an increase in dopamine secretion in the mesolimbic system (Delina-Stula *et al.*, 1988). It is possible, therefore, that, by mimicking the effects of antidepressant drugs on the mesolimbic dopamine system, nicotine indirectly evokes changes in brain 5-HTergic systems which, in the absence of the drug, could render an habitual smoker more susceptible to depressive states. Depression is, indeed, reported to be one of the symptoms experienced by tobacco smokers when they first abstain from smoking (West, 1988). Other studies have shown that depression is often associated with significant disturbances of pituitary–adrenal function which are reversed by treatment with antidepressant drugs (for review see File, 1990). These data provide some support for the speculative hypothesis that chronic nicotine administration evokes changes in the neural systems involved in the control of mood and that the psychopharmacological consequences of nicotine withdrawal could, in part, result from these changes.

5.4 Concluding comments

This chapter has sought to summarize the changes in brain neurochemistry which occur as a consequence of chronic nicotine administration and which have, at one time or another, been associated with the development of tolerance to and/or dependence upon nicotine. As with most psychotropic agents, the effects of chronic nicotine are complex and are, almost certainly, not yet fully documented. Nevertheless, there is clear evidence that nicotine stimulates the secretion of dopamine in the brain and that this effect mediates, at least in part, the rewarding properties of the drug which are sought by habitual smokers. However, when compared with the other psychostimulant drugs of dependence, environmental stimuli, especially stress, appear to contribute significantly to the development of nicotine dependence. Whilst a definitive explanation for this observation must await the results of further studies, the chapter has summarized data which support the speculative hypothesis that the apparent 'tranquillizing' properties of tobacco smoke may also be related to the increase in dopamine secretion evoked by nicotine and that this is the case because one or more of the dopamine-secreting pathways of the brain are involved in the neural systems used to 'cope' with stressful environments. Other data suggest that, in at least one experimental model of nicotine dependence, the animals may have become dependent upon the nicotine-evoked increase in dopamine secretion in order to continue coping with the stress of the test environment. The data currently available suggest that the effects of nicotine on hippocampal 5-HT may also be involved in the expression of nicotine withdrawal effects although, currently, their relationship to the specific symptoms of nicotine withdrawal must remain a matter of speculation.

Acknowledgements

The results from the author's laboratory which have been discussed in this chapter were obtained in collaboration with my colleagues, Drs Maureen Benwell, Alan Vale, John Anderson and Calum Graham, and I am happy to acknowledge their very significant contributions to the studies. The financial support for the studies from the MRC, the Wellcome Trust and the Scottish Home and Health Department is also gratefully acknowledged.

References

Abelin, T., Buehler, A., Muller, P., Veasnen, K. & Imhof, P.R. (1989) *Lancet* **I**, 7–10.

Abercrombie, E.D., Keefe, K.A., DiFischia, D.S. & Zigmond, M.J. (1989) *J. Neurochem.* **52**, 1655–1658.

Amano, H., Goshima, Y., Akema, N., Ueda, H., Kubo, T. & Misu, Y. (1989) *J. Pharmacobio-Dyn.* **12**, 18–23.

Andersson, K., Fuxe, K., Agnati, L.F. & Eneroth, P. (1981) *Med. Biol.* **59**, 170–176.

Balfour, D.J.K. (1973) *Eur. J. Pharmacol.* **23**, 19–26.

Balfour, D.J.K. (1984a) In *Nicotine and the Tobacco Smoking Habit* (International Encyclopedia of Pharmacology and Therapeutics, Section 114) (ed. Balfour, D.J.K.), pp 61–74. New York, Pergamon Press.

Balfour, D.J.K. (1984b) In *Nicotine and the Tobacco Smoking Habit* (International Encyclopedia of Pharmacology and Therapeutics, Section 114) (ed. Balfour, D.J.K.), pp 101–112. New York, Pergamon Press.
Balfour, D.J.K. (1990a) In *Psychotropic Drugs of Abuse* (International Encyclopedia of Pharmacology and Therapeutics, Section 130) (ed. Balfour, D.J.K.), pp 453–481. New York, Pergamon Press.
Balfour, D.J.K. (1990b) *J. Pharm. Pharmacol.* **42**, 257–260.
Balfour, D.J.K. (1991a) In *Addiction Controversies* (ed. Warburton, D.M.), pp 90–103. London, Harwood Academic Publishers.
Balfour, D.J.K. (1991b) *Br. J. Addict.* **86**, 489–493.
Balfour, D.J.K. & Benwell, M.E.M. (1979) *Psychoneuroendocrinology* **4**, 83–86.
Balfour, D.J.K., Khullar, K.A. & Longden, A. (1975) *Pharmacol. Biochem. Behav.* **3**, 179–184
Balfour, D.J.K., Benwell, M.E.M., Graham, C.A. & Vale, A.L. (1986a) *Br. J. Pharmacol.* **89**, 341–347.
Balfour, D.J.K., Graham, C.A. & Vale, A.L. (1986b) *Psychopharmacology* **90**, 528–532.
Benwell, M.E.M. & Balfour, D.J.K. (1979) *Psychopharmacology* **63**, 7–11.
Benwell, M.E.M. & Balfour, D.J.K. (1982a) *Psychopharmacology* **76**, 160–162.
Benwell, M.E.M. & Balfour, D.J.K. (1982b) *Eur. J. Pharmacol.* **84**, 71–77.
Benwell, M.E.M. & Balfour, D.J.K. (1985) *J. Pharm. Pharmacol.* **37**, 405–409.
Benwell, M.E.M. & Balfour, D.J.K. (1990) *Br. J. Pharmacol.* **99**, 259p.
Benwell, M.E.M., Balfour, D.J.K. & Anderson, J.M. (1988) *J. Neurochem.* **50**, 1243–1247.
Benwell, M.E.M., Balfour, D.J.K. & Anderson, J. M. (1990) *Psychopharmacology* **102**, 68–72.
Calabresi, P., Lacey, M.G. & North, R.A. (1989) *Br. J. Pharmacol.* **98**, 135–140.
Carroll, M.E., Lac, S.T., Asencio, M. & Keenan, R.M. (1989) *Life Sci.* **45**, 1381–1388.
Cervo, L. & Samanin, R. (1988) *J. Pharm. Pharmacol.* **40**, 155–156.
Clarke, P.B.S. (1987) *Psychopharmacology* **92**, 135–143.
Clarke, P.B.S. & Fibiger, H.C. (1987) *Psychopharmacology* **92**, 84–88.
Clarke, P.B.S. & Kumar, R. (1983) *Br. J. Pharmacol.* **78**, 329–337.
Clarke, P.B.S. & Pert, A. (1985) *Brain Res.* **348**, 355–358.
Clarke, P.B.S., Hommer, D.W., Pert, A. & Skirboll, L.R. (1985a) *Br. J. Pharmacol.* **85**, 827–835.
Clarke, P.B.S., Schwartz, R.D., Paul, S.M., Pert, C.B. & Pert, A. (1985b) *J. Neurosci.* **5**, 1307–1315.
Clarke, P.B.S., Fu, D.S., Jakubovic, A. & Fibiger, H.C. (1988) *J. Pharmacol. Exp. Ther.* **246**, 701–708.
Collins, A.C., Evans, C.B., Miner, L.L. & Marks, M.J. (1986) *Pharmacol. Biochem. Behav.* **24**, 1767–1773.
Collins, A.C., Romm, E. & Wehner, J.M. (1988) *Psychopharmacology* **96**, 7–14.
Copland, A.M. & Balfour, D.J.K. (1987) *Pharmacol. Biochem. Behav.* **27**, 619–624.
Corrigal, W.A., Herling, S. & Coen, K.M. (1989) *Pharmacol. Biochem. Behav.* **33**, 559–562.
Costa, L.G. & Murphy, S.D. (1983) *J. Pharmacol. Exp. Ther.* **226**, 392–397.
Costall, B., Kelly, M.E., Naylor, R.J., Onaivi, E.S. & Tyers, M.B. (1988) *Br. J. Pharmacol.* **96**, 325–332.
Costall, B., Kelly, M.E., Naylor, R.J. & Onaivi, E.S. (1989) *Pharmacol. Biochem. Behav.* **33**, 197–203.

Costall, B., Jones, B.J., Kelly, M.E., Naylor, R.J., Onaivi, E.S. & Tyers, M.B. (1990) *Pharmacol. Biochem. Behav.* **36**, 339–344.
Cox, B.M., Goldstein, A. & Nelson, W.T. (1984) *Br. J. Pharmacol.* **83**, 49–55.
Damsma, G., Day, J. & Fibiger, H.C. (1989) *Eur. J. Pharmacol.* **168**, 363–368.
Delini-Stula, A., Radeke, E. & von Reizen, H. (1988) *Neuropharmacology* **27**, 943–947.
De Sarno, P. & Giacobini, E. (1989) *J. Neurosci. Res.* **22**, 194–200.
Di Chiara, G. & Imperato, A. (1988) *Proc. Natl Acad. Sci. USA.* **85**, 5274–5278.
Edwards, J.A. & Warburton, D.M. (1984) In *Nicotine and the Tobacco Smoking Habit* (International Encyclopedia of Pharmacology and Therapeutics, Section 114) (ed. Balfour, D.J.K.), pp 113–131. New York, Pergamon Press.
Egan, T.M. & North, R.A. (1986) *Neuroscience* **19**, 565–571.
Emmett-Oglesby, M.W., Mathis, D.A., Moon, R.T.Y. & Lal, H. (1990) *Psychopharmacology* **101**, 292–309.
Engberg, G. (1989) *Life Sci.* **44**, 1535–1540.
Engberg, G. & Svensson, T.H. (1980) *J. Neural. Transm.* **49**, 137–150.
Fagerstrom, K.O. (1988) *Prog. Clin. Biol. Res.* **261**, 109–128.
File, S.E. (1990) *Pharmacol. Ther.* **46**, 357–375.
File, S.E., Curle, P.F., Baldwin, H.A. & Neal, M.J. (1987) *Neurosci. Lett.* **83**, 318–327.
FitzGerald, R.E., Oettinger, R. & Battig, K. (1985) *Pharmacol. Biochem. Behav.* **23**, 279–284.
Flynn, D.D. & Mash, D.C. (1986) *J. Neurochem.* **47**, 1948–1954.
Fudala, P.J., Teoh, K.W. & Iwamoto, E.T. (1985) *Pharmacol. Biochem. Behav.* **22**, 237–241.
Fung, Y.K. (1989) *J. Pharm. Pharmacol.* **41**, 66–68.
Fung, Y.K. & Lau, Y.-S. (1988) *Eur. J. Pharmacol.* **152**, 263–271.
Fung, Y.K. & Lau, Y.-S. (1989) *Pharmacol. Biochem. Behav.* **32**, 221–226.
Fuxe, K., Andersson, K., Harfstrand, A. & Agnati, L.F. (1986) *J. Neural. Transm.* **67**, 15–29.
Gilbert, D.G. (1979) *Psychol. Bull.* **86**, 643–661.
Giorguieff-Chesselet, M.F., Kemel, M.L., Wandscheer, D. & Glowinski, J. (1979) *Life Sci.* **25**, 1257–1262.
Goldberg, S.R., Spealmen, R.D. & Goldberg, D.M. (1981) *Science* **214**, 573–575.
Grenhoff, J. & Svensson, T.H. (1988) *Acta Physiol. Scand.* **133**, 595–596.
Haikala, H. & Ahtee, L. (1988) *Naunyn-Schmiedeberg's Arch. Pharmacol.* **338**, 169–173.
Hall, G.H. & Turner, D.M. (1972) *Biochem. Pharmacol.* **21**, 1829–1838.
Harris, C.M., Emmett-Oglesby, M.W., Robinson, N.G. & Lal, H. (1986) *Psychopharmacology* **90**, 85–89.
Herman, J.-P., Stinus, L. & Le Moal, M. (1984) *Psychopharmacology* **84**, 431–435.
Higgins, G.A., Bradbury, A.J., Jones, B.J. & Oakley, N.R. (1988) *Neuropharmacology* **27**, 993–1001.
Hutchinson, R.R. & Emley, G.S. (1985) *Psychol. Rec.* **35**, 491–502.
Imperato, A., Mulas, A. & Di Chiara, G. (1986) *Eur. J. Pharmacol.* **132**, 337–338.
Imperato, A., Puglisi-Allegra, S., Zocchi, A., Scrocco, M., Casolini, O. & Angelucci, L. (1990) *Eur. J. Pharmacol.* **175**, 211–214.
Iwamoto, E.T. (1990) *Psychopharmacology* **100**, 251–257.
Kellar, K.J., Whitehouse, P.J., Martino-Barrows, A.M., Marcus, K. & Price, D.L. (1987) *Brain Res.* **436**, 62–68.
Kelly, P.H., Seviour, P.W. & Iversen, S.D. (1975) *Brain Res.* **94**, 507–522.
Kirch, D.G., Gerhardt, G.A., Shelton, R.C., Freedman, R. & Watt, R.J. (1987) *Clin. Neuropharmacol.* **10**, 376–383.

Ksir, C., Hakan, R., Hall, D.P. & Kellar, K.J. (1985) *Neuropharmacology* **24**, 527–531.

Ksir, C., Hakan, R.L. & Kellar, K.J. (1987) *Psychopharmacology* **92**, 25–29.

Kubo, T., Amano, H., Kurahashi, K. & Misu, Y. (1989) *J. Pharmacobio-Dyn.* **12**, 107–112.

Lang, W.J., Latiff, A.A., McQueen, A. & Singer, G. (1977) *Pharmacol. Biochem. Behav.* **7**, 65–70.

Lapchak, P.A., Aruajo, D.M., Quirion, R. & Collier, B. (1989) *J. Neurochem.* **52**, 483–491.

Lapin, E.P., Maker, H.S., Sershen, H. & Lajtha, A. (1989) *Eur. J. Pharmacol.* **160**, 53–59.

London, E.D., Ball, M.J. & Waller, S.B. (1989) *Neurochem. Res.* **14**, 745–750.

Maj, J., Wedzony, K. & Klimek, V. (1987) *Eur. J. Pharmacol.* **140**, 179–185.

Marks, M.J. & Collins, A.C. (1982) *Mol. Pharmacol.* **22**, 554–564.

Marks, M.J., Burch, J.B. & Collins, A.C. (1983) *J. Pharmacol. Exp. Ther.* **226**, 817–825.

Marks, M.J., Romm, E., Gaffney, D.K. & Collins, A.C. (1986a) *J. Pharmacol. Exp. Ther.* **237**, 809–819.

Marks, M.J., Stitzel, J.A., Romm, E., Wehner, J.M. & Collins, A.C. (1986b) *Mol. Pharmacol.* **30**, 427–436.

Martino-Barrows, A.M. & Kellar, K.J. (1987) *Mol. Pharmacol.* **31**, 169–174.

Mason, S.T. & Fibiger, H.C. (1979) *Life Sci.* **25**, 2141–2147.

Mereu, G., Yoon, K.-W.P., Boi, V., Gessa, G.L., Naes, L. & Westfall, T.C. (1987) *Eur. J. Pharmacol.* **141**, 395–399.

Mifsud, J.-C., Hernandez, L. & Hoebel, B.G. (1989) *Brain Res.* **478**, 365–367.

Miner, L.L., Marks, M.J. & Collins, A.C. (1984) *J. Pharmacol. Exp. Ther.* **231**, 545–554.

Mitchell, S.N., Brazell, M.P., Joseph, M.H., Alavijeh, M.S. & Gray, J.A. (1989) *Eur. J. Pharmacol.* **167**, 311–322.

Mitchell, S.N., Brazell, M.P. & Gray, J.A. (1990) *Br. J. Pharmacol.* **99**, 266p.

Morrison, C.F. (1969) *Psychopharmacologia (Berl.)* **14**, 221–232.

Morrison, C.F. (1974) *Psychopharmacologia (Berl.)* **38**, 25–35.

Morrison, C.F. & Stephenson, J.A. (1970) *Psychopharmacologia (Berl.)* **18**, 133–143.

Morrison, C.F. & Stephenson, J.A. (1972) *Br. J. Pharmacol.* **46**, 151–156.

Nakamura, S., Sakaguchi, T. & Aoki, F. (1989) *Neurosci. Lett.* **100**, 147–152.

Nordberg, A., Wahlstrom, G., Arnelo, U. & Larsson, C. (1985) *Drug Alcohol. Depend.* **16**, 9–17.

Pellow, S., Chopin, P., File, S.E. & Briley, M. (1985) *J. Neurosci. Methods* **14**, 149–167.

Perry, E.K., Perry, R.H., Smith, C.J., Dick, D.J., Candy, J.M., Edwardson, J.A., Fairbairn, A. & Blessed, G. (1987) *J. Neurol. Neurosurg. Psychiatry* **50**, 806–809.

Pomerleau, C.S. & Pomerleau, O.F. (1987) *Psychophysiology* **24**, 278–285.

Pratt, J.A., Stolerman, I.P., Garcha, H.S., Giardini, V. & Feyerabend, C. (1983) *Psychopharmacology* **81**, 54–60.

Rapier, C., Lunt, G.G. & Wonnacott, S. (1988) *J. Neurochem.* **50**, 1123–1130.

Reavill, C. & Stolerman, I.P. (1990) *Br. J. Pharmacol.* **99**, 273–278.

Reavill, C., Jenner, P., Kumar, R. & Stolerman, I.P. (1988) *Neuropharmacology* **27**, 235–241.

Reavill, C., Walther, B., Stolerman, I.P. & Testa, B. (1990) *Neuropharmacology* **29**, 619–624.

Reilly, M.A., Lapin, E.P., Maker, H.S. & Lajtha, A. (1987) *J. Neurosci. Res.* **18**, 621–625.

Romanelli, L., Ohman, B., Adem, A. & Nordberg, A. (1988) *Eur. J. Pharmacol.* **148**, 289–291.

Romano, C. & Goldstein, A. (1980) *Science* **210**, 647–650.
Romano, C., Goldstein, A. & Jewell, J.P. (1981) *Psychopharmacology* **74**, 310–315.
Rosecrans, J.A. (1971a) *Eur. J. Pharmacol.* **14**, 29–37.
Rosecrans, J.A. (1971b) *Eur. J. Pharmacol.* **16**, 123–127.
Rowell, P.P. & Winkler, D.L. (1984) *J. Neurochem.* **43**, 1593–1598.
Rowell, P.P., Carr, L.A. & Garner, A.C. (1987) *J. Neurochem.* **49**, 1449–1454.
Russell, M.A.H. (1988) *Prog. Clin. Biol. Res.* **261**, 63–94.
Russell, M.A.H., Feyerabend, C. & Cole, P.V. (1976) *Br. Med. J.* **1**, 1043–1046.
Sakurai, Y., Takano, Y., Kohjimoto, Y., Honda, K. & Kamiya, H.-O. (1982) *Brain Res.* **242**, 99–106.
Schwartz, R.D. & Kellar, K.J. (1983) *Science* **220**, 214–216.
Schwartz, R.D. & Kellar, K.J. (1985) *J. Neurochem.* **45**, 427–433.
Singer, G., Wallace, M. & Hall, R. (1982) *Pharmacol. Biochem. Behav.* **17**, 579–581.
Smith, L.A. & Lang, W.J. (1980) *Pharmacol. Biochem. Behav.* **13**, 215–220.
Snell, L.D. & Johnson, K.M. (1989) *Synapse* **3**, 129–135.
Stolerman, I.P. (1988) *Pharmacol. Biochem. Behav.* **30**, 235–242.
Stolerman, I.P., Fink, R. & Jarvik, M.E. (1973) *Psychopharmacologia (Berl.)* **30**, 329–342.
Stolerman, I.P., Garcha, H.S., Pratt, J.A. & Kumar, R. (1984) *Psychopharmacology* **84**, 413–419.
Svensson, T.H. & Engberg, G. (1982) *Acta Physiol. Scand. (Suppl.)* **479**, 31–34.
Swerdlow, N.R., Vaccarino, F.J., Amalric, M. & Koob, G.F. (1986) *Pharmacol. Biochem. Behav.* **25**, 233–248.
Takayama, H., Majewska, M.D. & London, E.D. (1989) *J. Pharmacol. Exp. Ther.* **253**, 1083–1089.
Vale, A.L. & Balfour, D.J.K. (1989) *Pharmacol. Biochem. Behav.* **32**, 857–860.
Wesnes, K. & Warburton, D.M. (1983) *Neuropsychobiology* **9**, 223–229.
Wesnes, K. & Warburton, D.M. (1984) In *Nicotine and the Tobacco Smoking Habit* (International Encyclopedia of Pharmacology and Therapeutics, Section 114) (ed. Balfour, D.J.K.), pp 133–152. New York, Pergamon Press.
West, R. (1988) *Prog. Clin. Biol. Res.* **261**, 237–259.
Westfall, T.C. (1974) *Neuropharmacology* **13**, 693–700.
Westfall, T.C., Grant, H. & Perry, H. (1983) *Gen. Pharmacol.* **14**, 321–325.
Whitehouse, P.J., Martino, A.M., Antuono, P.G., Lowenstein, P.R., Coyle, J.T., Price, D.L. & Kellar, K.J. (1986) *Brain Res.* **371**, 146–151.
Willner, P. (1990) *Pharmacol. Ther.* **45**, 425–455.
Wise, R.A. (1990) In *Psychotropic Drugs of Abuse* (International Encyclopedia of Pharmacology and Therapeutics, Section 130) (ed. Balfour, D.J.K.), pp 23–58. New York, Pergamon Press.
Wise, R.A. & Bozarth, M.A. (1981) *Prog. Neuro-Psychopharmacol.* **5**, 467–474.
Wise, R.A. & Bozarth, M.A. (1987) *Psychol. Bull.* **94**, 469–492.
Wonnacott, S. (1987) *Human Toxicol.* **6**, 343–353.
Yoshida, K., Kato, Y. & Imura, H. (1980) *Brain Res.* **182**, 361–368.

CHAPTER 6

PSYCHOMOTOR STIMULANTS

Francis J. White and Marina E. Wolf

Wayne State University School of Medicine, Department of Psychiatry, Lafayette Clinic, 951 East Lafayette, Detroit, Michigan 48207, USA

Table of Contents

THE BIOLOGICAL BASES OF DRUG TOLERANCE AND DEPENDENCE
ISBN 0-12-564250-4

6.1 Introduction: psychomotor stimulants and reward processes

Use of psychomotor stimulants by humans as 'recreational drugs' can lead to dependence. Although many psychological and sociological variables are involved in the voluntary use of psychomotor stimulants, it is the powerful rewarding properties of these drugs which are primarily responsible for repeated use and abuse in humans. Self-administration studies conducted in laboratory animals have identified the mesolimbic dopamine (DA) system as a critical component of central reward circuitry. These same neurones are also intricately involved in the locomotor stimulating effects of psychomotor stimulants. This has led to a 'psychomotor stimulant theory of addiction' which argues that the underlying mechanisms of locomotor stimulation and reward are the same and a common denominator underlying the addictive qualities of a variety of substances is their ability to cause psychomotor activation. Accordingly, drugs which are not typically thought of as psychomotor stimulants (morphine, ethanol) are predicted to produce effects similar to those of amphetamine and cocaine, at least at certain doses.

This chapter reviews the anatomical, pharmacological, biochemical and electrophysiological evidence regarding the actions of amphetamine and cocaine, often comparing them to morphine in an attempt to address the evidence supporting the 'psychomotor stimulant theory of addiction'. It is hypothesized that a critical component of the rewarding effects of these various drugs is the ability to enhance mesolimbic DA transmission in the relative absence of compensatory decreases in DA neuronal activity. In addition, it is argued that a major effect of repeated psychomotor stimulant action is reverse tolerance or sensitization to their stimulant properties. Mechanisms underlying behavioural sensitization are reviewed. A comprehensive theory is presented in which sensitization is proposed to occur through a complex interplay between a number of neuronal adaptations, some of which may be necessary before others become manifest. Central to this theory is the enhanced activity of DA neurones following repeated psychomotor stimulants and resulting increases in DA release and D_1 DA receptor sensitivity. Finally, the question of sensitization to the rewarding effects of stimulants is addressed and the possible relevance of sensitization to human drug abuse is briefly discussed.

6.2 Neurochemical effects of psychomotor stimulants

Stimulants can be divided into two major classes, the amphetamine class and the non-amphetamine (cocaine or methylphenidate) class, based on the mechanism by which they elevate synaptic levels of DA and other monoamines. Although the amphetamines produce a number of effects on DA neurones, including inhibition of DA synthesis, inhibition of monoamine oxidase, and reuptake blockade, it is the ability to promote the release of DA which is of greatest importance to their stimulant properties. Considerable evidence indicates that amphetamine releases DA by facilitating the efflux of cytoplasmically located DA via reversal of the carrier-mediated DA uptake process (for review see Kuczenski, 1983). In contrast, cocaine and other stimulants in the non-amphetamine class act primarily to inhibit the reuptake of DA after its release from vesicular stores, but possess little direct releasing activity (Heikkila *et al.*, 1975).

Consistent with these mechanisms, the effects of amphetamine are blocked by inhibition of DA synthesis with α-methyl-*p*-tyrosine (Weissman *et al.*, 1966) but not disruption of vesicular DA stores with reserpine (Braestrup, 1977; Niddam *et al.*, 1985). In contrast, the effects of cocaine are blocked by reserpine but not α-methyl-*p*-tyrosine (Scheel-Kruger *et al.*, 1977; Van Rossum *et al.*, 1962). As would be predicted from these distinctions, amphetamine and cocaine differ in the dependence of their actions on impulse flow in DA neurones. The ability of amphetamine to release DA does not appear to require neuronal activity, since amphetamine-induced DA release is Ca^{2+}-independent (Carboni *et al.*, 1989; Westerink *et al.*, 1989) and can be maintained in the presence of tetrodotoxin (Westerink *et al.*, 1987). Furthermore, low doses of systemic apomorphine, which decrease DA neuronal activity through actions at somatodendritic DA autoreceptors (White and Wang, 1984c), do not alter the ability of amphetamine to increase DA release as measured by microdialysis (Kuczenski *et al.*, 1990). Another distinction between impulse-dependent and amphetamine-induced DA release is that the latter is insensitive to regulation by terminal autoreceptors that modulate DA release (Kamal *et al.*, 1981). Cocaine-induced increases in extracellular DA, however, are Ca^{2+}-dependent (Hurd and Ungerstedt, 1989; Pani *et al.*, 1990) and presumably impulse-dependent since they are blocked by tetrodotoxin (Nomikos *et al.*, 1990). These characteristics are consistent with the idea that cocaine does not release DA directly, but acts by blocking reuptake to potentiate the effects of DA released as a result of neuronal activity.

It should be noted that inhibition of impulse flow in DA neurones by low doses of apomorphine *does* inhibit the locomotor stimulant effects of amphetamine (Kuczenski *et al.*, 1990; Strombom and Liedman, 1982) even though amphetamine-induced increases in synaptic DA levels are not affected. Low 'autoreceptor-selective' doses of apomorphine have also been reported to prevent behavioural sensitization following repeated amphetamine administration (Riffee *et al.*, 1987). Thus, while the DA-releasing effects of amphetamine appear to be impulse-independent, it is not accurate to assume that all behavioural effects of amphetamine must also be impulse-independent. This discrepancy is but one of many suggesting that enhancement of synaptic DA levels does not provide a complete explanation for the locomotor activating effects of amphetamine (Kuczenski, 1986). The relationship between cocaine-induced increases in synaptic DA and behavioural activation has not been as thoroughly studied. However, these findings indicate that the possible role of other neurotransmitters as well as changes in the responsiveness of neurones postsynaptic to DA terminals cannot be neglected in attempting to understand the mechanism of psychostimulant action (White, 1990). Nevertheless, increases in synaptic DA levels following administration of amphetamine, cocaine, and other psychostimulants are clearly important to both acute responses to these agents and changes in responsiveness which accompany repeated administration.

The ability of cocaine to inhibit DA uptake is based upon binding of the drug to a site associated with the DA transporter (Kennedy and Hanbauer, 1983; Reith *et al.*, 1980). Moreover, the relative affinities of a series of cocaine congeners and other DA uptake blockers for the cocaine binding site (labelled with either [^{3}H]cocaine or [^{3}H]mazindol) correlate quite well with their ability to stimulate activity and maintain self-administration behaviour (Bergman *et al.*, 1989; Ritz *et al.*, 1987; Spealman *et al.*, 1989). These findings lend support to the psychomotor stimulant theory of addiction (Wise and Bozarth, 1987) in that these two behaviours might be mediated by the same system. In contrast, no such correlation exists between the affinities of amphetamine and related phenylethylamines for DA uptake sites and their reinforcing potencies (Ritz and Kuhar, 1989). This may suggest that amphetamine binds to a different site than cocaine in order to elicit its effects on the DA transporter. Attempts to correlate behavioural effects of psychostimulants with the results of binding studies must take into account the possible existence of multiple sites or allosterically linked sites on the DA transporter.

As might be predicted by their different mechanisms of action, amphetamine is more potent than cocaine at increasing extracellular DA levels within DA terminal fields after systemic administration (Di Chiara and Imperato, 1988; Moghaddam and Bunney, 1989). However, another group has reported comparable increases in extracellular DA levels if behaviourally equivalent doses of amphetamine and cocaine are compared (Maisonneuve *et al.*, 1990). Systemic administration of morphine also increases synaptic DA levels within DA terminal fields, presumably by exciting DA neurones in their cell body regions (Gysling and Wang, 1983; Matthews and German, 1984; see Section 6.3.2a), although local interactions at the level of the terminal fields may also play a role in morphine-induced DA release (Chesselet *et al.*, 1981; Iyengar *et al.*, 1989; see Chapter 7). The increase in extracellular DA levels produced by morphine is considerably less than that produced by amphetamine or cocaine (Di Chiara and Imperato, 1988), a finding which is not surprising since DA released by morphine, but not amphetamine or cocaine, would be subject to DA reuptake. Recent *in vivo* voltammetry experiments suggest that, due to the efficiency of the DA uptake mechanism, DA neurones need to be stimulated to fire at least three to four times faster than their basal rate (4–5 Hz) before increases in synaptic DA become detectable (Wightman and Zimmerman, 1990).

Recent *in vivo* microdialysis studies have sought to determine whether there are regional differences in the ability of amphetamine, cocaine and other psychomotor stimulants to increase extracellular concentrations of DA. Di Chiara and Imperato (1988) have argued that these and other drugs of abuse produce larger increases in extracellular DA levels in the nucleus accumbens (NAc) than the dorsal striatum, suggesting that preferential increases in mesolimbic DA turnover might be a fundamental property of drugs of abuse. However, Robinson and Camp (1990) have not observed preferential increases in extracellular DA levels in the NAc after systemic amphetamine administration, although they suggest that amphetamine might selectively influence mesolimbic DA activity through other mechanisms.

6.3 Psychomotor stimulant reward

6.3.1 Anatomy and pharmacology of reward

There is now abundant evidence that the rewarding properties of both the psychomotor stimulants and the opioids involve central DA-containing neuronal systems (Koob and Bloom, 1988; Wise and Rompre, 1989; Wise and Bozarth, 1987). Initial support for an involvement of DA was provided by the finding that DA receptor antagonists attenuate the rewarding effects of psychomotor stimulants (de Wit and Wise, 1977; Ettenberg *et al.*, 1982; Pettit *et al.*, 1984) and heroin (Bozarth and Wise, 1981; Spyraki *et al.*, 1983) (however, also see Ettenberg *et al.* (1982)). In addition, direct DA receptor agonists such as apomorphine and bromocriptine possess rewarding properties (Baxter *et al.*, 1974; Wise *et al.*, 1990; Woolverton *et al.*, 1984a; Yokel and Wise, 1978).

More precise anatomical and pharmacological manipulations identified the ventral tegmental area (VTA)–NAc dopaminergic pathway (meso-accumbens DA system) as being particularly important to psychomotor stimulant and opiate reward processes. Intravenous self-administration of cocaine is antagonized by infusion of the D_2 DA antagonist spiroperidol into the NAc, but not into the dorsal striatum, i.e. caudate-putamen (Phillips *et al.*, 1983a), the primary recipient of DA afferents from the substantia nigra. In addition, 6-OHDA lesions of DA neurones directed either at terminals within the NAc or at somata within the VTA attenuate the rewarding effects of amphetamine and cocaine (Lyness *et al.*, 1979; Roberts and Koob, 1982; Roberts *et al.*, 1977, 1980; Pettit *et al.*, 1984). Such lesions of the nigro-striatal DA system are ineffective. Similar effects of mesoaccumbens 6-OHDA lesions on opiate self-administration have been reported by some investigators (Phillips *et al.*, 1983b; Spyraki *et al.*, 1983) but not by others (Pettit *et al.*, 1984). Excitotoxin lesions of intrinsic neurones within the NAc block the rewarding effects of cocaine, apomorphine and heroin (Pettit *et al.*, 1984; Zito *et al.*, 1985), indicating that neurones postsynaptic to DA terminals are essential for self-administration of psychomotor stimulants. Finally, rats will self-administer amphetamine and morphine directly into the NAc (Hoebel *et al.*, 1983; Olds, 1982) and will work for direct injections of heroin or opioid peptides into the VTA (Bozarth and Wise, 1981).

The mesocortical DA system, in particular the VTA–medial prefrontal cortex (mPFC) projection, has also been implicated in the rewarding actions of cocaine. Direct infusions of cocaine into the mPFC, but not the NAc or VTA, will support self-administration in rats (Goeders and Smith, 1983), an effect which is blocked by co-infusion of the selective D_2 DA antagonist sulpiride (Goeders *et al.*, 1986). In addition, 6-OHDA lesions of DA terminals in the mPFC reduce self-administration of cocaine, but not DA, into this site (Goeders *et al.*, 1986). However, 6-OHDA lesions of the mPFC fail to block systemic self-administration of cocaine (Martin-Iverson *et al.*, 1986). To our knowledge, similar studies of amphetamine and opiates have not been conducted within the mPFC.

This contrasting evidence regarding the site at which cocaine exerts its rewarding effects has led to the proposal that the NAc and mPFC may play distinct roles in the process of cocaine reinforcement. The fact that rats will self-administer cocaine into the mPFC, but not the NAc, suggests that the mPFC may be involved in initiating the reinforcing effect of cocaine, whereas the NAc may be indirectly activated within the reward pathway and play an integral role in maintaining self-administration behaviour (Goeders *et al.*, 1986). This would explain why 6-OHDA lesions of the NAc in rats that had already established responding for systemic cocaine would disrupt the behaviour, whereas similar lesions of the mPFC would not.

6.3.2 Neurophysiology of reward

In addition to increasing DA transmission in DA terminal fields, amphetamine and cocaine also trigger compensatory decreases in DA neuronal activity by acting as indirect DA agonists at both somatodendritic autoreceptors and postsynaptic DA receptors on neurones involved in long-loop inhibitory feedback pathways. It would be predicted that the extent to which these compensatory mechanisms are successful in attenuating stimulant-induced increases in DA transmission would depend on the extent to which the effects of a particular stimulant are dependent on neuronal activity. As described in the following sections, electrophysiological studies have confirmed this hypothesis and provided considerable insight into the mechanisms by which psychomotor stimulants alter DA neuronal activity after both acute and repeated administration.

6.3.2.1 Dopamine neurones

In anaesthetized rats, intravenouly (i.v.) administered amphetamine causes a dose-dependent, DA antagonist-reversible suppression (ED_{50} values generally between 0.5 and 1.0 mg/kg) of the firing of VTA A10 DA neurones (Bunney *et al.*, 1973; Kamata and Rebec, 1984; Wang, 1981; White and Wang, 1984b). Using antidromic stimulation techniques to identify the projection sites of midbrain DA neurones, various investigators have demonstrated that amphetamine inhibits the firing of both mesoaccumbens and mesocortical DA neurones (Clark and Chiodo, 1988; Wang, 1981; White and Wang, 1984a, b), although the effect on mesocortical cells requires higher doses (ED_{50} value = 1.5 mg/kg), due to the fact that these neurones typically exhibit higher basal firing rates (White and Wang, 1984a).

In contrast to DA neurones within the substantia nigra, upon which amphetamine exerts inhibitory effects by both local autoreceptor and long-loop (striatonigral) feedback mechanisms (Bunney and Aghajanian, 1978; Groves *et al.*, 1975), the inhibition of mesoaccumbens and mesocortical DA neurones by amphetamine appears to involve only autoreceptor activation. Thus, excitotoxin lesions of the NAc or hemotransections rostral to the midbrain DA neurones fail to reduce the inhibitory effects of amphetamine on VTA DA neurones (Wang, 1981; White *et al.*, 1987). Furthermore, local administration of amphetamine to DA neurones by microiontophoresis results in considerably greater inhibition of VTA as compared to nigral DA neurones (Wang *et al.*, 1984). The inhibitory effects of amphetamine are not due to direct receptor stimulation but involve activation of autoreceptors by endogenous DA released by amphetamine. Thus, acute DA depletion produced by the tyrosine hydroxylase inhibitor α-methyl-*p*-tyrosine, in combination with reserpine, completely prevents the ability of systemic amphetamine to inhibit A10 DA cells (Wang *et al.*, 1984).

Cocaine also causes a dose-dependent ($ED_{50} = 0.75$ mg/kg) inhibition of the activity of antidromically identified mesoaccumbens DA neurones within the rat VTA (Einhorn *et al.*, 1988; White *et al.*, 1987). However, unlike amphetamine and most other DA agonists, cocaine-induced inhibition is usually only partial in that the maximal inhibition (at sub-lethal dose) seldom exceeds 70% of the basal firing rate. Thus, although the potencies of amphetamine and cocaine are similar, amphetamine is considerably more efficacious. In addition, the duration of amphetamine-induced inhibition (Clark and Chiodo, 1988) is considerably longer than that produced by cocaine (Einhorn *et al.*, 1988). The effect of cocaine on A10 DA cells is not due to its ability to inhibit the uptake of 5-HT or noradrenaline, since selective inhibitors of these transporters fail to mimic the effects of cocaine (Einhorn *et al.*, 1988). Likewise, the effect of cocaine cannot be attributed to its known local anaesthetic action since procaine and lidocaine, which are local anaesthetics possessing little to no psychomotor stimulant efficacy, fail to inhibit A10 DA cells. Thus, it is likely that the ability of cocaine to partially suppress the firing of VTA DA neurones results from blockade of the DA transporter and consequent increases in the level of DA available to interact with DA receptors. Support for this conclusion was obtained by demonstrating that haloperidol reversed the inhibition of A10 DA neurones produced by cocaine (Einhorn *et al.*, 1988). The effect of cocaine is dependent upon endogenous DA since it is attenuated by acute DA depletion (Einhorn *et al.*, 1988; White, 1990).

Microiontophoretic studies indicate that cocaine only weakly inhibits DA neurones following local application to the VTA, an effect that can be blocked by iontophoretic administration of the D_2 receptor antagonist sulpiride (Einhorn *et al.*, 1988). Simultaneous iontophoretic administration of cocaine and DA significantly enhances the inhibitory effects of DA, indicating further that cocaine acts by blocking the uptake of DA within the VTA (Einhorn *et al.*, 1988). The relatively weak effects of local, as compared to systemic, cocaine administration suggest that systemic cocaine might inhibit A10 DA neuronal activity by a mechanism besides potentiation of DA autoreceptor activation. In fact, unlike the effects of amphetamine, the inhibition of A10 DA cells by cocaine appears to involve a NAc–VTA negative feedback pathway. Thus, both excitotoxin lesions of the NAc and acute hemitransections significantly attenuate the partial inhibitory effects of cocaine on A10 DA neurones (Einhorn *et al.*, 1988). The difference between amphetamine and cocaine was postulated (White *et al.*, 1991) to involve the greater extracellular concentrations of DA within the VTA produced by amphetamine-induced DA release as compared to cocaine-induced uptake inhibition as recently confirmed with microdialysis techniques (Kalivas *et al.*, 1989; Bradberry and Roth, 1989). Accordingly, it was hypothesized that effects of the NAc–VTA feedback pathway are only observable (i.e. not redundant) when autoreceptor-induced inhibition of A10 DA neurones is incomplete (Einhorn *et al.*, 1988; White *et al.*, 1987).

Antidromically identified mesocortical DA neurones exhibit little to no inhibition following systemic cocaine administration (White *et al.*, 1987; White, 1990). This reduced responsiveness of mesocortical, as compared to mesoaccumbens, DA neurones is not surprising given the relative paucity of impulse-regulating somatodendritic autoreceptors on mesocortical DA neurones and their higher basal firing rate (Chiodo *et al.*, 1984; White and Wang, 1984a). In view of the fact that a feedback projection seems instrumental in mediating the effects of cocaine on mesoaccumbens DA neurones, the lack of effect of this stimulant on mesocortical DA cells might also indicate the lack of a similar long-loop regulatory system from the mPFC to the VTA. In fact, there is evidence that such a pathway does exist but is primarily excitatory (aspartate) in nature, unlike the inhibitory GABAergic NAc–VTA projection (Christie *et al.*, 1985); see White (1991) for further discussion.

In contrast to amphetamine and cocaine, systemic administration of morphine increases the firing of A10 DA neurones within the VTA (Gysling and Wang, 1983; Matthews and German, 1984). Morphine therefore differs from these agents in that it produces stimulatory effects on DA transmission without invoking compensatory autoregulatory processes to decrease DA cell firing. As with the decreases in cell firing observed with amphetamine, cocaine and other DA agonists (White and Wang, 1984c), the increases observed with morphine are dependent upon basal firing rate, with slower cells responding more robustly (Gysling and Wang, 1983). Comparative studies in anaesthetized and paralysed rats indicate that anaesthesia dampens the responsiveness of A10 DA neurones to morphine (Matthews and German, 1984). The opioid antagonist naloxone readily reverses morphine-induced excitation (Gysling and Wang, 1983; Matthews and German, 1984). Iontophoretic administration of morphine also enhances the firing of A10 DA cells (Gysling and Wang, 1983; Matthews and German, 1984). Non-DA neurones within the VTA are potently inhibited by either systemic or local morphine in a naloxone-sensitivie manner (Gysling and Wang, 1983). This last finding led Gysling and Wang (1983) to speculate that the increases in DA unit activity were indirectly mediated by a loss of inhibition typically provided by the non-DA cells within the VTA. Intracellular studies support this notion since opioids fail to affect DA cells but hyperpolarize and inhibit the activity of non-DA neurones (Lacey *et al.*, 1989).

6.3.2.2 Nucleus accumbens neurones

Systemic administration of either amphetamine (Rebec and Zimmerman, 1980) or cocaine (White, 1990; White *et al.*, 1987) suppresses the firing of

NAc neurones in anaesthetized rats. To date, careful dose–response studies of amphetamine effects of NAc neurones have not been reported. As for cocaine, i.v. administration inhibits NAc neurones with a similar potency ($ED_{50} = 0.67$) to that obtained with A10 DA cells ($ED_{50} = 0.71$). However, cocaine is much more effective at inhibiting NAc neurones as compared to mesoaccumbens A10 DA cells (Figure 1). These inhibitory effects of cocaine on NAc neurones are reversed by both D_1 and D_2 selective antagonists, although D_1 DA receptor antagonists are both more potent and efficacious than D_2 antagonists (White, 1990).

NAc neurones, like their neighbours in the dorsal striatum (Nisenbaum *et al.*, 1988; Skirboll and Bunney, 1979), can be divided into at least two subtypes, based primarily on their extracellular waveform (White *et al.*, 1987). The majority of NAc neurones exhibit a negative–positive waveform, are seldom spontaneously active and are typically inhibited by 5-HT. These cells are

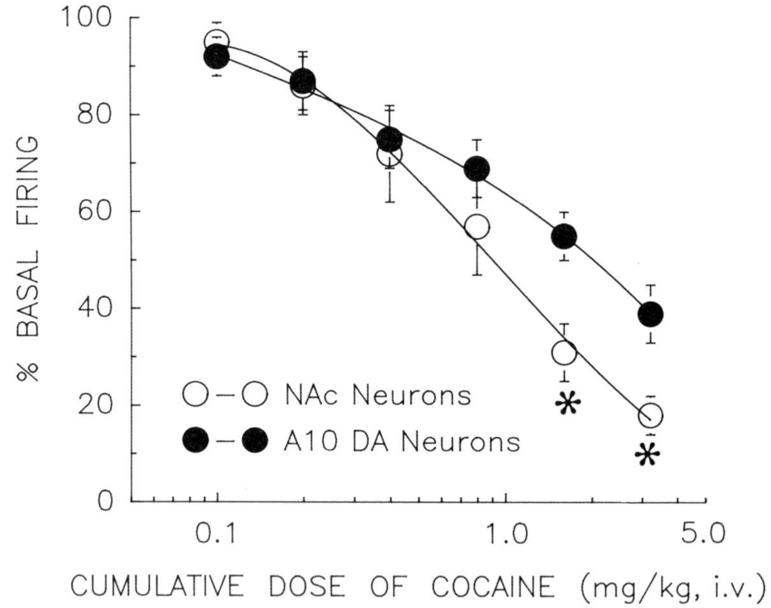

Figure 1 Comparison of the inhibitory effects of i.v. cocaine on A10 dopamine (DA) neurones in the rat ventral tegmental area and on neurones within the rat nucleus accumbens (NAc). Cocaine was administered to chloral hydrate-anaesthetized rats in a cumulative dose regimen in which each dose doubled the previous dose. Injections were separated by 60–90 s. Each point represents the mean ± SEM for 8 A10 DA cells and 12 NAc neurones. Asterisks represent the doses at which cocaine was more effective at inhibiting NAc neurones as compared to A10 DA neurones ($p < 0.01$).

referred to as type I NAc cells. In contrast, type II NAc neurones exhibit positive–negative waveforms, are more often spontaneously active and are usually excited by 5-HT. To study quiescent NAc neurones, iontophoretic administration of the excitatory amino acid glutamate is typically used to 'drive' cellular activity.

When applied locally to NAc cells by microiontophoresis, cocaine inhibits neuronal firing (Qiao *et al.*, 1990; White, 1990; White *et al.*, 1987). Low sub-inhibitory currents of cocaine also markedly potentiate the rate-suppressant effects of DA on NAc neurones. As with i.v. administration, the inhibitory effects of iontophoretic cocaine on NAc cells are blocked by either D_1 (White *et al.*, 1987) or D_2 selective antagonists (Qiao *et al.*, 1990; White *et al.*, 1987). When type I and II NAc neurones are compared, cocaine is considerably more potent on type I cells (White *et al.*, 1987). In contrast, DA is equipotent at inhibiting the two subtypes of NAc cells. Cocaine is less potent than DA at inhibiting type II NAc cells but is more potent than DA on type I NAc cells (White, 1990; White *et al.*, 1987).

This latter finding might be related to the differential effect of 5-HT on type I (inhibitory) and II (excitatory) NAc neurones (White *et al.*, 1987). Since cocaine inhibits the reuptake of 5-HT, it is possible that enhanced activation of both DA and 5-HT receptors might account for the potent inhibition of type I NAc neurones. On the other hand, since most type II neurones are typically excited by iontophoretic 5-HT, the effect of cocaine on 5-HT uptake would oppose the simultaneous inhibitory action of DA. This hypothesis was supported by the finding that combined administration of the selective DA uptake inhibitor GBR 12909 and the selective 5-HT uptake blocker fluoxetine was necessary to achieve the degree of inhibition of type I NAc cells typically observed with cocaine alone (White *et al.*, 1987). In addition, GBR 12909 was slightly more effective than cocaine at inhibiting type II NAc neurones whereas fluoxetine produced small excitatory effects (White, 1990). Thus, the potent inhibitory effects of cocaine on type I NAc neurones reflects simultaneous potentiation of both DA- and 5-HT-mediated inhibition while the weaker inhibition of type II neurones results from competing inhibitory and excitatory influences of DA and 5-HT, respectively (White *et al.*, 1987).

As noted above, cocaine is much more effective at inhibiting NAc neurones than mesoaccumbens A10 DA neurones when administered systemically. Similarly, iontophoretic cocaine inhibits NAc neurones to a much greater extent than A10 DA neurones (Figure 2). This is in contrast to results obtained with directly acting DA agonissts in that A10 DA cells are typically much more sensitive than NAc neurones, presumably due to the greater sensitivity of D_2 autoreceptors as compared to postsynaptic D_2 receptors (White and Wang, 1986; White *et al.*, 1987). It has been suggested (White, 1990) that

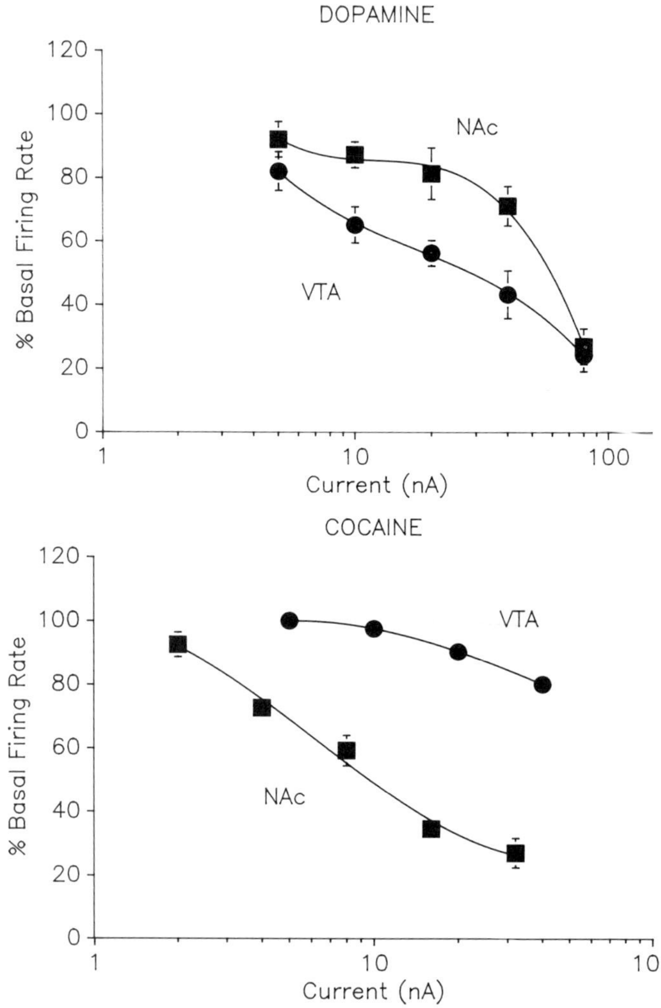

Figure 2 Comparison of the effects of both DA and cocaine, administered iontophoretically, on nucleus accumbens (NAc) neurones and A10 DA neurones in the rat ventral tegmental area (VTA). Both type I and type II neurones are included in the NAc data. Note that while DA is more potent on A10 DA neurones, cocaine is more potent on NAc neurones. Adapted from White (1990) with permission.

this apparent discrepancy might be due to greater concentrations of DA released by nerve terminals as compared to dendrites (Kalivas *et al.*, 1989). Thus, inhibition of DA reuptake in the NAc would probably have greater functional consequences than inhibiting the reuptake of DA in the VTA.

Microdialysis studies support this hypothesis since i.v. cocaine results in a maximal increase in extracellular DA levels of 300% in the NAc as compared to a 180% increase in the VTA (Bradberry and Roth, 1989). However, because basal extracellular DA levels are considerably higher in the NAc than the VTA, it seems unlikely that a relatively small difference in the percentage increase in DA levels in response to cocaine can completely account for the greater sensitivity of postsynaptic DA receptors. An alternative hypothesis might involve differences between the NAc and the VTA with respect to the proximity of uptake sites to the relevant DA receptors.

Systemic (s.c.) administration of morphine and heroin produces heterogeneous effects on NAc neurones, including excitation, inhibition and no effect (Hakan and Henriksen, 1987). In contrast, microinjections of morphine into the VTA uniformly inhibit NAc neurones (Hakan and Henriksen, 1989), an effect which is at least partially reversed by DA antagonists, suggesting mediation via activation of DA firing. In addition, iontophoretic administration of morphine and enkephalin analogues inhibits both spontaneously active NAc neurones and cells driven to fire by iontophoretic administration of excitatory amino acids (Hakan and Henriksen, 1989). The mixed effects of systemic opioids on NAc activity appear to be mediated by opposing effects on NAc neurones and on other afferents to the NAc, such as the hippocampus (Hakan *et al.*, 1989).

Taken together, these findings suggest that a common mechanism of psychomotor stimulant and opiate action involves inhibition of NAc neurones. Amphetamine and cocaine do so by acting at the DA transporter to elevate synaptic DA levels in the NAc. Morphine also appears to exert its inhibitory effects on NAc neurones via elevation of synaptic DA levels in the NAc, although it appears to do so indirectly via actions on DA neuronal activity within the VTA. A common mechanism of action involving inhibition of NAc neurones is consistent with the well-documented role of NAc projection neurones in mediating locomotor responses (Mogenson and Yim, 1991; Pulvirenti *et al.*, 1991).

6.3.2.3 Medial prefrontal cortex neurones

Preliminary studies within the rat mPFC have indicated that cocaine inhibits the firing of neurones within layers V and VI and that, like the NAc, both DA and 5-HT mechanisms may be involved (White, 1990). Iontophoretic application of cocaine onto glutamate-driven single cells within the mPFC produces a partial inhibition of activity. The effect of iontophoretic cocaine on mPFC cells is less pronounced than that observed within the NAc. This differential effectiveness may be related to the fact that cocaine causes larger increases in synaptic DA within the NAc as compared to the mPFC

(Moghaddam and Bunney, 1989). As with NAc neurones, 5-HT mechanisms may also play a role in cocaine's effects on mPFC cells (White, 1990). Thus, cocaine potentiates the inhibitory effects of both DA and 5-HT. Similar pharmacological studies of amphetamine and morphine within the mPFC have not been reported.

6.3.3 Psychomotor stimulants and DA transmission

Although it is clear that the rewarding effects of psychomotor stimulants involve enhanced transmission in the mesoaccumbens and mesocortical DA systems, any comprehensive theory as to the precise neuronal mechanisms responsible for reward must take into account the fact that directly acting DA agonists, which also enhance DA transmission, are not serious drugs of abuse, despite mild reinforcing effects in animals (Section 6.3.1). Thus, the psychomotor stimulants (including opioids) must differ from direct DA agonists in some fundamental way with respect to their overall effects on DA neurotransmission. One such difference may be that direct DA agonists produce untoward side-effects (e.g. emesis) not shared by the psychomotor stimulants. Another possibility is that psychomotor stimulants differ from directly acting DA agonists in that postsynaptic DA receptor stimulation by the latter class of drugs is provided by endogenous DA. Exogenous agonists may have access to DA receptors which are not normally stimulated by endogenous DA and may have effects at non-DA receptors not normally influenced by DA.

6.3.3.1 Effects on compensatory mechanisms in DA neurones

Another important aspect of the action of psychomotor stimulants is the extent to which they trigger compensatory autoregulatory processes in DA neurones that may serve to offset their stimulatory effect on DA transmission. It must first be appreciated that, although apparently contradictory, the *decrease* of firing of mesoaccumbens A10 DA cells produced by cocaine and amphetamine is, in fact, consistent with the hypothesis that enhanced DA transmission is involved in reward mechanisms. Amphetamine- and cocaine-induced decreases in firing rate represent a compensatory, homeostatic response to enhanced DA neurotransmission within the primary target site of these cells, the NAc. However, as will be discussed below, the compensatory processes induced by psychostimulants are relatively weak in comparison with their overall stimulatory effects on DA transmission within the NAc. It is argued that this may account for their rewarding properties as well as many of the changes in DA transmission that accompany their repeated administration.

As described in Section 6.3.2.2, cocaine is more effective at suppressing the firing of postsynaptic cells within the NAc than inhibiting the DA cells themselves. This is presumably due to an additive potentiation of DA and 5-HT effects on the majority of NAc cells. By inhibiting NAc neurones, cocaine also activates long-loop feedback inhibitory processes which serve to decrease the firing rate of DA neurones. Yet even the combination of somatodendritic autoreceptor stimulation and long-loop feedback regulation is apparently insufficient to suppress DA cell firing completely. Thus, the net effect of cocaine on the mesoaccumbens DA system is an initial increase in synaptic levels of DA within the NAc, as a result of blocking DA uptake, followed by continued impulse-dependent release of DA, as a result of incomplete suppression of neuronal activity. In summary, cocaine causes considerable enhancement of mesoaccumbens DA neurotransmission due to the relatively poor compensatory response of DA cells and the resulting build-up of synaptic DA.

Unlike cocaine, amphetamine produces a total inhibition of DA unit activity. However, the resulting decrease in impulse-dependent DA release within the NAc does not prevent the DA-releasing effects of amphetamine, which are independent of impulse flow (Section 6.2). Similarly, since amphetamine-induced DA release is not under the control of release-modulating nerve terminal autoreceptors, stimulation of nerve terminal autoreceptors by increased synaptic DA levels does not alter the releasing effects of amphetamine. Thus, despite compensatory decreases in DA neuronal activity, DA release continues unabated following amphetamine administration.

Amphetamine and cocaine are even less effective at inhibiting the firing rate of mesocortical DA cells than mesoaccumbens DA cells. Two factors may account for this: (1) the relative paucity of somatodendritic autoreceptors on mesocortical DA neurones (Chiodo *et al.*, 1984; White and Wang, 1984a); (2) differences in the efficacy of long-loop feedback pathways (White, 1991). Thus, enhanced DA release within cortical terminal fields may be even less well compensated by diminished impulse flow than is the case for the mesoaccumbens DA projection. Whether this is related to the postulated role of the mPFC in initiating reward processes is an important question for future research.

In contrast to amphetamine and cocaine, opiates and other compounds with rewarding properties (e.g. nicotine, ethanol) increase A10 unit firing. The ability of morphine to stimulate mesoaccumbens DA cells leads to enhanced release of DA within the NAc (Di Chiara and Imperato, 1988), and, in general, an inhibition of NAc neuronal activity (Hakan and Henriksen, 1987; Hakan *et al.*, 1989). Morphine may also directly inhibit NAc neurones by stimulating μ-type opioid receptors within the NAc (Hakan and Henriksen, 1989). Thus, morphine acts to inhibit NAc neurones through both dopaminergic and non-dopaminergic mechanisms, resulting in an even greater effect on the activity of NAc projection neurones than would be obtained from DA receptor stimulation alone. Moreover, morphine seems to do so without activating many of the compensatory processes which result from cocaine or amphetamine administration. Because of long-loop NAc–VTA feedback, the inhibition of NAc cells should activate (i.e. disinhibit) inhibitory, GABAergic interneurones within the VTA and thereby compensate for enhanced DA transmission within the NAc by shutting down A10 DA neurones. Yet this does not occur. Although the reasons for a lack of compensation are unknown, it is likely that the direct inhibitory effects of morphine on the VTA interneurones (Gysling and Wang, 1983; Lacey *et al.*, 1989) override the disinhibition produced by the NAc–VTA pathway. Thus, DA neurones remain activated. This model would explain why opioids which are μ-receptor agonists would greatly activate the mesoaccumbens DA system, i.e. they might override homeostatic mechanisms which would normally compensate for enhanced DA transmission within the NAc.

To summarize, the hypothesis being presented here is that psychomotor stimulants and perhaps other drugs of abuse derive their rewarding properties from their ability to enhance DA transmission through the mesoaccumbens and mesocortical DA systems in the presence of weak or absent compensatory decreases in DAergic activity. This is similar to the hypothesis of Di Chiara and Imperato (1988), who argued that a common feature of all drugs of abuse is their ability to increase preferentially synaptic concentrations of DA within the NAc. The present hypothesis extends that of Di Chiara and Imperato (1988) by placing additional emphasis on the effects of synaptic DA on its receptors and the overall change in activity within the DA systems. Other important contributions would include the extent to which NAc neurones possessing relevant DA receptors are receiving other inputs and the interactions between enhanced DA receptor occupation and information flow through the NAc (Mogenson and Yim, 1991).

6.4 Effects of repeated psychomotor stimulant administration: sensitization

Psychomotor stimulant dependence is, by definition, a problem of long-term, compulsive drug self-administration. Therefore, elucidation of the neurobiological effects of repeated psychomotor stimulant administration is essential for understanding drug dependence. One of the fundamental principles of pharmacology is that the effects of drugs may change when they are administered repeatedly. With respect to the psychomotor stimulants, such changes can be categorized into two distinct, and opposite, types. Tolerance refers to the reduced efficacy of a given dose of a drug following repeated administration. Tolerance has long been studied within the contact of physical dependence and withdrawal and is often an important determinant of persistent drug use, particularly with the opioids (Koob and Bloom, 1988). In direct opposition to tolerance is *sensitization*, or 'reverse tolerance', in which the effects of a drug actually increase following repeated administration (Robinson and Becker, 1986). Of particular interest is the fact that sensitized drug effects can be quite persistent, even permanent, under appropriate conditions of psychomotor stimulant administration. In the second half of this chapter, we will focus on the neuronal mechanisms which have been hypothesized to underly stimulant-induced sensitization. Because this area has recently been extensively reviewed (Robinson and Becker, 1986) our approach will be to review the more recent literature, establish accepted neurobiological correlates of sensitization and attempt to integrate newer hypotheses into a coherent perspective.

Behavioural sensitization has most often been studied with repeated amphetamine administration, although, in recent years, a substantial literature has evolved from studies of other stimulants, notably cocaine and morphine. Augmentation of stimulant-induced behaviour is most often studied in rats and is typically quantified as increased horizontal or vertical locomotion and induction of repetitive stereotyped sniffing, licking and gnawing. During repeated intermittent injections of a constant dose of stimulants, these behaviours become progressively enhanced. The intermittent nature of the administration schedule is crucial since continuous administration of the drug fails to produce sensitization to a subsequent challenge (Robinson and Becker, 1986). A number of other variables impact upon the expression of sensitization and the degree to which it persists. It is beyond the scope of the present discussion to enumerate all of these in detail. The interested reader should refer to Robinson and Becker (1986). However, it is important to note that the expression of sensitization is dependent upon the number of injections, the time interval between injections, the age and sex of the animal and the withdrawal period following drug discontinuation. One other variable which has received little attention, but which may have a large impact on the phenomenon, is the extent to which drug administration is controlled by the investigator or the animal (i.e. self-administration). Given the potential importance of this variable to human drug abuse, it is likely that it will receive significant attention in future studies.

6.4.1 Anatomy of sensitization

Several investigators have utilized intracerebral microinjection techniques in an effort to localize the brain sites involved in the development of behavioural sensitization. The mesoaccumbens DA system is known to be primarily involved in the locomotor stimulating effects of psychomotor stimulants. Direct microinjection of DA and DA agonists into the nucleus accumbens elicits locomotor activity (for review see Kelly, 1977). However, early studies indicated that the locomotor activity elicited by microinjections of amphetamine into the NAc was not increased following repeated administration to this area

(Dougherty and Ellinwood, 1981; Hitzemann *et al.*, 1980). Similar results were obtained with opiates (Vezina *et al.*, 1987). Later studies have confirmed this finding and also demonstrated that repeated injections of amphetamine or opioids into the NAc fail to sensitize rats to subsequent systemic injections of these agents (Kalivas and Weber, 1988; Vezina and Stewart, 1990). Thus, although the NAc is an essential structure for the locomotor stimulating effects of psychostimulants, drug actions in this area are not sufficient to produce sensitization.

In contrast, it appears that the VTA may play an important role in the initiation of sensitization to psychomotor stimulants. Repeated microinjections of amphetamine into the VTA result in sensitization to the locomotor stimulating effects observed in response to systemic administration of this drug (Kalivas and Weber, 1988). Moreover, sensitized responses are also observed when these rats are pretreated with intra-VTA amphetamine and challenged with systemic cocaine (Kalivas and Weber, 1988) or morphine (Vezina and Stewart, 1990). This is despite the fact that intra-VTA injections of amphetamine fail to elicit locomotion. Repeated injections of opioids into the VTA also produce sensitization to the acute stimulating effects of such treatment (Joyce and Iversen, 1979; Kalivas, 1985; Vezina and Stewart, 1984). Taken together, these findings indicate that alterations of neuronal activity within the VTA are essential for the initiation of behavioural sensitization. In addition, they suggest that the mechanisms responsible for sensitization are, to some extent, independent of the actual production of locomotor activity.

6.4.2 Pharmacology of sensitization and conditioned locomotion

6.4.2.1 Pharmacology of sensitization

Attempts to characterize the pharmacology of sensitization have primarily employed DA receptor blockers. Early studies using non-selective DA antagonists indicated that pretreatment with haloperidol prevented the development of amphetamine sensitization (Kuczenski and Leith, 1981). More recent studies which have employed selective D_2 DA receptor antagonists have produced somewhat inconsistent results. Ujike *et al.* (1989) reported that the D_2 selective antagonist YM-09151-2 completely prevented the development of sensitization to methamphetamine. In contrast, several groups have found that D_2 DA receptor antagonists do not block sensitization. For example, Gale (1984) reported that the D_2 selective antagonist droperidol failed to prevent cocaine sensitization. Similarly, Vezina and Stewart (1989) reported that the D_2 selective antagonists Ro22-2586 and sulpiride, at doses which blocked the acute locomotor stimulating effects of either systemic amphetamine or intra-VTA morphine, failed to block sensitization to repeated administration of these agents. Pimozide, another purported selective D_2 antagonist, blocked the development of sensitization to intra-VTA morphine, but not to systemic amphetamine (Vezina and Stewart, 1989). These authors argued that the pimozide–morphine interaction may have been due to depolarization inactivation of A10 DA cells produced by overexcitation of the neurones. The results for discrepancies in the literature regarding the ability of D_2 antagonists to block sensitization remain unclear.

Unlike the situation with D_2 antagonists, there is near uniform agreement regarding the ability of the D_1 selective antagonist SCH 23390 to prevent the development of sensitization to amphetamine. This D_1 receptor blocker prevents the development of sensitization to both methamphetamine (Ujike *et al.*, 1989) and *d*-amphetamine (Drew and Glick, 1990; Vezina and Stewart, 1989). However, SCH 23390 failed to block the development of sensitization to intra-VTA morphine (Vezina and Stewart, 1989).

In a study of considerable potential importance, Stewart and Vezina (1989) recently observed that intra-VTA microinjections of SCH 23390 blocked sensitization to systemic amphetamine injections. Thus, these authors argued that a critical event in the development of sensitization to amphetamine is an alteration in the activation of D_1 DA receptors by endogenous DA released from the dendrites of midbrain DA cells. Unfortunately, we currently have no idea as to the functional roles of D_1 receptors within the VTA. In fact, there is some controversy about their existence. Receptor autoradiographic analyses using radiolabelled SCH 23390 have reported that D_1 receptors are moderate (Mansour *et al.*, 1990), sparse (Boyson *et al.*, 1986; Dawson *et al.*, 1986; Dubois *et al.*, 1986; Savasta *et al.*, 1986) or absent (Altar and Hauser, 1987) within the VTA. In addition, neither DA-stimulated adenylate cyclase nor DARPP-32 (dopamine and adenylate cyclase related phosphorotein), both markers for D_1 receptors, have been detected in the area (Beart and McDonald, 1980; Lorez and Burkard, 1979; Walaas and Greengard, 1984). Certainly VTA DA neurones do not possess D_1 receptors (Mansour *et al.*, 1990; Wachtel *et al.*, 1989; White and Wang, 1984b). In light of these inconsistent reports and recent electrophysiological studies showing that local administration of SCH 23390 inactivates midbrain DA neurones in a brain slice preparation (Suppes and Pinnock, 1987), there is need for caution in interpreting the findings of Stewart and Vezina (1989). Certainly, additional studies are needed to determine whether the effect observed by Stewart and Vezina (1989) resulted from D_1 receptor antagonism or from other, perhaps local anaesthetic-like effects on neuronal activity.

While stimulation of DA receptors appears necessary for the *development* of behavioural sensitization, this may not be the case for the *expression* of sensitization. Thus, haloperidol does not block the expression of sensitization when administered to amphetamine-sensitized animals prior to a challenge dose of amphetamine (Kuribara *et al.*, 1986). Similarly, haloperidol does not block the expression of sensitization in the one-day high-dose cocaine sensitization paradigm (Post *et al.*, 1991). This may suggest that sensitization results in lasting changes in the brain that are subsequently able to influence behavioural responses to psychostimulants even when DA receptors are blocked.

6.4.2.2 Pharmacology of conditioned locomotion

It is well known that the behavioural activating effects of amphetamine and other psychostimulants are controlled by environmental stimuli and that repeated pairing of psychostimulant administration with a particular set of environmental stimuli can result in the production of locomotion by exposure to the stimuli alone (Stewart and Vezina, 1988). This is known as conditioned locomotion, and is studied by administering repeated injections of a psychostimulant and then measuring locomotion on a subsequent test day when animals are placed in the testing environment without drug. The relationship between conditioned locomotion and behavioural sensitization is complex; see Stewart and Vezina (1988) and Martin-Iversen and McManus (1990) for discussion. However, it should be noted that conditioning alone cannot account for the phenomenon of behavioural sensitization (Robinson and Becker, 1986).

It has been reported that pimozide blocks the development of conditioned locomotion resulting from repeated pairing of amphetamine or cocaine administration with a particular test environment (Beninger and Hahn, 1983; Beninger and Herz, 1986). Results obtained with haloperidol in a one-day high-dose cocaine sensitization paradigm may support this conclusion (Post *et al.*, 1991). In contrast to these findings, a more recent report suggests that DA receptor stimulation may not be required for the development of conditioned locomotion. In this study, both SCH 23390 and haloperidol, as well as the combination of both drugs, failed to block the development of amphetamine-conditioned locomotion (Martin-Iverson and McManus, 1990). These results suggest that the establishment of conditioned locomotion may involve different neurochemical events than the establishment of behavioural sensitization. Different mechanisms are also suggested by the observation that pimozide blocks the development of amphetamine-conditioned locomotion even though most investigators find that it fails to block the development of behavioural sensitization to amphetamine (see above). This issue deserves further examination, since environmental stimuli clearly play an important role in drug-taking behaviour (Stewart *et al.*, 1984).

It remains unclear whether DA antagonists prevent the *expression* of conditioned locomotion when administered on the saline test day. Pimozide pretreatment did not alter the expression of environment-specific conditioned locomotion induced by repeated administration of cocaine (Beninger and Herz, 1986) or amphetamine (Beninger and Hahn, 1983). In contrast, another study reported that haloperidol and sulpiride blocked the expression of amphetamine-conditioned locomotion over the same range of doses effective at blocking unconditioned locomotor stimulatory effects of amphetamine; for pimozide, however, higher doses were required to block the expression of conditioned locomotion than unconditioned locomotion (Poncelet *et al.*, 1987). However, the doses of pimozide which blocked the expression of conditioned locomotion in this study were almost identical to the dose reported to be ineffective by Beninger and Hahn (1983).

6.4.3 Neurochemistry of sensitization

Both the behavioural and neurochemical changes which accompany behavioural sensitization to amphetamine and other psychostimulants are extremely complex. Kuzcenski and Segal (1988) have pointed out that it is incorrect to view sensitization merely as a shift to the left in the dose–response curve for psychostimulants. Particularly with respect to amphetamine, which has been most thoroughly studied, behavioural responses to repeated administration include components of both tolerance and sensitization and are unlikely to be explained by a single neurochemical change. While changes in DA activity clearly occur, alterations in non-dopaminergic neurones are also likely to play important roles (Kuczenski and Segal, 1988; see also Section 6.4.3.6). Thus, different neurochemical changes may trigger and accompany different phases of behavioural sensitization.

6.4.3.1 Changes in DA release

The neurochemical change most clearly associated with sensitization is an augmentation of stimulant-induced DA release in the striatum and NAc. This phenomenon was first noted in studies of *in vitro* DA release in which the ability of amphetamine to induce DA release was found to be augmented in striatal slices obtained from sensitized rats (Kolta *et al.*, 1985; Robinson and Becker, 1982). This finding was subsequently confirmed in a number of postmortem and *in vitro* studies of DA turnover in sensitized rats (Robinson and Becker, 1986). Similar results have been obtained with respect to cocaine-, opioid- and stressor-induced sensitization (Kalivas *et al.*, 1988; Kalivas and Duffy, 1988; Peris and Zahniser, 1987, 1989; Robinson *et al.*, 1987; Wilcox *et al.*, 1986). With the introduction of *in vivo* microdialysis techniques, increased release of DA within the NAc and striatum of sensitized rats has been observed in response to acute challenge with either amphetamine (Robinson *et al.*,

1988; Patrick *et al.*, 1991) or cocaine (Akimoto *et al.*, 1989; Kalivas and Duffy, 1990; Pettit *et al.*, 1990) following their repeated administration.

Augmentation of DA release shares a number of features with sensitization of the behavioural response. First of all, alterations in DA release are relatively persistent, having been observed 30 days after completing an escalating dosage regimen of amphetamine (Robinson *et al.*, 1988). Less is known about the persistence of neurochemical sensitization to cocaine. It should be noted, however, that augmentation of DA release is not always observable immediately after withdrawal of cocaine or amphetamine; in some cases, this is also true for sensitization to the motor stimulant effects of acute psychostimulant challenge (Kalivas and Stewart, 1991). Second, treatments which cross-sensitize in behavioural studies also appear to cross-sensitize with respect to neurochemical studies of DA-releasing effects. For example, neurochemical cross-sensitization has been demonstrated between cocaine and methamphetamine (Kazahaya *et al.*, 1989; Akimoto *et al.*, 1990) and between footshock stress and psychostimulants (Kalivas and Duffy, 1989; Robinson *et al.*, 1987; Wilcox *et al.*, 1986). Finally, altered DA releasability also resembles locomotor sensitization in terms of its dependence on dose and temporal parameters of the drug treatment schedule (Robinson and Becker, 1986; Robinson, 1991).

The mechanism underlying augmentation of DA release following intermittent psychostimulant administration remains unknown. The most trivial explanation for sensitization and accompanying increases in DA release is a change in the pharmacokinetics of psychostimulants such that higher effective concentrations in the brain are achieved after repeated administration. It has been suggested that this may contribute to cocaine sensitization since increased concentrations of cocaine in plasma and in the NAc, as measured by microdialysis, are associated with chronic cocaine administration (Pettit *et al.*, 1990). However, cocaine is cleared from brain too rapidly for this to account fully for the long-lasting nature of sensitization. Also arguing against this explanation are the observations that increased bioavailability does not occur as a result of repeated administration of morphine (Kalivas and Duffy, 1987) or amphetamine (Robinson and Becker, 1986) and that cross-sensitization occurs between structurally different drugs. Furthermore, pharmacokinetic explanations do not account for the fact that some effects of repeated psychostimulant administration show sensitization while others show tolerance (Robinson and Becker, 1986).

Sensitization to amphetamine has been reported to increase the amount of DA released by electrical stimulation or K^+ depolarization, leading to the proposal that sensitization leads to a change in the intracellular distribution of DA such that it is more readily releasable by such diverse stimuli as amphetamine and depolarization (Castañeda *et al.*, 1988; Robinson and

Becker, 1986). It is not clear whether repeated administration of cocaine results in an enhancement of the ability of depolarizing stimuli to release DA. An enhancement of K^+-stimulated DA release in the striatum and NAc has been reported, but only at certain concentrations of K^+ and only after certain doses of cocaine (Kalivas and Duffy, 1988). Yi and Johnson (1990b) reported no change in [^{3}H]DA release from striatal slices following repeated cocaine treatment. In addition, the intracellular compartmentalization of [^{3}H]DA in synaptosomes was unchanged by repeated cocaine administration, although subsequent effects of amphetamine on the subcellular distribution and release of [^{3}H]DA were altered (Yi and Johnson, 1990b). Other possible explanations for sensitization-induced increases in DA release include changes in DA synthesis, the DA uptake mechanism, or DA autoreceptor function (see below). Interestingly, the ability of cocaine treatment to enhance releasability of DA from striatal slices is prevented by either D_1 or D_2 DA receptor antagonists, suggesting that long-loop feedback regulation may play a role in the initiation of enhanced releasability (Peris and Zahniser, 1989).

To date, increased DA releasability following repeated psychostimulant administration has been reported only in the dorsal striatum and NAc. Other DA projection areas have not been examined. It is interesting to note, however, that increased somatodendritic DA release has been reported in the VTA after acute administration of amphetamine, cocaine, and morphine (Bradberry and Roth, 1989; Kalivas *et al.*, 1989; Klitenick and Kalivas, 1990) as well as following acute stress (Deutch *et al.*, 1985). In contrast to results obtained in striatum and NAc, repeated daily cocaine or morphine treatment has been reported to *decrease* DA release and turnover in the VTA (Kalivas and Duffy, 1988; Kalivas *et al.*, 1988). K^+-stimulated DA release was found to be decreased in VTA slices prepared from rats treated with cocaine or morphine as compared to slices prepared from saline rats, while amphetamine-stimulated DA release was decreased in slices prepared from cocaine- but not morphine-treated rats (Kalivas and Duffy, 1988). These investigators have suggested that altered somatodendritic DA release may play an important role in the initiation of sensitization. Decreased somatodendritic DA release in the VTA following repeated psychostimulant administration is proposed to result in less somatodendritic autoreceptor stimulation and a resultant increase in DA neuronal activity (Kalivas and Duffy, 1988; Kalivas and Stewart, 1991). This hypothesis is consistent with the results of electrophysiological studies discussed below.

6.4.3.2 Changes in DA synthesis

An increase in DA synthesis, with a resulting increase in the availability of releasable DA, could account for an augmentation of DA release in sensitized rats. There is no evidence, however, for an increase in DA synthesis following repeated amphetamine administration (Kuczenski and Leith, 1981; Kaneno *et al.*, 1986; Robinson and Becker, 1986). Some changes in DA metabolie levels have been noted; however, these changes did not exactly parallel in time-course the behavioural changes associated with amphetamine sensitization (Kuczenski and Leith, 1981). In a recent study, chronic cocaine administration was reported to decrease basal DA synthesis in the NAc as measured using microdialysis in combination with local perfusion of the decarboxylase inhibitor NSD-1015 (Brock *et al.*, 1990). This could reflect supersensitivity of synthesis-modulating autoreceptors (see Section 6.4.3.3). It might also be consistent with an increase in basal DA release following repeated cocaine and a resultant increase in the tonic level of synthesis-modulating autoreceptor stimulation. Although changes in basal DA release following repeated cocaine are not detected by microdialysis, it is possible that this may reflect limitations of the technique (see Section 6.2) and the efficiency of the DA uptake system (Wightman and Zimmerman, 1990).

6.4.3.3 Changes in nerve terminal autoreceptors

It is possible that the augmentation of DA releasability which accompanies sensitization could result in changes in the sensitivity of synthesis-modulating and release-modulating DA autoreceptors located on DA nerve terminals. Conversely, changes in autoreceptor sensitivity could be proposed to account for changes in DA releasability. However, while several studies have examined the effect of repeated psychostimulant administration on nerve terminal autoreceptors, no clear consensus has emerged.

Changes in the sensitivity of release-modulating autoreceptors are unlikely to account for the augmentation of amphetamine-induced DA release after repeated administration, since amphetamine-induced DA release is not subject to autoreceptor control (see Section 6.2). Cocaine differs from amphetamine in that it increases extracellular DA levels in a calcium-dependent, tetrodotoxin-sensitive manner by acting on vesicular storage pools which are presumably released in response to neuronal activity (see Section 6.2). The level of autoreceptor stimulation might therefore be expected to influence cocaine-induced increases in extracellular DA levels, although this has not been examined directly.

Repeated cocaine administration has been reported to both increase (Dwoskin *et al.*, 1988; Peris *et al.*, 1990) and decrease (Yi and Johnson, 1990a) the sensitivity of release-modulating DA autoreceptors. In the first study, male rats were given injections of cocaine (10 mg/kg) or saline once a day for 8 or 14 days and striatal slices were prepared 24 h after the last injection. Pergolide, a D_2 agonist, was found to produce a greater inhibition of electrically stimulated DA release in slices prepared from cocaine-treated rats (Dwoskin *et al.*, 1988). In the second study, female rats were given daily injections of cocaine (15 mg/kg twice a day) or saline for 7 days and striatal slices were prepared 7 days after the last injection. The D_2 selective agonist N-0437 was able to inhibit calcium-stimulated DA release from synaptosomes prepared from saline rats but not cocaine-treated rats (Yi and Johnson, 1990a). Obviously, many procedural differences could account for the discrepancy between results obtained in these studies. It is possible, however, that autoreceptors are supersensitive immediately following cocaine withdrawal and that autoreceptor subsensitivity develops more gradually. This may parallel the observation that the magnitude of both behavioural sensitization and augmentation of DA release increases as the time between the last exposure to sensitizing drug and the test for sensitized response is increased (reviews: Robinson, 1988; Kalivas and Stewart, 1991). A gradual increase in DA releasability might account for the gradual appearance of autoreceptor subsensitivity, or vice versa.

Autoreceptors on DA nerve terminals also modulate DA synthesis. However, little is known about how autoreceptor regulation of DA synthesis may change during sensitization. Several studies have examined the sensitivity of synthesis-modulating autoreceptors *in vivo* after repeated amphetamine using the gamma butyrolactone (GBL) model (see Wolf and Roth (1987) for details). Two studies reported no difference in the potency of apomorphine in the GBL model following either twice-daily injections of amphetamine (5 mg/kg × 5 days, tested 3 days after the last dose) (Conway and Uretsky, 1982) or daily injection of amphetamine (6 mg/kg × 14 days, tested 10 days after the last dose) (Kaneno *et al.*, 1986). However, a recent study (Tyler *et al.*, 1989) indicated that the inhibitory effects of quinpirole were enhanced after treatment of female rats with an escalating dose regimen of amphetamine (1–10 mg/kg × 30 days, tested 8 days after last dose).

Other studies have examined the effects of repeated cocaine or amphetamine treatment on basal DA synthesis rates (see Section 6.4.3.2) or cocaine-induced decreases in DA synthesis. One study examined the effects of 3 days of cocaine pretreatment on DA synthesis in the striatum, NAc, and A10 region (Kalivas *et al.*, 1988). Acute cocaine depressed DA synthesis (measured as DOPA formation after injection with the DOPA decarboxylase inhibitor NSD-1015) in all brain regions. Fourteen days following the end of treatment, the effects of acute cocaine on DOPA formation were enhanced in the striatum and NAc but not in A10 (Kalivas *et al.*, 1988). These results could reflect autoreceptor supersensitivity in the striatum or NAc, or an increase in basal synaptic levels of DA such that uptake inhibition by cocaine becomes more efficacious following repeated treatment. Increased basal synaptic levels of DA would also explain the finding that basal DOPA synthesis, measured *in vivo* using microdialysis, is decreased in the NAc following repeated cocaine administration (see Section 6.4.3.2; Brock *et al.*, 1990).

6.4.3.4 Changes in DA uptake

There is considerable precedent for changes in the sensitivity of neurotransmitter receptors as a result of persistent changes in occupation, but comparatively little information about the ability of neurotransmitter transporters to undergo similar compensatory changes. Results regarding changes in the number of DA uptake sites or their affinity for substrate following repeated amphetamine or cocaine treatment have been inconsistent. Izenwasser and Cox (1990) reported a substantial increase in the K_m for dopamine uptake in the NAc of cocaine-treated rats (15 mg/kg × 3 days, tested 24 h after last injection) with no change in the V_{max}. No change in striatal DA uptake was found. In contrast, Yi and Johnson (1990b) reported a 30% increase in the V_{max} with no change in the affinity of the uptake carrier for DA or cocaine in striatal tissue from rats treated daily with 15 mg/kg for 7 days and then challenged with cocaine 30 min before sacrifice. Chronic cocaine treatment without the cocaine challenge failed to increase the V_{max}. Another group has reported no differences in striatal [^{3}H]DA uptake measured one day after either a single injection or after 8 days of repeated injections (Peris *et al.*, 1990). In two of the above studies, binding of tritiated ligands to the DA uptake site was evaluated in the same rats. No differences in striatal [^{3}H]nomifensine binding (Peris *et al.*, 1990) or [^{3}H]GBR-12935 binding (Yi and Johnson, 1990b) were reported. Similarly, Allard *et al.* (1990) reported no change in K_d or B_{max} values for [^{3}H]GBR-12935 binding after chronic treatment (twice daily × 21 days, tested 3 days after last injection) with amphetamine (2.5 mg/kg) or cocaine (10 mg/kg), as well as after chronic administration of directly acting DA agonists and antagonists. Obviously, further studies are necessary using treatment regimens and withdrawal times known to produce behavioural sensitization.

6.4.3.5 Changes in postsynaptic DA receptor sensitivity

If an increase in DA receptor number or sensitivity is responsible for enhanced responsiveness of the DA system to psychomotor stimulants following sensitization, one might expect sensitized animals to exhibit either hypersensitivity to the behavioural effects of directly acting DA agonists or changes in DA receptor binding. In fact, neither has been observed consistently (Robinson and Becker, 1986). Thus, the majority of studies prior to 1986 did not report hypersensitivity to apomorphine and other directly acting DA agonists in amphetamine-sensitized animals. Similarly, although reports of both upregulation and downregulation of DA receptors has been published, the bulk of the evidence was not in favour of increased DA receptor number as a mechanism of behavioural sensitization to amphetamine. In fact, most binding studies reported either a decrease or no change in DA receptor number (Robinson and Becker, 1986). It should be noted that, since that review, more specific radioligands for DA receptors, particularly D_1 DA receptors, have become available, as have more sophisticated quantitative autoradiographic techniques. However, there are still no compelling reports of enhanced D_1 or D_2 DA receptor binding following repeated amphetamine administration (Kuczenski and Segal, 1988).

A number of recent studies have examined the effects of repeated cocaine administration on D_1 and D_2 DA receptors within the rat striatal complex. One report indicated enhanced densities of D_2 DA receptors within the NAc but diminished densities within the caudate-putamen, with no changes in affinity, following repeated cocaine administration (Goeders and Kuhar, 1987). In this study, binding experiments were performed immediately after the last cocaine injection. Similar changes in striatal and NAc D_2 DA receptors were reported by Kleven *et al.* (1990), although this study demonstrated that D_2 receptor number returned to normal within 2 weeks of the last cocaine injection. This study also found an increase in D_1 receptors within the mPFC but a decrease in D_1 receptors in the NAc and striatum. The density of NAc D_1 receptors returned to normal within 2 weeks whereas the increased level initially observed within the mPFC was replaced by a decrease following the 2-week withdrawal period. The decrease in striatal D_1 receptors persisted for at least 2 weeks. Peris *et al.* (1990) also reported a selective increase in D_2 receptors in the NAc after repeated cocaine, but noted that receptor number normalized within one week while behavioural sensitization persisted during this period. In summary, reports of changes in DA receptor number following repeated cocaine are inconsistent and, in most cases, far too transient to account fully for behavioural sensitization

Despite an apparent lack of change in receptor number, evidence obtained from electrophysiological studies suggests an increase in D_1 receptor sensitivity after repeated cocaine administration (Henry *et al.*, 1989; White *et al.*, 1991; see Section 6.4.4). This may suggest that neurochemical changes downstream from receptor occupation play a role in behavioural sensitization. The idea that cocaine administration might result in functional DA receptor supersensitivity as a result of enhanced receptor–effector coupling was originally proposed by Memo *et al.* (1981), who reported augmented adenylate cyclase stimulation by DA and an increase in membrane-bound calmodulin in striatal membrane preparations from rats treated with cocaine. The results of more recent studies suggest that the ability of D_1 agonists to stimulate adenylate cyclase is unchanged immediately after withdrawal from chronic amphetamine treatment (Robinson and Becker, 1986; Barnett *et al.*, 1987) or 2 weeks after withdrawal (Roseboom *et al.*, 1990) but *is* enhanced 4 weeks after withdrawal (Roseboom *et al.*, 1990). Since behavioural sensitization is apparent within 2 weeks using the paradigm employed by Roseboom *et al.*, the increased sensitivity of the D_1 receptor-coupled adenylate cyclase seen after 4 weeks of withdrawal does not appear to be directly related to behavioural sensitization.

Exposure to D_1 agonists, including amphetamine, produces desensitization of D_1 receptor-coupled adenylate cyclase activity (Barton and Sibley, 1990; Roseboom and Gnegy, 1989). Two studies have suggested that this process undergoes sensitization after repeated amphetamine pretreatment in the sense that amphetamine becomes more potent at eliciting desensitization of D_1 receptor-coupled adenylate cyclase activity (Roseboom *et al.*, 1990; Barnett *et al.*, 1987). For example, a dose of 2.5 mg/kg amphetamine is not sufficient to produce acute desensitization of D_1-coupled adenylate cyclase or to elicit oral stereotypies. However, following repeated administration of amphetamine, this dose becomes capable of eliciting both effects (Barnett *et al.*, 1987). Similarly, Roseboom *et al.* (1990) reported that repeated amphetamine injections, administered according to an escalating dose regimen known to produce behavioural sensitization, produced an increase in the potency of amphetamine at desensitizing D_1 receptor-coupled adenylate cyclase in striatum but not NAc. This study also found that repeated amphetamine treatment resulted in a translocation of calmodulin from membranes to cytosol and a loss of the ability of calmodulin to potentiate D_1 receptor-stimulated adenylate cyclase activity. These results, and others (Roberts-Lewis *et al.*, 1986), suggest that desensitization of D_1 receptor-coupled adenylate cyclase may be linked to the production of intense stereotypies and that this process appears to undergo sensitization with a time-course which, for the most part, parallels that of behavioural sensitization (Roseboom *et al.*, 1990). In considering these data, it is informative but not necessarily helpful to note that chronic amphetamine pretreatment has been reported to produce no change in the intensity of stereotyped behaviour produced by apomorphine challenge (Conway and Uretsky, 1982; Robinson and Becker, 1986).

Some D_2 DA receptors are coupled in an inhibitory manner to adenylate cyclase activity; acute desensitization of this response occurs after exposure to D_2 agonists (Bates *et al.*, 1991). Acute pretreatment with high doses of amphetamine also results in desensitization of D_2 receptor-coupled inhibition of adenylate cyclase activity (Roseboom and Gnegy, 1988). However, the effect of chronic amphetamine pretreatment on this process has not been examined. Nestler and colleagues have reported increased forskolin-stimulated adenylate cyclase activity and cAMP-dependent protein kinase activity in the NAc following repeated cocaine treatment. In addition, there was a reduction in levels of the α-subunits of the inhibitory GTP binding proteins G_i and G_o (Nestler *et al.*, 1990; Terwilliger *et al.*, 1991). These results suggest that changes in both signal transduction mechanisms and in the regulation of specific G protein subunits may play important roles in long-term adaptive processes such as behavioural sensitization.

6.4.3.6 Changes in other transmitter systems

Recent studies suggest that behavioural sensitization may require stimulation of the *N*-methyl-D-aspartate (NMDA) class of glutamate receptors. Thus, the noncompetitive NMDA antagonist MK-801 has been reported to block the development of behavioural sensitization to both amphetamine (Karler *et al.*, 1989, 1990; Wolf and Khansa, 1991) and cocaine (Karler *et al.*, 1989). Further studies will be necessary to determine whether competitive NMDA receptor antagonists mimic the effect of MK-801 and to identify the location of the glutamate receptors involved in sensitization. However, these results suggest that behavioural sensitization may resemble certain forms of long-term potentiation in its requirement for NMDA receptor stimulation (Collingridge and Bliss, 1987; Nicoll *et al.*, 1988). A role for non-dopaminergic systems in sensitization is also supported by a recent report that corticosteroid receptor activation is necessary for behavioural sensitization to amphetamine (Rivet *et al.*, 1989). Interestingly, female rats have been reported to exhibit greater behavioural responses following an initial administration of amphetamine, more robust behavioural sensitization following repeated administration, and greater and more persistent elevations of plasma corticosterone in response to stress (Robinson and Becker, 1986).

6.4.4 Neurophysiology of sensitization

Electrophysiological experiments have also investigated possible neuronal correlates of behavioural sensitization. One of the earliest hypotheses regarding the mechanisms underlying behavioural sensitization was subsensitivity of DA autoreceptors (Martres *et al.*, 1977; Muller and Seeman, 1979). Antelman and Chiodo (1981) first demonstrated a subsensitivity of nigral (A9) DA neurones to the rate-suppressant effects of relatively low (i.v.) doses of apomorphine following repeated amphetamine administration. Subsequent studies extended this observation to A10 DA neurones within the VTA (Kamata and Rebec, 1984; White and Wang, 1984b). When injected either once (5.0 mg/kg, i.p.) or twice (1.0–10.0 mg/kg) daily for one week, A10 DA neurones were significantly less sensitive to i.v. amphetamine (Kamata and Rebec, 1984; White and Wang, 1984b) and apomorphine (White and Wang, 1984b). In addition, a direct demonstration of subsensitive

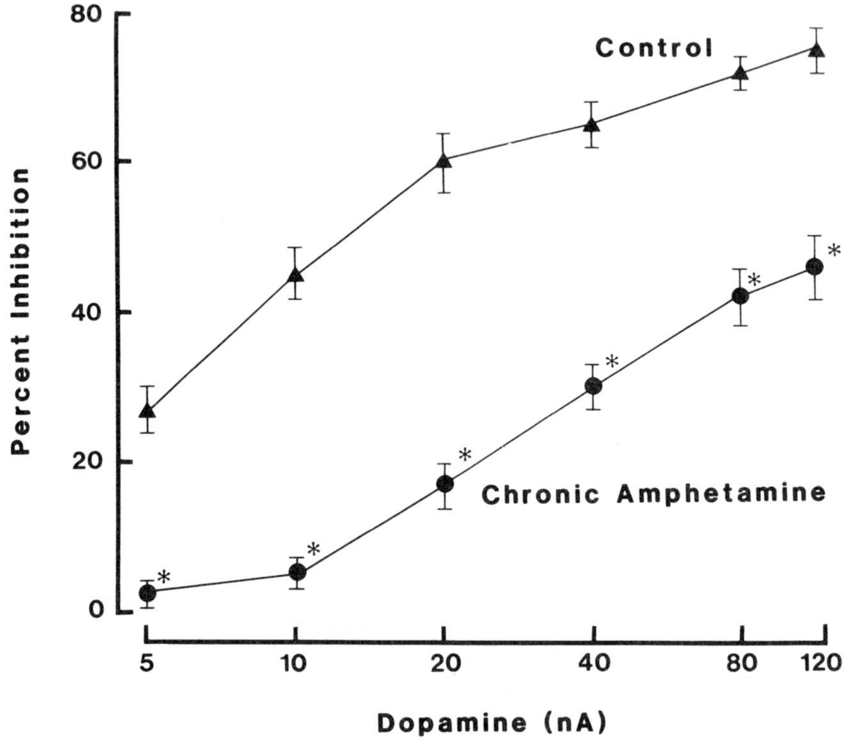

Figure 3 Comparison of the effects of dopamine, administered iontophoretically, on A10 DA neurones recorded from saline control rats and rats that had received repeated amphetamine (5 mg/kg, b.i.d. for 7 days) and were tested 1 day after the last injection. Each point represents the mean ± standard error of 20 cells recorded from six rats in each group. Asterisks represent points that were significantly different from control ($p < 0.01$). The ordinate indicates microiontophoretic current in nanoamperes (nA). From White and Wang (1984b) with permission.

somatodendritic DA autoreceptors was provided since A10 DA neurones in amphetamine-treated rats were subsensitive to the inhibitory effects of iontophoretically administered DA (Figure 3). Their subsensitivity was reduced but still evident 8 days following the discontinuation of amphetamine injections (White and Wang, 1984b).

A similar subsensitivity of impulse-regulating somatodendritic autoreceptors has been reported following repeated cocaine injections. Following twice-daily injections (10 mg/kg, i.p.) for 2 weeks, A10 DA neurones were significantly less sensitive to the inhibitory effects of i.v. apomorphine when compared to control animals (Ackerman and White, 1990; Henry *et al.*, 1989). Acute administration of cocaine 12–24 hours prior to testing failed to produce this subsensitivity. This, it appears that repeated cocaine decreased the sensitivity of DA autoreceptors by enhancing the degree of stimulation by the endogenous transmitter. Further evidence supporting this conclusion was provided by iontophoretic studies indicating that repeated cocaine administration reduced the responsiveness of A10 DA cells to DA, but not to GABA (Henry *et al.*, 1989). Despite the fact that $GABA_B$ receptors and D_2 DA autoreceptors share the same K^+ conductance in midbrain DA neurones (Lacey *et al.*, 1988), the locus of cocaine-induced desensitization would appear to be restricted to D_2 DA autoreceptors.

Because the basal activity of A10 DA cells is dependent on the density or sensitivity of A10 DA autoreceptors (White and Wang, 1984a), autoreceptor subsensitivity might be expected to increase the firing rate of spontaneously active A10 DA neurones and activate normally quiescent DA neurones. As shown in Table 1, repeated administration of either cocaine or amphetamine significantly increases both the number and the mean basal firing rate of spontaneously active A10 DA cells (Henry *et al.*, 1989; White and Wang, 1984b). When tested 4 or 8 days following the last injection of a cocaine treatment regimen, the subsensitivity of DA autoreceptors was observed to return to normal. Thus, after a 4-day withdrawal period, subsensitivity to apomorphine was less apparent and by 8 days after treatment was no longer evident (Ackerman and White, 1990). Thus, autoreceptor subsensitivity

Table 1 Repeated administration of amphetamine (5 mg/kg, b.i.d. for 7 days, tested 24 h after the last injection) or cocaine (10 mg/kg, b.i.d. for 14 days, tested 24 h after the last injection) caused an increase in the number of spontaneously active A10 DA cells recorded per electrode track and in the average basal firing rate of those cells. Data are from White and Wang (1984b) (amphetamine) and Henry *et al.* (1989) (cocaine) with permission. All data are means ± standard errors. Asterisks represent values which were significantly different from appropriate saline control groups. Note that two different control groups are included because the studies were conducted several years apart and used different lengths of drug administration (above).

Group	Number of rats	DA cells/track	Mean firing rate (spikes/s)
Control	6	1.48 ± 0.07	3.24 ± 0.05
Amphetamine	6	2.11 ± 0.11*	4.01 ± 0.14*
Control	6	1.45 ± 0.09	4.19 ± 0.22
Cocaine	5	2.08 ± 0.14*	5.58 ± 0.16*

induced by repeated cocaine administration is not a persistent effect (Figure 4). This raises questions as to the relevance of this change to behavioural sensitization which is known to be a long-lasting phenomenon.

Careful pharmacological studies regarding possible alterations in NAc neurones following repeated amphetamine have not been reported. Alloway and Rebec (1983) first demonstrated that the typical inhibitory effects of i.p. amphetamine on NAc neurones were either slightly reduced or unaltered by repeated amphetamine administration. However, the receptors responsible for the effects of amphetamine within the NAc have not been investigated using electrophysiological techniques.

In a series of studies, White and colleagues have determined the effects of repeated cocaine on NAc neurones (Henry *et al.*, 1989; White *et al.*, 1991). In contrast to the effects of repeated cocaine treatment on VTA DA neurones, the responses of NAc neurones to iontophoretic cocaine were enhanced one day after the cessation of cocaine treatment (Henry *et al.*, 1989). Recently, these findings were extended by the demonstration that NAc cells were significantly more sensitive to the inhibitory effects of the D_1 selective agonist SKF 38393 following repeated cocaine treatment (Figure 5). In contrast, there was no significant increase in the inhibitory effects of the selective D_2 agonist quinpirole. Thus, the sensitization of NAc neurones to iontophoretic DA observed in the previous studies appears to be due primarily to enhanced sensitivity of the D_1 DA receptor.

Unlike D_2 DA autoreceptor subsensitivity, the sensitization of D_1 receptors within the NAc persisted for 8 days following the cessation of cocaine injections (Figure 5). In addition, D_1 receptor supersensitivity was still evident following a one-month withdrawal period. Normosensitivity was restored 2 months after the last injection. Thus, the sensitization of D_1 DA postsynaptic receptors within the NAc appears to be a relatively long-lasting adaptation produced by the repeated administration of cocaine and, therefore, may be related to behavioural sensitization. Behavioural studies are necessary to determine the persistence of behavioural sensitization following this cocaine treatment regimen.

▶

Figure 4 Inhibition of VTA DA neurones by apomorphine following repeated cocaine treatment. The dose–response curve for apomorphine is shown for rats given 10 mg/kg cocaine or 1 ml/kg saline i.p. twice daily for 14 days and tested (A) 1 day, (B) 4 days or (C) 8 days after the last injection. Each point represents the mean ± SEM. The ID_{50} was calculated by linear regression analysis for individual cells, and statistical significance was determined by ANCOVA using basal firing rate as covariate. A significant difference between points in the dose–response curve was determined by Dunnett's test. An asterisk indicates $p < 0.05$. From Ackerman and White (1990) with permission.

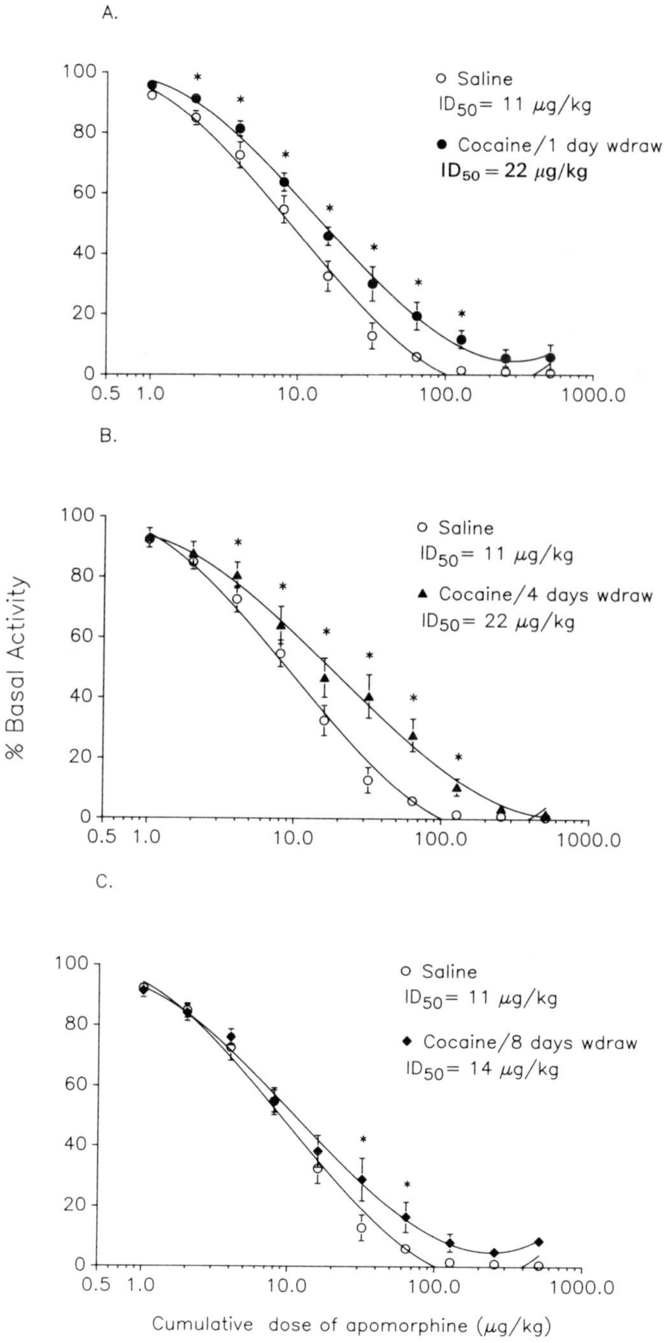
A.
100
80
60
40
20
0
0.5 1.0 10.0 100.0 1000.0
○ Saline
ID50= 11 μg/kg
● Cocaine/1 day wdraw
ID50 = 22 μg/kg
B.
% Basal Activity
○ Saline
ID50= 11 μg/kg
▲ Cocaine/4 days wdraw
ID50= 22 μg/kg
C.
○ Saline
ID50= 11 μg/kg
◆ Cocaine/8 days wdraw
ID50= 14 μg/kg
Cumulative dose of apomorphine (μg/kg)

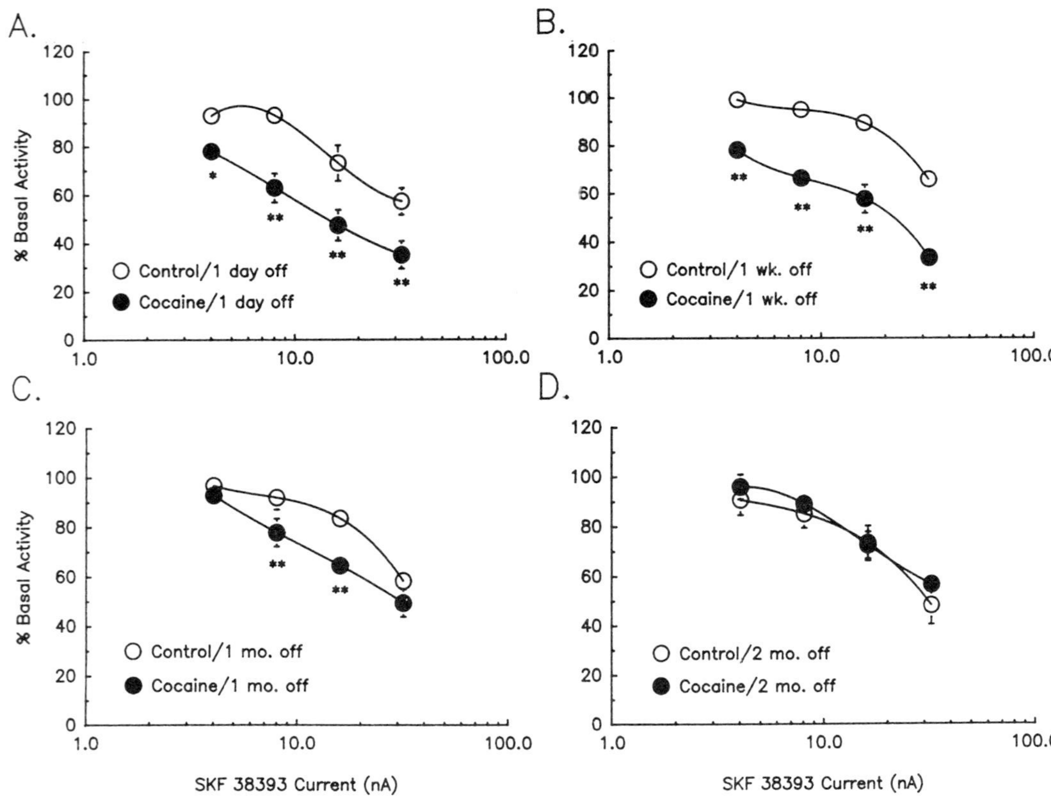

Figure 5 Nucleus accumbens (NAc) neurones from cocaine-treated rats were sensitized to iontophoretically applied SKF 38393. Current response curves illustrating the effects of microiontophoretically applied SKF 38393 on NAc neurones from rats receiving twice-daily injections of either vehicle or cocaine, and tested either: (A) 16–24 h ($n = 12$ cells, control; $n = 14$ cells, cocaine); (B) 1 week ($n = 13$ cells, control; $n = 15$ cells, cocaine); (C) 1 month ($n = 15$ cells/group); or (D) 2 months ($n = 10$ cells/group) after the final injection. Each point represents the mean ± SEM (*$P < 0.05$, **$P < 0.01$).

The finding of an enhanced D_1, but not D_2, receptor-mediated electrophysiological response following repeated cocaine administration is surprising in view of other studies regarding the effects of similar treatment regimens on D_1 receptor density, as discussed above. Recall that increases in D_1 receptor density within the NAc or caudate-putamen of rats following repeated cocaine administration have not been observed (Kleven *et al.*, 1990; Peris *et al.*, 1990). A similar dissociation exists between electrophysiological and ligand binding studies of D_1 receptors following 6-OHDA lesions of nigro-striatal DA neurones. Although such denervation results in a highly supersensitive response of caudate-putamen neurones to SKF 38393 (Hu *et al.*, 1990), D_1 receptor density is generally reported to be unchanged or decreased (Altar and Marien, 1987; Ariano, 1988; Filloux *et al.*, 1987; Leslie and Bennett, 1987; Marshall *et al.*, 1989). Taken together, these findings suggest that D_1 receptor supersensitivity probably occurs beyond the level of the recognition site (see Section 6.4.3.5).

6.4.5 Mechanisms of sensitization: a synthesis

Repeated administration of psychomotor stimulants, including morphine, results in an enhancement of transmission through the mesoaccumbens neuronal system as compared to the first exposure to the drug. Anatomical and pharmacological experiments have identified important sites where sensitization may occur while biochemical and electrophysiological studies have identified several potential components of the sensitized response. Each of these components may be essential for the development of behavioural sensitization accompanying repeated exposure to cocaine.

The most widely accepted neuronal alteration which has been demonstrated to occur in sensitized rats is the increased releasability of DA upon acute challenge with a psychomotor stimulant or other depolarizing stimulus. Many of the features of the altered releasability produced by repeated amphetamine administration match those of the enhanced behavioural response. It is persistent, it is influenced by the period of withdrawal following drug discontinuation and it is influenced by the dose and temporal parameters of the drug treatment schedule (Robinson, 1991). Similar comparative parametric studies of either cocaine- or morphine-induced sensitization and increased releasability have not been reported.

Increased releasability appears to be maintained by mechanisms operative at the level of the DA nerve terminal since it can be demonstrated in striatal slices taken from amphetamine- or cocaine-sensitized rats (Kolta *et al.*, 1985, 1989; Peris and Zahniser, 1989; Robinson and Becker, 1982). It is not clear, however, where this alteration is initiated. Thus, while studies have shown that repeated administration of amphetamine into the NAc fails to produce sensitization to the locomotor activating effects of amphetamine, it is not known whether this type of treatment is capable of producing increased DA releasability in the NAc. If so, it would argue for a dissociation between increased releasability and sensitization. If not, it would imply that the process of sensitization is initiated elsewhere and somehow 'transferred' to the NAc. This notion is consistent with the observation that rats sensitized by systemic amphetamine administration are also supersensitive to the locomotor stimulating effects of intra-NAc amphetamine (Kolta *et al.*, 1989).

Recent work suggests that the VTA may play an important role in the initiation of sensitization, as evidenced by the ability of repeated intra-VTA microinjections of amphetamine and morphine to cause enhanced behavioural activation to subsequent systemic challenge. In future studies of sensitization, it will be vital to address the mechanisms by which repeated administration of psychomotor stimulants alters events within the VTA and how that alteration is subsequently expressed within the NAc. One such mechanism may involve the development of somatodendritic autoreceptor subsensitivity following repeated psychostimulant administration. Subsensitivity of impulse-regulating somatodendritic autoreceptors on A10 DA cells results in an increase in the number of spontaneously active DA cells and their average basal firing rate. Although autoreceptor subsensitivity does not persist during withdrawal from the chronic treatment regimen, it has been argued that the resulting hyperactivity of DA cells may be a necessary triggering stimulus for other, more persistent, neuronal alterations relevant to sensitization (Ackerman and White, 1990).

Consistent with this proposal is the hypothesis that intracranial administration of opioids or amphetamine into the VTA produces sensitization because these compounds increase dendritic release of DA within the VTA (Kalivas and Duffy, 1987; Kalivas *et al.*, 1989). Enhanced extracellular DA levels within the VTA might lead to desensitization of A10 somatodendritic autoreceptors and a subsequent increase in basal DAergic activity within the VTA. Alternatively, reduced dendritic DA release, which has been reported following repeated administration of opioids and cocaine (Kalivas and Duffy, 1987, 1988), might also result in enhanced DA neuronal activity, due to reduced autoreceptor stimulation, independent of changes in autoreceptor sensitivity.

Is it possible that the increase in the firing rate of DA neurones brought about by reduced somatodendritic DA release and/or autoreceptor subsensitivity might serve as an initiating stimulus for more persistent changes in dopaminergic function? Certainly, a link between increased neuronal activity and increased releasability seems plausible. However, in spite of the electrophysiological evidence indicating increased firing of DA neurones, it has been argued that sensitization fails to produce an increase in basal DA turnover in DA projection fields. This conclusion is based primarily on dialysis studies indicating normal levels of extracellular DA in the rat NAc following repeated amphetamine or cocaine administration; an augmentation of DA release is evident only upon challenge with the sensitizing drug (Robinson *et al.*, 1988; Kalivas and Duffy, 1990). However, such studies would not be expected to detect increased DA release induced by modest increases in impulse flow such as the 25–33% increase produced by repeated psychostimulant administration (Henry *et al.*, 1989; White and Wang, 1984b). As noted above, changes in extracellular DA are only detectable when DA neurones are stimulated at frequencies of 10–20 Hz, or 100–400% over basal firing rates (4–5 Hz) when the DA uptake system becomes saturated; see Wightman and Zimmerman (1990) for discussion. Thus, although not detectable by microdialysis or voltammetric techniques, synaptically relevant increases in DA release could accompany the increases in neuronal firing rate produced by repeated amphetamine or cocaine. An increase in basal DA release would probably result in significantly enhanced stimulation of postsynaptic DA receptors as well as possible alterations in DA nerve terminal function. Indeed, repeated cocaine administration has been reported to decrease DA synthesis in the NAc, as determined by *in vivo* microdialysis studies employing local perfusion with the DOPA decarboxylase inhibitor NSD-1015 (Brock *et al.*, 1990). Increased DA release might also account for some of the neurochemical changes discussed in previous sections, such as alterations in the sensitivity of nerve terminal autoreceptors or the activity of the DA transporter. Each of these alterations could be viewed as a homeostatic response to enhanced impulse flow in DA neurones.

Autoreceptor subsensitivity following repeated psychomotor stimulant administration might also be a necessary trigger for the persistent enhancement of D_1 receptor sensitivity within the NAc. Like cocaine, repeated administration of the D_1 selective agonist SKF 38393 results in supersensitive D_1 inhibitory responses in both the caudate-putamen (White *et al.*, 1990), and NAc (Henry and White, 1990), as well as enhanced behavioural responses to D_1 selective agonists (Braun and Chase, 1988; White *et al.*, 1990). However, neither of these alterations endures beyond 8 days post-injection. Importantly, D_1 selective agonists do not directly influence impulse-regulating DA autoreceptors which are exclusively of the D_2 subtype (Wachtel *et al.*, 1989; White and Wang, 1984b), and thus do not cause diminished autoreceptor sensitivity following repeated administration (Henry and White, 1990). Obviously, the lack of autoreceptor subsensitivity following repeated SKF 38393 treatment is not necessarily the cause of a less persistent (as compared to cocaine) D_1 supersensitivity within the NAc, which might also be due to other differences between the effects of these two compounds. However, it is an interesting possibility worthy of further study.

Based upon recent receptor antagonism studies, Vezina and Stewart (1989) have argued against a role for autoreceptor subsensitivity in behavioural sensitization. The failure of selective D_2 antagonists to prevent sensitization to repeated amphetamine was suggested to indicate a lack of autoreceptor involvement based upon the notion that blocking D_2 autoreceptors should prevent the ability of repeated amphetamine to cause subsensitivity (Vezina and Stewart, 1989). However, blockade of D_2 receptors increases the firing of A10 DA neurones (White and Wang, 1984b), as does autoreceptor subsensitivity, suggesting further that increases in DA neuronal activity might be a critical alteration required to initiate sensitization.

In summary, it is likely that behavioural sensitization results from a complex interplay between a number of neuronal adaptations, some of which may be necessary before others become manifest. Given the capacity of the brain DA system to overcome and compensate for various perturbations, it is not surprising that some alterations produced by repeated psychostimulant administration may not persist upon withdrawal. However, this should not eliminate them from consideration as potential necessary events in a time-dependent chain of adaptations eventually leading to altered behavioural responsiveness. It is also possible that individual differences exist between animals, or within the same animal at different times, with respect to the mechanisms underlying sensitization. Finally, it is conceivable that, despite obvious similarities and cross-sensitization between the various psychostimulants, there exist subtle differences in the mechanisms underlying sensitization to their behavioural effects. Only with continued investigations using a variety of approaches will a clear picture of the neurobiology of sensitization emerge.

6.5 Sensitization of drug reward: implications for the psychomotor stimulant theory of addiction

The psychomotor stimulant theory of addition argues that the neuronal mechanisms underlying locomotor stimulation are the same as those underlying reward processes (Wise and Bozarth, 1987). Since the locomotor stimulating effects of psychostimulants exhibit sensitization following repeated administration, it should be the case that the rewarding effects of psychomotor stimulants should also show sensitization. Surprisingly little attention has been paid to this question. Woolverton *et al.* (1984b) reported that repeated non-contingent administration of methamphetamine sensitized rhesus monkeys to the rewarding effects of low doses of this psychostimulant. Similar studies have been conducted in rats. Thus, it was recently reported that repeated administration of amphetamine increased the likelihood that rats would self-administer low doses of amphetamine (Piazza *et al.*, 1989). Horger *et al.* (1990) have reported similar effects of repeated non-contingent cocaine administration on the subsequent probability of rats self-administering low, typically non-reinforcing doses of cocaine. Finally, Lett (1989) used the conditioned place preference paradigm to demonstrate that repeated administration of either amphetamine, cocaine or morphine prior to preference conditioning resulted in greater place preferences for the drugs than did control saline injections. Moreover, there was cross-sensitization between the various drugs.

The above findings contrast with the generally accepted notion that the euphorigenic properties of drugs of abuse wane with repeated exposure and that increased dosing is necessary to maintain desired levels of the 'high'. Obviously, self-administration of drugs depends upon a wide variety of environmental and experimental variables, including schedules of reinforcement, limited versus unlimited access, the dose of drug administered per infusion and the previous drug history of the subject. Unfortunately, studies of drug self-administration have not typically addressed the issue of sensitization to response-contingent injections. Note that all of the studies cited above used non-contingent exposure to sensitize animals to the rewarding effects of psychomotor stimulants.

One recent study examined the ability of self-administered cocaine to increase DA levels within the NAc using *in vivo* microdialysis in freely moving rats (Hurd *et al.*, 1989). Rats that had 9 days of exposure to the cocaine self-administration procedure were compared to yoked control rats that received either saline or cocaine injections at the same time as the groups self-administering cocaine. The ability of cocaine to elevate DA levels within the NAc was considerably *reduced* in the cocaine-experienced rats as compared to the yoked controls which received cocaine for the first time. Thus, rather than an enhanced ability of cocaine to elevate synaptic DA, as would be expected in sensitized rats, tolerance to this effect was observed. Although not directly addressed by these studies, the findings may have considerable relevance to the issues of sensitization to rewarding efficacy and contingent versus non-contingent cocaine administration. It seems probable that cocaine-experienced rats were sensitized to cocaine, or to DA, since lower synaptic levels of DA were able to maintain reinforcement. However, the mechanism of sensitization was more likely to be enhanced postsynaptic DA receptor responsiveness to lower levels of synaptic DA, as suggested by the findings of White and colleagues (Henry *et al.*, 1989; White *et al.*, 1991).

Future research is needed to determine whether contingent psychomotor stimulant administration impacts differently on dopaminergic or other neurobiological substrates as compared to non-contingent administration. This variable may be important for the demonstration of sensitization of reward as well as locomotor stimulation. It is already known that rats receiving non-contingent cocaine injections while yoked to rats self-administering the drug are more susceptible to cardiotoxic effects (Dworkin and Smith, 1988). The potential relevance of such findings to human drug abuse is obvious. Robinson (1991) has recently suggested that experienced drug users may take larger doses of drugs not because they are tolerant to the euphoric effects, but because they desire to achieve more intense 'highs' and can do so with the development of tolerance to the untoward and aversive 'side-effects'. Sensitization to the rewarding effects of psychomotor stimulants and related issues such as the interchangeability of stress and drug exposure in sensitization and the influence of conditioned stimulus control over such mechanisms are all likely to be major contributing factors to both the vulnerability of drug dependence and possible relapse following attempted withdrawal (Robinson, 1991).

References

Ackerman, J.A. & White, F.J. (1990) *Neurosci. Lett.* **117**, 181–187.

Akimoto, K., Hamamura, T. & Otsuki, S. (1989) *Brain Res.* **490**, 339–344.

Akimoto, K., Hamamura, T., Kazahaya, Y., Akiyama, K. & Otsuki, S. (1990) *Brain Res.* **507**, 344–346.

Allard, P., Eriksson, K., Ross, S.B. & Marcusson, J.O. (1990) *Psychopharmacology* **102**, 291–294.

Alloway, K.D. & Rebec, G.V. (1983) *Brain Res.* **283**, 71–79.

Altar, C.A. & Hauser, K. (1987) *Brain Res.* **410**, 1–11.

Altar, C.A. & Marien, M.R. (1987) *J. Neurosci.* **7**, 213–222.

Antelman, S.M. & Chiodo, L.A. (1981) *Biol. Psychiatry* **16**, 717–722.

Ariano, M.A. (1988) *Brain Res.* **443**, 204–214.

Barnett, J.V., Segal, D.S. & Kuczenski, R. (1987) *J. Pharmacol. Exp. Ther.* **242**, 40–47.

Barton, A.C. & Sibley, D.R. (1990) *Mol. Pharmacol.* **38**, 531–541.

Bates, M.D., Senogles, S.E., Bunzow, J.R., Liggett, S.B., Civelli, O. & Caron, M.G. (1991) *Mol. Pharmacol.* **39**, 55–63.

Baxter, B.L., Gluckman, M.I., Stein, L. & Scerni, R.A. (1974) *Pharmacol. Biochem. Behav.* **2**, 387–391.

Beart, P.M. & McDonald, D. (1980) *J. Neurochem.* **34**, 1622–1629.

Beninger, R.J. & Hahn, B. (1983) *Science* **220**, 1304–1306.

Beninger, R.J. & Herz, B. (1986) *Life Sci.* **38**, 1425–1431.

Bergman, J., Madras, B.K., Johnson, S.E. & Spealman, R.D. (1989) *J. Pharmacol. Exp. Ther.* **251**, 150–155.

Boyson, S.J., McGonigle, P. & Molinoff, P.B. (1986) *J. Neurosci.* **6**, 3177–3188.

Bozarth, M.A. & Wise, R.A. (1981) *Life Sci.* **29**, 1881–1886.

Bradberry, C.W. & Roth, R.H. (1989) *Neurosci. Lett.* **103**, 97–102.

Braestrup, C. (1977) *J. Pharm. Pharmacol.* **29**, 464–472.

Braun, A.R. & Chase, T.N. (1988) *Eur. J. Pharmacol.* **147**, 441–451.

Brock, J.W., Ng, J.P. & Justice, J.B., Jr (1990) *Neurosci. Lett.* **117**, 234–239.

Bunney, B.S. & Aghajanian, G.A. (1978) *Naunyn-Schmiedeberg's Arch. Pharmacol.* **304**, 255–261.

Bunney, B.S., Walters, J.R., Roth, R.H. & Aghajanian, G.K. (1973) *J. Pharmacol. Exp. Ther.* **135**, 560–571.
Carboni, E., Imperato, A., Perezzani, L. & Di Chiara, G. (1989) *Neuroscience* **28**, 653–661.
Castañeda, E., Becker, J.B. & Robinson, T.E. (1988) *Life Sci.* **42**, 2447–2456.
Chesselet, M.F., Chéramy, A., Reisine, T.D. & Glowinski, J. (1981) *Nature* **291**, 320–322.
Chiodo, L.A., Bannon, M.J., Grace, A.A., Roth, R.H. & Bunney, B.S. (1984) *Neuroscience* **12**, 1–16.
Christie, M.J., Bridge, S., James, L.B. & Beart, P.M. (1985) *Brain Res.* **333**, 169–172.
Clark, D. & Chiodo, L.A. (1988) *Synapse* **2**, 474–485.
Collingridge, G.L. & Bliss, T.V.P. (1987) *Trends Neurosci.* **10**, 288–293.
Conway, P.G. & Uretsky, N.J. (1982) *J. Pharmacol. Exp. Ther.* **221**, 650–655.
Dawson, T.M., Gehlert, D.R., McCabe, R.T., Barnett, A. & Wamsley, J.K. (1986) *J. Neurosci.* **6**, 2352–2365.
Deutch, A.Y., Tam, S.-Y. & Roth, R.H. (1985) *Brain Res.* **333**, 143–146.
deWit, H. & Wise, R.A. (1977) *Can. J. Psychol.* **31**, 195–203.
Di Chiara, G. & Imperato, A. (1988) *Proc. Natl Acad. Sci. USA* **85**, 5274–5278.
Dougherty, Jr, G.G. & Ellinwood, Jr, E.E. (1981) *Life Sci.* **28**, 2295–2298.
Drew, K.L. & Glick, S.D. (1990) *Psychopharmacology* **101**, 465–471.
Dubois, A., Savasta, M., Curet, O. & Scatton, B. (1986) *Neuroscience* **19**, 125–137.
Dworkin, S.I. & Smith, J.E. (1988) In *Problems of Drug Abuse* (ed. Harris, L.S.), pp 266–274. NIDA Research Monographs 90. Washington, DC, US Government Printing Office.
Dwoskin, L.P., Peris, J., Yasuda, R.P., Philpott, K. & Zahniser, N.R. (1988) *Life Sci.* **42**, 255–262.
Einhorn, L.C., Johansen, P.A. & White, F.J. (1988) *J. Neurosci.* **8**, 100–112.
Ettenberg, A., Pettit, H.O., Bloom, F.E. & Koob, G.F. (1982) *Psychopharmacology* **78**, 204–209.
Filloux, F.M., Wamsley, J.K. & Dawson, T.M. (1987) *Brain Res.* **408**, 205–209.
Gale, K. (1984) In *Mechanisms of Tolerance and Dependence: 1984* (ed. Sharp, C.W.), pp 323–332. NIDA Research Monograph 54. Washington, DC, US Government Printing Office.
Goeders, N.E. & Kuhar, M.J. (1987) *Alcohol Drug Res.* **7**, 207–216.
Goeders, N.E. & Smith, J.E. (1983) *Science* **221**, 773–775.
Goeders, N.E. & Smith, J.E. (1986) *Pharmacol. Biochem. Behav.* **25**, 191–199.
Goeders, N.E., Dworkin, S.I. & Smith, J.E. (1986) *Pharmacol. Biochem. Behav.* **24**, 1429–1440.
Groves, P.M., Wilson, C.J., Young, S.J. & Rebec, G.V. (1975) *Science* **210**, 654–656.
Gysling, K. & Wang, R.Y. (1983) *Brain Res.* **277**, 119–127.
Hakan, R.L. & Henriksen, S.J. (1987) *Neurosci. Lett.* **83**, 307–312.
Hakan, R.L. & Henriksen, S.J. (1989) *J. Neurosci.* **9**, 3538–3546.
Hakan, R.L., Callaway, C. & Henriksen, S.J. (1989) *Neurosci. Lett.* **101**, 163–168.
Heikkila, R.E., Orlansky, H. & Cohen, G. (1975) *Biochem. Pharmacol.* **103**, 241–248.
Henry, D.J. & White, F.J. (1990) *Soc. Neurosci. Abstr.* **16**, 1051.
Henry, D.J., Greene, M.A. & White, F.J. (1989) *J. Pharmacol. Exp. Ther.* **251**, 833–839.
Hitzemann, R., Wu, J., Hom, D. & Loh, J. (1980) *Psychopharmacology* **72**, 93–101.
Hoebel, B.G., Monaco, A.P., Hernandez, L., Aulisi, E.F., Stanley, B.G. & Lenard, L. (1983) *Psychopharmacology* **81**, 158–163.
Horger, B.A., Shelton, K. & Schenk, S. (1990) *Pharmacol. Biochem. Behav.* **37**, 707–711.

Hu, X.-T., Wachtel, S.R., Galloway, M.P. & White, F.J. (1990) *J. Neurosci.* **10**, 2318–2329.
Hurd, Y.L. & Ungerstedt, Y. (1989) *Eur. J. Pharmacol.* **166**, 261–269.
Hurd, Y.L., Weiss, F., Koob, G.F., Anden, N.-E. & Understedt, U. (1989) *Brain Res.* **498**, 199–203.
Iyengar, S., Kim, H.S., Marien, M.R., McHugh, D. & Wood, P.L. (1989) *Neuropharmacology* **28**, 123–128.
Izenwasser, S. & Cox, B.M. (1990) *Brain Res.* **531**, 338–341.
Joyce, E.M. & Iversen, S.D. (1979) *Neurosci. Lett.* **14**, 207–212.
Kalivas, P.W. (1985) *J. Pharmacol. Exp. Ther.* **235**, 544–550.
Kalivas, P.W. & Duffy, P. (1987) *J. Pharmacol. Exp. Ther.* **241**, 204–212.
Kalivas, P.W. & Duffy, P. (1988) *J. Neurochem.* **50**, 1498–1504.
Kalivas, P.W. & Duffy, P. (1989) *Biol. Psychiatry* **25**, 913–928.
Kalivas, P.W. & Duffy, P. (1990) *Synapse* **5**, 48–58.
Kalivas, P.W. & Stewart, J. (1991) *Brain Res. Rev.* (in press).
Kalivas, P.W. & Weber, B. (1988) *J. Pharmacol. Exp. Ther.* **245**, 1095–1102.
Kalivas, P.W., Duffy, P., Abhold, R. & Dilts, R.P. (1988) In *Sensitization in the Nervous System* (eds Kalivas, P.W. & Barnes, C.D.), pp 119–143. Caldwell, NJ, Telford Press.
Kalivas, P.W., Bourdelais, A., Abhold, R. & Abbott, L. (1989) *Neurosci. Lett.* **100**, 215–220.
Kamal, L.A., Arbilla, S. & Langer, S.Z. (1981) *J. Pharmacol. Exp. Ther.* **216**, 592–598.
Kamata, K. & Rebec, G.V. (1984) *Life Sci.* **34**, 2419–2427.
Kaneno, S., Watanabe, A. & Takahashi, R. (1986) *Eur. J. Pharmacol.* **123**, 287–294.
Karler, R., Calder, L.D., Chaudhry, I.A. & Turkanis, S.A. (1989) *Life Sci.* **45**, 599–606.
Karler, R., Chaudhry, I.A., Calder, L.D. & Turkanis, S.A. (1990) *Brain Res.* **537**, 76–82.
Kazahaya, Y., Akimoto, K. & Saburo, O. (1989) *Biol. Psychiatry* **25**, 902–912.
Kelly, P.H. (1977) In *Handbook of Psychopharmacology*, Vol. 8 (eds Iversen, L.L., Iversen, S.D. & Snyder, S.H.), pp 295–331. New York, Plenum Press.
Kennedy, L.T. & Hanbauer, I. (1983) *J. Neurochem.* **41**, 172–178.
Kleven, M.S., Perry, B.D., Woolverton, W.L. & Seiden, L.S. (1990) *Brain Res.* **532**, 265–270.
Klitenick, M.A. & Kalivas, P.W. (1990) *Soc. Neurosci. Abstr.* **16**, 382.18.
Kolta, M.G., Shreve, P., De Souza, V. & Uretsky, N.J. (1985) *Neuropharmacology* **24**, 823–829.
Kolta, M.G., Shreve, P. & Uretsky, N.J. (1989) *Neuropharmacology* **28**, 9–14.
Koob, G.F. & Bloom, F.E. (1988) *Science* **242**, 715–723.
Kuczenski, R. (1983) In *Stimulants: Neurochemical, Behavioral and Clinical Perspectives* (ed. Creese, I.), pp 31–61. New York, Raven Press.
Kuczenski, R. (1986) *J. Neurochem.* **46**, 1605–1611.
Kuczenski, R. & Leith, N.J. (1981) *Pharmacol. Biochem. Behav.* **15**, 405–413.
Kuczenski, R. & Segal, D.S. (1988) In *Sensitization in the Nervous System* (eds Kalivas, P.W. & Barnes, C.D.), pp 175–205. Caldwell, NJ, Telford Press.
Kuczenski, R., Segal, D.S. & Manley, L.D. (1990) *J. Neurochem.* **54**, 1492–1499.
Kuribara, H., Asami, T. & Tadokoro, S. (1986) *Jpn. J. Psychopharmacol.* **6**, 127–128.
Lacey, M.G., Mercuri, N.B. & North, R.A. (1988) *J. Physiol.* **401**, 437–453.
Lacey, M.G., Mercuri, N.B. & North, R.A. (1989) *J. Neurosci.* **9**, 1233–1241.
Leslie, C.A. & Bennett, J.P. (1987) *Brain Res.* **415**, 90–97.
Lett, B.T. (1989) *Psychopharmacology* **98**, 357–362.
Lorez, H.P. & Burkard, W.P. (1979) *Experientia* **35**, 744–746.

Lyness, W.H., Friedle, N.M. & Moore, K.E. (1979) *Pharmacol. Biochem. Behav.* **11**, 553–556.
Maisonneuve, I.M., Keller, R.W. & Glick, S.D. (1990) *Brain Res.* **535**, 221–226.
Mansour, A., Meador-Woodruff, J.H., Bunzow, J.R., Civelli, O., Akil, H. & Watson, S.J. (1990) *J. Neurosci.* **10**, 2587–2600.
Marshall, J.F., Navarrete, R. & Joyce, J.N. (1989) *Brain Res.* **493**, 247–257.
Martin-Iverson, M.T. & McManus, D.J. (1990) *Brain Res.* **521**, 175–184.
Martin-Iverson, M.T., Szostak, C. & Fibiger, H.C. (1986) *Psychopharmacology* **88**, 310–314.
Martres, M.P., Constentin, J., Baudry, M., Marcais, H., Protrais, P. & Schwartz, J.C. (1977) *Brain Res.* **136**, 319–337.
Matthews, R.T. & German, D.C. (1984) *Neuroscience* **11**, 617–625.
Memo, M., Pradhan, S. & Hanbauer, I. (1981) *Neuropharmacology* **20**, 1145–1150.
Mogenson, G.J. & Yim, C.C. (1991) In *The Mesolimbic Dopamine System: From Motivation to Action* (eds Willner, P. & Scheel-Kruger, J.), pp 106–130. New York, John Wiley and Sons.
Moghaddam, B. & Bunney, B.S. (1989) *Synapse* **4**, 156–161.
Muller, P. & Seeman, P. (1979) *Eur. J. Pharmacol.* **55**, 149–157.
Nestler, E.J., Terwilliger, R.Z., Walker, J.R., Sevarino, K.A. & Duman, R.S. (1990) *J. Neurochem.* **55**, 1079–1082.
Nicoll, R.A., Kauer, J.A. & Malenka, R.C. (1988) *Neuron* **1**, 97–103.
Niddam, R., Arbilla, S., Scatton, B., Dennis, T. & Langer, S.Z. (1985) *Naunyn-Schmiedeberg's Arch. Pharmacol.* **329**, 123–127.
Nisenbaum, E.S., Orr, W.B. & Berger, T.W. (1988) *J. Neurosci.* **8**, 4138–4150.
Nomikos, G.G., Damsma, G., Wenkstern, D. & Fibiger, H.C. (1990) *Synapse* **6**, 106–112.
Olds, M.E. (1982) *Brain Res.* **237**, 429–440.
Pani, L., Carboni, S., Kusmin, A., Gessa, G.L. & Rossetti, Z.L. (1990) *Eur. J. Pharmacol.* **176**, 245–246.
Patrick, S.L., Thompson, T.L., Walker, J.M. & Patrick, R.L. (1991) *Brain Res.* **538**, 343–346.
Peris, J. & Zahniser, N.R. (1987) *Pharmacol. Biochem. Behav.* **27**, 533–535.
Peris, J. & Zahniser, N.R. (1989) *Pharmacol. Biochem. Behav.* **32**, 71–76.
Peris, J., Boyson, S.J., Cass, W.A., Curella, P., Dwoskin, L.P., Larson, G., Lin, L.-Hl., Yasuda, R.P. & Zahniser, N.R. (1990) *J. Pharmacol. Exp. Ther.* **253**, 38–44.
Pettit, H.O., Ettenberg, A., Bloom, F.E. & Koob, G.F. (1984) *Psychopharmacology* **84**, 167–173.
Pettit, H.O., Pan, H.-T., Parsons, L.H. & Justice, J.B., Jr, (1990) *J. Neurochem.* **55**, 798–804.
Phillips, A.G., Broekkamp, C.L.E. & Fibiger, H.C. (1983a) *Prog. Neuro-Psychopharmacol. Biol. Psychiatry* **7**, 585–591.
Phillips, A.G., LePaine, F.G. & Fibiger, H.C. (1983b) *Life Sci.* **33**, 2505–2511.
Piazza, P.V., Deminiere, J., Le Moal, M. & Simon, H. (1989) *Science* **245**, 1511–1513.
Poncelet, M., Dangoumau, L., Soubrie, P. & Simon, P. (1987) *Psychopharmacology* **92**, 393–397.
Post, R.M., Weiss, S.R.B. & Pert, A. (1991) In *Cocaine: Pharmacology, Physiology and Clinical Strategies* (eds Lakoski, J., Galloway, M.P. & White, F.J.) New Jersey, The Telford Press (in press).
Pulvirenti, L., Swerdlow, N.R., Hubner, C.B. & Koob, G.F. (1991) In *The Mesolimbic Dopamine System: From Motivation to Action* (eds Willner, P. & Scheel-Kruger, J.), pp

131–140. New York, John Wiley and Sons.
Qiao, J.-T., Dougherty, P.M., Wiggins, R.C. & Dafny, N. (1990) *Neuropharmacology* **29**, 379–385.
Rebec, G.V. & Zimmerman, K.S. (1980) *Brain Res.* **201**, 485–491.
Reith, M.E.A., Sershen, H. & Lajtha, A. (1980) *Life Sci.* **27**, 1055–1062.
Riffee, W.H., Wanek, E. & Wilcox, R.E. (1987) *Eur. J. Pharmacol.* **135**, 255–258.
Ritz, M.C. & Kuhar, M.J. (1989) *J. Pharmacol. Exp. Ther.* **248**, 1010–1017.
Ritz, M.C., Lamb, R.J., Goldberg, S.R. & Kuhar, M.J. (1987) *Science* **237**, 1219–1223.
Rivet, J.-M., Stinus, L., LeMoal, M. & Mormede, P. (1989) *Brain Res.* **498**, 149–153.
Roberts, D.C.S. & Koob, G.F. (1982) *Pharmacol. Biochem. Behav.* **17**, 901–904.
Roberts, D.C.S., Corcoran, M.E. & Fibiger, H.C. (1977) *Pharmacol. Biochem. Behav.* **6**, 615–620.
Roberts, D.C.S., Koob, G.F., Klonoff, P. & Fibiger, H.C. (1980) *Pharmacol. Biochem. Behav.* **12**, 781–787.
Roberts-Lewis, J.M., Roseboom, P.H., Iwaniec, L.M. & Gnegy, M.E. (1986) *J. Neurosci.* **6**, 2245–2251.
Robinson, T.E. (1988) In *Sensitization in the Nervous System* (eds Kalivas, P.W. & Barnes, C.D.), pp 145–173. Caldwell, NJ, Telford Press.
Robinson, T.E. (1991) In *The Biological Basis of Substance Abuse* (eds Barchas, J. & Korenman, S.) Oxford University Press.
Robinson, T.E. & Becker, J.B. (1982) *Eur. J. Pharmacol.* **85**, 253–254.
Robinson, T.E. & Becker, J.B. (1986) *Brain Res. Rev.* **11**, 157–198.
Robinson, T.E. & Camp. D.M. (1990) *Neuropsychopharmacology* **3**, 163–173.
Robinson, T.E., Becker, J.B., Young, E.A., Akil, H. & Castandea, E. (1987) *Neuropharmacology* **26**, 679–691.
Robinson, T.E., Jurson, P.A., Bennett, J.A. & Bentgen, K.M. (1988) *Brain Res.* **462**, 211–222.
Roseboom, P.H. & Gnegy, M.E. (1988) *Mol. Pharmacol.* **34**, 148–156.
Roseboom, P.H. & Gnegy, M.E. (1990) *Mol. Pharmacol.* **34**, 148–156.
Roseboom, P.H., Hewlett, G.H.K. & Gnegy, M.E. (1990) *J. Pharmacol. Exp. Ther.* **255**, 197–203.
Savasta, M., Dubois, A. & Scatton, B. (1986) *Brain Res.* **375**, 291–301.
Scheel-Kruger, J., Braestrup, C., Nielson, M., Golembiowski, K. & Mogilnicka, E. (1977) In *Cocaine and Other Stimulants* (eds Ellinwood, E., Jr & Kilby, M.), pp 373–407. New York, Plenum.
Skirboll, L.R. & Bunney, B.S. (1979) *Life Sci.* **25**, 1419–1434.
Spealman, R.D., Madras, B.K. & Bergman, J. (1989) *J. Pharmacol. Exp. Ther.* **251**, 142–149.
Spyraki, C., Fibiger, H.C. & Phillips, A.G. (1983) *Psychopharmacology* **79**, 278–283.
Stewart, J. & Vezina, P. (1988) In *Sensitization in the Nervous System* (eds Kalivas, P.W. & Barnes, C.D.), pp 207–224. Caldwell, NJ, Telford Press.
Stewart, J. & Vezina, P. (1989) *Brain Res.* **495**, 401–406.
Stewart, J., deWit, H. & Eikelboom, R. (1984) *Psychol. Rev.* **91**, 251–268.
Strombom, U.H. & Liedman, B. (1982) *Psychopharmacology* **78**, 271–276.
Suppes, T. & Pinnock, R.D. (1987) *Neuropharmacology* **26**, 331–337.
Terwilliger, R.Z., Beitner-Johnson, D., Sevarino, K.A., Crain, S.M. & Nestler, E.J. (1991) *Brain Res.* **548**, 100–110.
Tyler, C.V., Keegan, M.J. & Galloway, M.P. (1989) *Soc. Neurosci. Abstr.* **25**, 432.
Ujike, H., Onoue, T., Akiyama, K., Hamamura, T. & Otsuki, S. (1989) *Psychopharmacology* **98**, 89–92.

Van Rossum, J., Van Schoot, J. & Hurkman, J. (1962) *Experientia* **18**, 229–230.
Vezina, P. & Stewart, J. (1984) *Pharmacol. Biochem. Behav.* **20**, 925–934.
Vezina, P. & Stewart, J. (1989) *Brain Res.* **499**, 108–120.
Vezina, P. & Stewart, J. (1990) *Brain Res.* **516**, 99–106.
Vezina, P., Kalivas, P.W. & Stewart, J. (1987) *Brain Res.* **417**, 51–58.
Wachtel, S.R., Hu, X.-T., Galloway, M.P. & White, F.J. (1989) *Synapse* **4**, 327–346.
Walaas, S.I. & Greengard, P. (1984) *J. Neurosci.* **4**, 84–98.
Wang, R.Y. (1981) *Brain Res. Rev.* **3**, 153–165.
Wang, R.Y., White, F.J. & Voigt, M.M. (1984) In *Neurology and Neurobiology*, Vol. 8B: *Catecholamines: Neuropharmacology and Central Nervous System—Theoretical Aspects* (eds Usdin, E., Carlsson, A., Dahlstrom, A. & Engel, J.), pp 319–369. New York, Alan R. Liss, Inc.
Weissman, A., Koe, B. & Tenen, S. (1966) *J. Pharmacol. Exp. Ther.* **151**, 339–352.
Westerink, B.H.C., Tuntler, J., Damsma, G., Rollema, H. & de Vries, J.B. (1987) *Arch. Pharmacol.* **336**, 502–507.
Westerink, B.H.C., Hofsteede, R.M., Tuntler, J. & de Vries, J.B. (1989) *J. Neurochem.* **52**, 722–729.
White, F.J. (1990) *Behav. Pharmacol.* **1**, 303–315.
White, F.J. (1991) In *The Mesolimbic Dopamine System: From Motivation to Action* (eds Willner, P. & Scheel-Kruger, J.), pp 61–103. New York, John Wiley and Sons.
White, F.J. & Wang, R.Y. (1984a) *Life Sci.* **34**, 1161–1170.
White, F.J. & Wang, R.Y. (1984b) *Brain Res.* **309**, 283–292.
White, F.J. & Wang, R.Y. (1984c) *J. Pharmacol. Exp. Ther.* **231**, 275–280.
White, F.J. & Wang, R.Y. (1986) *J. Neurosci.* **6**, 274–280.
White, F.J., Einhorn, L.C., Johansen, P.A. & Wachtel, S.R. (1987) In *Neurophysiology of Dopaminergic Systems: Current Status and Clinical Perspectives* (eds Chiodo, L.A. & Freeman, A.S.), pp 317–365. Detroit, Lakeshore Publishing Co.
White, F.J., Hu, X.-T. & Brooderson, R.J. (1990) *Eur. J. Pharmacol.* **191**, 497–499.
White, F.J., Henry, D.J., Hu, X.-T., Jeziorski, M. & Ackerman, J.M. (1991) In *Cocaine: Pharmacology, Physiology and Clinical Strategies* (eds Lakoski, J.M., Galloway, M.P. & White, F.J.). Boca Raton, FL, CRC Press.
Wightman, R.M. & Zimmerman, J.B. (1990) *Brain Res. Rev.* **15**, 135–144.
Wilcox, R.A., Robinson, T.E. & Becker, J.B. (1986) *Eur. J. Pharmacol.* **124**, 375–376.
Wise, R.A. & Bozarth, M.A. (1987) *Psychol. Rev.* **94**, 469–492.
Wise, R.A. & Rompré, P.-P. (1989) *Annu. Rev. Psychol.* **40**, 191–225.
Wise, R.A., Murray, A. & Bozarth, M.A. (1990) *Psychopharmacology* **100**, 355–360.
Wolf, M.E. & Khansa, M.R. (1991) *Brain Res.* (in press).
Wolf, M.E. & Roth, R.H. (1987) In *Dopamine Receptors* (eds Creese, I. & Fraser, C.M.), pp 45–96. New York, Alan R. Liss.
Woolverton, W.L., Goldberg, L.I. & Ginos, J. (1984a) *J. Pharmacol. Exp. Ther.* **230**, 678–683.
Woolverton, W.L., Cervo, L. & Johanson, C.E. (1984b) *Pharmacol. Biochem. Behav.* **21**, 737–741.
Yi, S.-J. & Johnson, K.M. (1990a) *Pharmacol. Biochem. Behav.* **36**, 457–461.
Yi, S.-J. & Johnson, K.M. (1990b) *Neuropharmacology* **29**, 475–486.
Yokel, R.A. & Wise, R.A. (1978) *Psychopharmacology* **58**, 289–296.
Zito, K.A., Roberts, D.C.S. & Vickers, G. (1985) *Pharmacol. Biochem. Behav.* **23**, 1029–1036.

CHAPTER 7

OPIOID TOLERANCE AND DEPENDENCE

Brian M. Cox[1] and Linda L. Werling[2]

[1] *Department of Pharmacology, F. Edward Hébert School of Medicine, Uniformed Services University of the Health Sciences, Bethesda MD 20814, USA*
[2] *Department of Pharmacology, George Washington University School of Medicine, Washington DC 20037, USA*

Table of Contents

7.1 Introduction

In this chapter, we have summarized current views on the mechanisms underlying opioid tolerance and dependence. A brief overview of the pharmacology of opiate drugs and opioid peptides is presented and the heterogeneity of opioid receptors is discussed. The general characteristics of opioid tolerance and dependence at the single cell level and in the whole animal are described, and experiments characterizing modifications in cell function associated with

THE BIOLOGICAL BASES OF DRUG TOLERANCE AND DEPENDENCE
ISBN 0-12-564250-4

tolerance and dependence are considered. Changes in the rates of metabolism or elimination of opiate drugs are probably of little significance in opiate tolerance. Alterations in receptor properties are more clearly implicated, and evidence is accumulating suggesting that adaptive changes in the function of effector systems play significant roles in opiate tolerance and dependence. The importance of behavioural factors in the loss of opioid sensitivity and in the development of the dependent state in the whole animal is also reviewed briefly.

The last sections of the chapter consider the effects of acute and chronic opioid exposure on three functional systems subject to regulation by opioids. The first system considered is the spinal and supraspinal system regulating sensitivity to noxious stimuli. The primary clinical use of opiate drugs is in the relief of pain, and tolerance to this action is a significant clinical problem. A greater understanding of the mechanisms underlying tolerance to opioid analgesia might lead to improved treatment regimens in the relief of severe pain. We next consider the role of the locus coeruleus in the genesis and expression of opioid withdrawal symptoms. Finally, the processes implicated in opiate drug-induced reinforcement with emphasis on opioid action in the ventral tegmental area (VTA) and in the mesolimbic dopaminergic projection system are discussed. Opiate-induced reward is presumed to be a primary factor leading to sustained self-administration of opiate drugs in animals and man.

7.2 Pharmacology of opioid drugs and opioid peptides

Numerous substances with diverse chemical structures produce pharmacological effects similar to those of morphine, the major alkaloid produced by the opium poppy, *Papaver somniferum.* In addition to the naturally occurring alkaloids, morphine and codeine, semi-synthetic agents such as heroin (diacetylmorphine) and etorphine, and simpler synthetic compounds such as methadone, meperidine (pethidine), fentanyl and their congeners, can all induce effects similar to those of morphine. The structure of morphine was determined more than a century ago, and by that time it was known that tolerance and dependence resulted from the repeated use of opium extracts. Many synthetic opiate drugs were developed during the five decades from 1920 through 1970 as a result of a major effort to identify substances that would provide the effective relief of severe pain that is uniquely characteristic of opiate drugs of the morphine type, while avoiding the problems of tolerance and abuse liability (Archer, 1986). It was not until the mid-1970s that several peptides of neural or endocrine origin with actions similar to those of morphine were identified. Most of the pharmacological actions of opiate drugs are now thought to arise from an interaction of the drug with receptors normally activated by endogenous opioid peptides (Evans *et al.*, 1988).

It is now known that in mammals endogenous opioids arise from at least three genes each coding for a precursor peptide for a different family of endogenous opioids. The first opioid peptides to be characterized were the enkephalins, methionine- and leucine-enkephalin (Hughes *et al.*, 1975). Their precursor peptide, proenkephalin, contains six copies of the methionine-enkephalin sequence, and one copy of the leucine-enkephalin sequence. Enkephalins are widely distributed in the brain and peripheral nervous system, in the endocrine and reproductive systems, and in some cells of the immune system. At many sites in the nervous system, enkephalins probably function as neurotransmitters (or neuromodulators); their functions in the endocrine, reproductive and immune systems are less well understood. The dynorphins (dynorphin A, dynorphin B, α-neo-endorphin and shorter related peptides) derived from prodynorphin (also known as proenkephalin B) are also found in neural, endocrine and reproductive tissues, although their concentrations are lower, and they are less widely distributed than the enkephalins. The dynorphins are also presumed to function as neurotransmitters or neuromodulators at selected synapses in brain and spinal cord (Khachaturian *et al.*, 1985).

The third family of opioid peptides, β-endorphin and shorter peptides derived from β-endorphin, are synthesized as part of the multifunctional precursor peptide, pro-opiomelanocortin (POMC). This peptide is a precursor for adrenocorticotrophic hormone (ACTH) and melanocyte stimulating hormone (MSH) in addition to β-endorphin. POMC and its products are found in cells in two brain nuclei, the arcuate nucleus of hypothalamus and the nucleus tractus solitarius of medulla. However, much higher concentrations of POMC and its products are present in the anterior and intermediate lobes of the pituitary. β-Endorphin is released together with its co-synthesized peptides from both endocrine and neural cells. Processing of the precursor peptide differs among tissues; thus in the anterior lobe of the pituitary, activation by CRF results in release of ACTH, β-endorphin and its immediate precursor, β-lipotropin. In the intermediate lobe of the pituitary the ACTH region of POMC is further processed to release α-MSH upon stimulation, while the β-endorphin region of the precursor is released mainly as β-endorphin and its *N*-acetylated and C-terminally truncated forms, with little β-lipotropin being secreted (Akil *et al.*, 1984). As with the other opioid peptides, β-endorphin and related peptides are also found in cells of the reproductive and immune systems but their functions in this system are uncertain (Douglass *et al.*, 1987; Sibinga and Goldstein, 1988).

A major therapeutic action of opiates is their ability to provide symptomatic relief of pathological pain. Despite years of searching for alternative drugs with less abuse potential, the opiates remain the drugs of choice for the relief of severe pain. With the advent of improved methods of artificial respiration and the development of drugs with a short duration of action, opiates have also become important anaesthetic agents, especially for patients with impaired cardiovascular function (Yaksh *et al.*, 1988). Fentanyl and related drugs are generally the preferred opiates for anaesthesia, in part because of their rapid elimination from the body making it possible for anaesthesia to be maintained by intravenous infusion of the drug with relatively rapid recovery following termination of the infusion. Opiates are also valued for their ability to provide symptomatic relief of diarrhoea and dysentery; drugs like loperamide and diphenoxylate offer significant advantages over the prototypic opiate, morphine, for this purpose (Kromer, 1988). In relation to these therapeutic actions, tolerance is most significant with respect to pain relief. Many patients suffer from conditions resulting in moderate or severe pain which continues for days, weeks or months. Opiate drugs provide relief but do not cure the underlying condition; hence repeated use of the drug is necessary.

Most therapeutically useful opiates also induce a euphoric effect that may support self-administration of the drug both in human populations and in laboratory animals (Koob and Bloom, 1988). In dependent individuals, it is this reinforcing effect of opiates and the desire to avoid the unpleasant withdrawal symptoms that are the main factors which contribute to the maintenance of drug-taking behaviour.

7.3 Opioid receptors and their effector systems

7.3.1 Opioid receptor types

There are three classes of opioid receptor for which associated function has been well defined. Two of these were originally described in the chronic spinal dog model of Martin *et al.* (1976). The μ-receptor, so named because of its activation by morphine, mediated analgesia, miosis, bradycardia, and hypothermia. The κ-receptor, activated by ketocyclazocine, appeared responsible for sedation, and depression of flexor reflexes, but had no involvement in skin twitch reflex or pulse rate. A third class of receptors described by this group was named σ for its activation by SKF 10,047 (*N*-allylnormetazocine). For an effect to be considered consequent to opioid receptor activation, the effect must be reversed by the classical opioid antagonist naloxone or its more potent analogue, naltrexone. While the μ- and κ-receptor-mediated events observed by Martin *et al.* were readily reversible by naltrexone, later evidence indicated that physiological events effected by σ-receptors were not reversed by naltrexone (Vaupel, 1983), and this class of receptors is now not generally considered to be opioid in nature. An additional class of opioid receptor identified by Lord *et al.* (1977) was activated by the enkephalins and was named δ. The existence of multiple opioid receptors has been demonstrated in binding studies using either radiolabelled ligands selective for receptor types, or non-selective radiolabelled ligands in the presence of site-selective concentrations of blocking agents.

Other receptors considered to be opioid on the basis of their sensitivity to naloxone have been identified in binding studies, but a clear functional significance associated with these receptors is thus far lacking. Among these receptors are the subtypes of μ, called μ_1 and μ_2. μ_1-receptors have been proposed to mediate analgesia, and μ_2-receptors to mediate respiratory depression (Pasternak and Wood, 1986). These assumptions are based upon the observation that naloxonazine antagonized analgesia but not the respiratory depression induced by morphine. Unfortunately, there is to date no antagonist that can reverse the respiratory depression without affecting the analgesia. Nevertheless, if selective μ_1-agonists can be developed, they may be promising agents for the relief of pain with fewer side-effects than non-selective μ-agonists.

Subtypes of κ-receptors have also been proposed (Gouarderes *et al.*, 1986; Zukin *et al.*, 1988). There may be as many as four subtypes of the κ-receptor based upon evidence from radioligand binding studies (Clark *et al.*, 1989). The functional significance of these sites remains to be elucidated.

Opioid receptors termed ε were originally identified as those that mediated inhibition of electrically evoked twitch in rat vas deferens (Lemaire *et al.*, 1978). These receptors were believed to be selectively activated by β-endorphin. Whether the characteristics of this receptor type are really distinctly different from those of μ-receptors remains to be determined. Finally, λ-receptors, first described in binding studies in rat brain (Grevel and Sadee, 1983), were defined as having high affinity for naloxone, but low affinity for another opioid antagonist, diprenorphine. A functional role for this class of receptor has not been proposed as yet.

7.3.2 Functional assays

Model systems for studying opioid receptor function have been developed for the three major classes of opioid receptor, μ, δ, and κ, and have assisted in the elucidation of the second messenger systems activated by opioid agonist binding. The enzyme adenylate cyclase, responsible for the conversion of ATP to cAMP, was the first second messenger system shown to be affected by

Table 1 Well-characterized opioid receptor types.

Receptor type	Prototypic agonist	Selective agonists	Selective antagonists	Functions
μ	Morphine	DAMGO PL-017 Sufentanil	Naloxone (low concentrations) CTOP, CTAP	Activation of G_i, G_o; open K^+ channels; inhibition of adenylate cyclase
δ	DADLE	DPDPE	Naltrindole ICI 174864	Activation of G_i, G_o; open K^+ channels; inhibition of adenylate cyclase
κ	Ketocyclazocine EKC	U69593 CI-977 (PD117302 U50488H)	nor-BNI	Activation of unknown G protein; close some Ca^{2+} channels

References: Martin *et al.* (1976), Lord *et al.* (1977), North and Williams (1985), Watson and Abbott (1990), Werz and Macdonald (1984).

CI-977, (5R)-(5α,7α,8β)-*N*-methyl-*N*-[7-(1-pyrrolidinyl)-1-oxaspiro[4,5]dec-8-yl]-4-benzofuranacetamide monohydrochloride; CTAP, cyclic D-Phe-Cys-Tyr-D-Trp-Arg-Thr-Pen-Thr-NH_2; CTOP, cyclic D-Phe-Cys-Tyr-D-Trp-Orn-Thr-Pen-Thr-NH_2; DADLE, [D-Ala^2, D-Leu^5]enkephalin; DAMGO, Tyr-D-Ala-Gly-(Me)Phe-Gly-ol; DFDPE, [D-Pen^5, D-Pen^5] enkephalin; EKC, ethylketocyclazocine; ICI 174864, $allyl_2$-Tyr-(α-aminoisobutyric acid)$_2$-Phe-Leu-OH; nor-BNI, nor-binaltorphimine; PD117302, (±)-*trans*-*N*-methyl-*N*-[2-(1-pyrrolodinyl)-cyclohexyl]benzo[b]thiophene-4-acetamide; PL-017, [*N*-(Me)Phe^3, D-Pro^4]morphiceptin; U50488H, *trans*-(±)3,4-dichloro-*N*-methyl-*N*-[2-(1-pyrrolodinyl)cyclohexyl] benzene-acetamide methanesulphonate; U69593, (5α,7α,8β)-(−)-*N*-methyl-*N*-[7-(1-pyrrolidinyl)-1-oxaspiro[4,5]dec-8-yl]-4-benzene-acetamide.

Table 2 Other proposed opioid receptor types and subtypes.

Receptor subtype	Unique characteristic	Proposed functions	Refs
μ	(Readily blocked by naloxone)		
μ_1	Irreversibly occupied by naloxonazine	Analgesia	(1)
μ_2	Not irreversibly blocked by naloxonazine	Respiratory depression, etc.	(1)
κ	(Less sensitive to inhibition by naloxone; high affinity for EKC)		
κ_1^*	High affinity for arylacetamides (e.g U69593)	Analgesia, etc.	(2)
κ_2^*	Low affinity for U69593 High affinity for bremazocine	Unknown	(3)
κ_3	High affinity for naloxone benzoylhydrazine	Analgesia	(4)
ε	Highly sensitive to β-endorphin; in rat vas deferens	Inhibition of neurally evoked contractions	(5)
λ	Very high affinity for naloxone	Unknown	(6)

References: 1, Pasternak and Wood (1986); 2, Clark *et al.* (1988); 3, Zukin *et al.* (1988), Tiberi and Magnan (1990); 4, Clark *et al.* (1989); 5, Wuster *et al.* (1978); 6, Grevel and Sadee (1983).

* Rothman *et al.* (1990) have suggested that both κ_1 and κ_2 sites can be subdivided into κ_{1a}, κ_{1b}, and κ_{2a}, κ_{2b}, respectively, on the basis of their affinities for α-neoendorphin and other dynorphin-derived peptides. The proposed κ_{2b} sites of Rothman *et al.* (1990) may be similar to the proposed κ_3 subtype of Clark *et al.* (1989).

opioids. Early observations using specialized cell types revealed that the activity of this enzyme could be stimulated by certain neurotransmitters or hormones and inhibited by others. Opioid receptors with characteristics of the δ-receptor have been shown to be negatively linked to adenylate cyclase in brain (Childers, 1988). Because of the relatively high concentrations of naloxone required to reverse agonist inhibition, as well as the stringent incubation conditions necessary to observe the opioid inhibition of the enzyme, it is unclear whether the receptors mediating this action are truly δ. However, δ-receptors are responsible for inhibition of adenylate cyclase in NG108-15 neuroblastoma × glioma hybrid cells (Loh *et al.*, 1988). The NG108-15 cell has been a particularly useful model in this regard since it bears opioid receptors only of the δ type.

Receptor-mediated stimulation or inhibition of adenylate cyclase has been shown to be dependent upon the presence of a guanyl nucleotide binding protein (G protein). G proteins are heterotrimeric structures composed of α-, β-, and γ-subunits. The G protein couples the receptor to the cyclase. G proteins mediating inhibition of adenylate cyclase or other negative regulation of physiological response appear to be of at least two types, termed G_i and G_o. Both these G proteins are sensitive to pertussis toxin, an exotoxin produced by *Bordetella pertussis*. Pertussis toxin ADP ribosylates the G protein, resulting in the inability of the G-protein to interact with its normally associated transduction system (Katada and Ui, 1982). Pertussis toxin abolished the ability of opioid agonists to inhibit adenylate cyclase activity in NG108-15 cells (Kurose *et al.*, 1983).

The interactions of agonist, receptor and G proteins were initially proposed by Gilman (1986) for the β-adrenergic system, and can be applied to the opioid receptor system. When agonist binds with receptor, the agonist–receptor complex can interact with the G protein. In the resting state, the G protein is bound to GDP, but upon agonist binding to the receptor, the GDP is

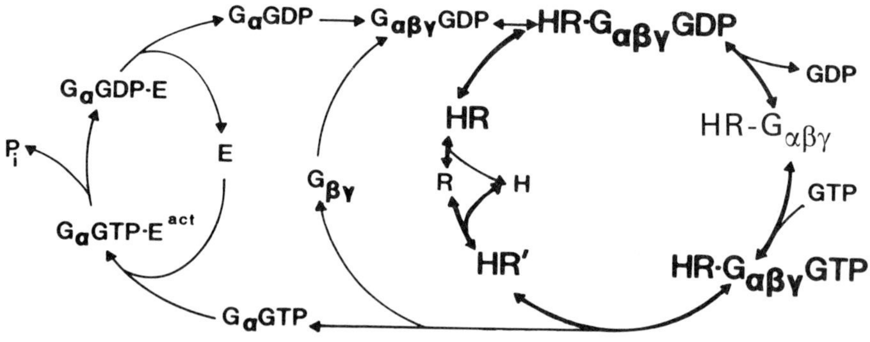

Figure 1 Proposed scheme for the interactions of agonists, receptors, and G protein(s). The agonist (H) binds to free receptor (R), which leads to the association of the HR complex with the G protein (G). The G protein is composed of three subunits, α, β and γ. In the unstimulated state, the G protein is bound to GDP, but upon association with the HR complex, if GTP is available, the GTP replaces the bound GDP, resulting in the formation of the complex $HR.G_{\alpha\beta\gamma}.GTP$. The $G_\alpha.GTP$ complex is then released and can activate an effector system, E. The activation of the effector system (E^{act}) is associated with the release of free inorganic phosphate (P_i) and the $G_\alpha.GDP.E$ complex. Free $G_\alpha.GDP$, $G_{\beta\gamma}$, and E are then available for recycling through the system. After Gilman (1986).

replaced by GTP. The opioid agonist affinity for the receptor is reduced by the interaction of the G protein with GTP, resulting in one or more low-affinity states of the receptor (Werling *et al.*, 1988a). The association of GTP with the agonist–receptor–G protein complex results in dissociation of the complex. This dissociation allows liberated GTP-activated α-subunit of the G protein to inhibit adenylate cyclase. When membranes prepared from brain or other opioid receptor-bearing tissue are treated with pertussis toxin, GTP no longer reduces the affinity of opioid agonist for receptors that are coupled to pertussis toxin-sensitive G proteins. Among opioid receptors, those most clearly shown to be linked to pertussis toxin-sensitive G proteins are of the μ and δ types.

The 7315c rat pituitary tumour cell has provided a fortuitous model of opioid action because it bears opioid receptors only of the μ type, analogous to the δ-receptor model developed in NG108-15 cells. The μ-receptors in 7315c cells are negatively linked to adenylate cyclase (Frey and Kebabian, 1984; Puttfarcken *et al.*, 1988). Pretreatment of these cells with pertussis toxin abolished the ability of GTP to reduce the affinity of μ opioid agonists for their receptors (Puttfarcken *et al.*, 1988).

Mu opioid receptors have been associated with an increase in potassium conductance in guinea-pig myenteric plexus (Morita and North, 1982), mouse dorsal root ganglion cells (Werz and Macdonald, 1983), and rat locus coeruleus (North *et al.*, 1987). Intracellular application of a non-hydrolysable analogue of GTP produced similar effects to application of opioid agonist to locus coeruleus cells (North *et al.*, 1987), and prior intracerebroventricular injection of pertussis toxin prevented the hyperpolarizing action of opioid (Agajanian and Wang, 1986) on these cells. These findings support a role for a G protein in the activation of the potassium conductance linked to μ opioid receptors.

In the guinea-pig submucous plexus (North *et al.*, 1987) and in mouse dorsal root ganglion cells (Werz and Macdonald, 1983), agonist binding at δ-receptors activates a potassium conductance with characteristics similar to those associated with activation of μ-receptors. In the submucous plexus, intracellular injections of a non-hydrolysable GTP analogue potentiated opioid agonist effects, again suggesting that potassium channel activity linked to opioid receptors was G protein linked (North *et al.*, 1987).

Delta opioid receptors have also been shown to be coupled to calcium channels in NG108-15 cells (Hescheler *et al.*, 1987). A δ opioid agonist inhibited the voltage-dependent inward calcium current in these cells, and this inhibition was prevented by pretreatment with pertussis toxin. Inhibition of calcium current could be completely restored by infusion with low concentrations of the α-subunit of G_o. Calcium conductance was also reduced by κ opioid agonists in dispersed mouse dorsal root ganglion cells in culture (Werz and Macdonald, 1984, 1985).

7.4 Effects of chronic agonist exposure on receptor–effector function

Chronic agonist exposure results in a decreased effectiveness of the agonist or related drugs as measured by the ability of that drug to produce some physiological response. Among the first biochemical changes sought in opioid systems were differences in receptor properties occurring after sustained agonist exposure. In early studies, these changes were not observed (Klee and Streaty, 1973; Hollt *et al.*, 1975). However, at this time the heterogeneity of opioid receptors was not appreciated. Since most drugs used for chronic studies were relatively selective for one of these subtypes, but ligands used to measure receptor properties were non-selective, changes in one receptor population may have been too small to detect against a background of radiolabelled ligand binding to all receptor types. Recent studies have taken advantage of the development of more selective radioligands for measurement of receptor properties, as well as an increasing understanding of the processes of signal transduction initiated by opioid agonist action, to gain insight into some of the mechanisms associated with the development of tolerance. Also, the availability of tissue models in which a single type of opioid receptor is expressed has helped to clarify changes in the properties of individual receptor types.

The NG108-15 neuroblastoma × glioma hybrid cells express opioid receptors only of the δ type. Activation of these receptors by opioid agonist results in inhibition of the enzyme adenylate cyclase, and therefore a reduced accumulation of cAMP. After exposure of the cells to morphine or etorphine, opioids were much less able to inhibit adenylate cyclase (Sharma *et al.*, 1975; Loh *et al.*, 1988). When the very efficacious agonist etorphine was used for chronic treatment, the loss of agonist effect was within one hour. Downregulation in receptor number was observable at a later time point, indicating that the loss in effectiveness of opioid agonist was a two-step process involving both a desensitization and a downregulation. Downregulation in NG108-15 cells has been shown to be dependent upon agonist concentration, length of exposure and temperature.

Agonists producing tolerance and dependence in humans are relatively μ-selective. For this reason, the availability of the 7315c pituitary tumour cell provides an especially useful model for examining the changes in μ-receptor properties and function in a population of cells that bears opioid receptors only of the μ type. Incubation of these cells with morphine in primary culture resulted in a complete loss of the ability of morphine or other μ-agonists to inhibit adenylate cyclase. Loss of this ability occurred within hours, and before any reduction in receptor number could be detected. After 24 hours, a loss in μ-receptor number became apparent, and after 72 hours total μ-receptor density was reduced to about 40% (Puttfarcken *et al.*, 1988). As with

δ-receptors in NG108-15 cells, the development of tolerance appeared to involve the two-step process of desensitization followed by downregulation. In addition to the reduction in receptor number, there was also a loss in the ability of guanyl nucleotides to alter binding affinity. In membranes prepared from untreated cells, GTP or its non-hydrolysable analogue GTPγS induced a very low affinity state of the μ-receptor. In contrast, no very low affinity sites were measured in the presence of GTPγS in membranes prepared from morphine-treated cells. The affinity of radiolabelled μ-agonist for its receptor after chronic morphine exposure was very similar to its affinity after treatment of the 7315c cells with pertussis toxin. As discussed in Section 7.3.2, pertussis toxin ADP ribosylates the G protein such that it can no longer interact with the receptor, resulting in a functional uncoupling from the effector system. The similarity of chronic opioid effects and pertussis toxin treatment suggests that tolerance to both may involve a functional uncoupling of receptor from effector system.

Early experiments were unsuccessful in elucidating changes in receptor properties in brain after chronic opioid agonist exposure, in part due to the non-selective nature of the available ligands. More recent efforts have used newer receptor type-selective ligands to quantitate binding parameters. Changes in the binding properties of μ opioid receptors can be measured in brain tissue after the induction of tolerance to morphine. In cortical tissue from guinea-pigs that had received a constant infusion of morphine from a subcutaneously implanted osmotic pump for 6 days, the affinity of agonist for μ-receptors was reduced overall, but the most striking alteration was the loss in the ability of non-hydrolysable GTP analogues to induce a very low affinity state of the μ-receptor (Werling *et al.*, 1989). This loss in guanyl nucleotide regulation was identical to that found in 7315c pituitary tumour cells after chronic morphine exposure. Prior treatment of the membranes with pertussis toxin caused a similar loss in guanyl nucleotide regulation of μ-agonist binding, consistent with functional uncoupling of receptor from effector in tolerance. In guinea-pig brain membranes, there was also a reduction of about 20% in total μ-receptor density. This is much lower than the 60% reduction in receptor number observed in the pituitary tumour cells after 48 hours of morphine exposure. This may be explained by the inability to achieve as high morphine concentrations in the brain of tolerant animals as that applied directly to the 7315c cells.

The tolerance induced in guinea-pig brain tissue was shown to be selective, since no changes were observed in δ or κ binding properties. The same tolerance-inducing regimen has also been shown to be selective in a functional assay. Mu- and κ-receptors are both able to inhibit the potassium-stimulated release of preloaded radiolabelled noradrenaline from slices of guinea-pig cortex. However, in tissue taken from animals exposed to chronic morphine for 6 days, the ability of μ opioid agonists to inhibit release was significantly reduced, while the ability of κ opioid agonists to inhibit release was unaffected (Werling *et al.*, 1988b).

7.5 Effects of chronic exposure to opioids

7.5.1 Tolerance to the various pharmacological effects

Repeated exposure to opiate drugs results in the development of tolerance. The magnitude of the observed tolerance depends on the dose of opiate drug given and the interval between doses. Tolerance also appears to develop more rapidly to some actions of opiates than to others. Anecdotal evidence suggests that there is very rapid tolerance to the nauseant and emetic actions of opiates which are very prominent in ambulant humans given their first dose of opiate drug. Nausea and emesis appear less frequently in subjects receiving a second or subsequent dose reasonably soon after the first dose. Quantitative measurements of the rates of tolerance development have been made in laboratory animals for the analgesic and locomotor stimulant actions of opiate drugs. Measurable tolerance to these actions can be observed after a single large dose of the drug, but tolerance continues to develop further during frequent repeated administration of the same dose of drug and is also apparent after repeated administration of lower doses of drug which may not induce demonstrable tolerance after a single administration. In some experimental systems, the opiate dose–response curve may be shifted to the right to the extent that the drug dose must be increased 100-fold or more to produce an effect equal to that initially produced by the drug. Eventually, if the drug is given frequently enough and in adequate dose, the effect of the drug (e.g. analgesia or locomotor stimulation) is virtually eliminated. In most cases, the effect of the opiate drug can be restored by increasing the dose of the drug. In several assays of opiate drugs, tolerance is initially manifest as a shift to the right in the opiate drug dose–response curve with no reduction in the maximum response to the drug if a sufficiently high dose is given. When large doses are given repeatedly, a reduction in the maximum effect may occur (Blasig *et al.*, 1979; Christie *et al.*, 1987).

Careful studies of the rates of metabolism and elimination of opiate drugs after chronic treatment with morphine have failed to find evidence of changes in the rates of drug absorption, metabolism or excretion of sufficient magnitude to account for the degree of tolerance developed. For a few synthetic opiates, including methadone, there is a measurable induction of liver cytochrome P-450 enzymes (Misra *et al.*, 1973), but, in general, enzyme induction is not a significant factor in opiate drug tolerance. Behavioural factors are likely to contribute significantly to the level of observed tolerance to opiate drugs in intact animals and in man (Goudie and Emmett-Oglesby, 1989), but cannot account for the reduced response to opiate drugs observed in cells or isolated tissues maintained in culture (Sharma *et al.*, 1975). Many experiments point to changes in the sensitivities of cells on which the opiates act as a mechanism of primary importance in the generation of the opiate-tolerant state.

The initial parallel shift in the opioid dose–response curve, with a subsequent reduction in maximum response with more intensive tolerance-inducing treatments, is similar to the changes in dose–response curves when receptors are partially occupied by irreversible antagonists in a system where there is a substantial receptor reserve (i.e. where a maximum response can be induced when only a small fraction of the receptors present are occupied by agonist). Recently, detailed studies of receptor function (described in Section 7.4) suggest that tolerance arises from a temporary inactivation (manifest as an inability to activate effector systems) of the receptor as a result of occupation and activation by agonist. *In vivo* studies of analgesic tolerance and tolerance to the locomotor stimulant actions of morphine are consistent with this interpretation.

One implication of the hypothesis that tolerance results from a temporary inactivation of receptors responsible for opiate drug effects is that the magnitude of the observed tolerance will depend in part on the magnitude of the receptor reserve in each neural system. Increasing the dose of opiate drug will overcome tolerance in systems where there is a large excess of opiate receptors (e.g. in pain-regulating pathways where opiates exert their analgesic actions) but will be ineffective in overcoming tolerance in systems in which occupation of most of the receptors present in the system is necessary for an effect to be observed. To our knowledge, no attempt has been made to estimate the magnitude of the opiate receptor reserve in the pathways mediating the nauseant and emetic actions of morphine, but one possible explanation of the rapid tolerance observed to the nauseant and emetic actions of opiates is the lack of receptor reserve in these pathways.

A second implication of the receptor inactivation model of tolerance is that the rate of recovery from tolerance will depend not only on the rate of elimination of the tolerance-inducing drug but also on the rate at which functional opiate receptors again become available for activation by opiate drug. The time-course for return of the pharmacological response will reflect the rate of recovery of inactivated receptors and the rate at which newly synthesized receptors are inserted into the cell membrane. It is probable that the receptor synthesis rate will vary among physiological systems regulated by opioids, and also among species. In the rat, measurements of the rate of recovery from analgesic tolerance have demonstrated that at least two components of the recovery rate can be identified; an initial rapidly decaying component with a half-time of less than 24 hours (perhaps related to the rate of drug elimination) and a more slowly decaying component with a half-time of 12 to 14 days (Cox *et al.*, 1975). It remains to be determined if this slowly decaying component of analgesic tolerance is related to a recovery of receptor function or if other factors are also involved.

Tolerance induced by morphine also extends to all other drugs activating the same receptors as morphine. Animals tolerant to the analgesic actions of morphine are also tolerant to the analgesic actions of fentanyl, methadone or meperidine. There is also cross-tolerance to the actions of endogenous opioid peptides in systems where these act on the same receptors as morphine. However, as noted in Section 7.3.1, endogenous opioid peptides and some synthetic opiate drugs such as etorphine can activate types of opioid receptors that are not normally activated by morphine. In systems where more than one type of opioid receptor can regulate the measured response there may be significantly less tolerance to peptides or synthetic agonists with good potency at several types of receptor (e.g. enkephalins, β-endorphin, dynorphins, etorphine) than to drugs like morphine or fentanyl that act predominantly at one type of opioid receptor (in this case, at μ-receptors).

7.5.2 Opiate dependence

Chronic exposure to opiate agonists also leads to the development of a state of dependence on the opiate drug. In this state essentially normal function is maintained as long as an opiate agonist is still present in the system. On removal of the drug, either by discontinuation of administration or by displacement of the drug from opioid receptors by administration of an antagonist such as naloxone, a disturbed physiological state known as a withdrawal syndrome develops.

The opiate drug withdrawal syndrome in man is characterized by an initial period of restlessness, intense craving for the drug, yawning, rhinorrhoea, lacrimation, and piloerection (gooseflesh; 'cold turkey'). Additional symptoms gradually become more predominant, including insomnia, loss of appetite, nausea, vomiting, hyperthermia, hypotension, muscle aches and pains, muscle jerks ('kicking the habit'), abdominal cramping, defecation and weight loss. Some male subjects experience ejaculation, some female subjects orgasms. Seizures are uncommon, and the syndrome is not usually life-threatening in reasonably healthy individuals. In laboratory animals many of the same features are observed although the most prominent symptoms may vary among species. Martin *et al.* (1976) have characterized the opiate withdrawal syndrome in dogs. In rats and mice defecation and escape jumping are prominent and readily quantifiable features of morphine withdrawal (Cicero and Meyer, 1973; Fernandes *et al.*, 1977).

The time-course of the development of opiate dependence and recovery from the dependent state have been extensively characterized in studies conducted at the Addiction Research Center in Lexington, Kentucky, from the 1930s through to the 1970s (Kolb and Himmelsbach, 1938; Andrews and Himmelsbach, 1944). These studies provide quantitative support for the clinical observation that the acute symptoms of withdrawal from morphine or heroin begin to be apparent 6–8 hours after the last morphine or heroin dose, and continue to increase in severity until about 72 hours after the last dose when the symptoms begin to decline in severity over a period of several days. By 7–10 days the symptoms of acute withdrawal from morphine have disappeared. However, signs of protracted abstinence, including intense drug craving and sleep disturbances, may persist for months or even years. Protracted abstinence symptoms vary considerable in intensity, apparently waxing and waning in response both to internal cues and to environmental and social factors (Martin and Jasinski, 1969).

Naloxone treatment initiates a withdrawal syndrome that is more rapid in onset than withdrawal initiated by cessation of drug administration. In the 2–3-hour period following naloxone administration to subjects dependent on morphine or heroin, the major symptoms of opiate withdrawal described above are observed. The ability of antagonists to elicit withdrawal symptoms in opiate-dependent subjects has been used in a diagnostic test for opiate dependence in man. Low doses of naloxone induce yawning, rhinorrhoea and gooseflesh. In laboratory rats or mice, vertical jumping to escape from an open-topped container or jumping off an elevated platform are characteristic behaviours associated with naloxone-precipitated opiate withdrawal. These behaviours are seldom seen in drug-free animals or in dependent animals before withdrawal and therefore are also reliable indicators of the dependent state (Fernandes *et al.*, 1977). Another measure of the intensity of opiate dependency in rats is the induction of defecation by naloxone. Opiate-dependent rats experience significant weight loss during naloxone-precipitated withdrawal caused by cessation of food intake and almost complete evacuation of the lower abdominal tract (Wei *et al.*, 1973b). Both in laboratory animals and in man the severity of the opiate-dependent state is increased when higher doses of opiate are administered to induce dependence, when the frequency at which the opiate drug is administered is increased, and when the duration of drug treatment is increased. However, studies in man suggest that with frequent administration of very high doses of opiate drug there may be a ceiling on the degree of dependence that can be achieved (Andrews and Himmelsbach, 1944). It is not clear if the failure to observe more severe withdrawal after very high drug doses reflects saturation of the dependence induction processes or is artifactually imposed by the abstinence scale used to quantify withdrawal.

Withdrawal symptoms induced by discontinuation of drug treatment can readily be suppressed by the administration of another dose of opiate drug. However, the additional drug treatment reinforces the dependent state, further sensitizing the animal to naloxone-induced withdrawal (Cheney *et al.*, 1972). The interactions between opiate agonists and antagonists in opiate-dependent animals are still not fully understood. In laboratory rats or mice, recovery from morphine dependence as measured by sensitivity to naloxone-induced escape jumping occurs within 24–36 hours (Cox *et al.*, 1975; Brase *et al.*, 1976). However, administration of a single dose of morphine to rats withdrawn from morphine at any time within the preceding 2 or 3 weeks exposes a state of protracted dependence as indicated by their continued high sensitivity to naloxone-induced escape jumping when tested one hour after the priming dose of morphine. The state of protracted dependence exposed by the single priming dose of morphine decays following morphine treatment with a half-time of about 15 days, a half-time very similar to that reported for a component of tolerance to the analgesic actions of morphine (see above; Cox *et al.*, 1975). These results suggest that an underlying state of protracted dependence may persist in rats for weeks or months after discontinuation of opiate drug treatment, although acute withdrawal symptoms are no longer apparent after a day or two. In man, the acute symptoms of morphine or heroin discontinuation are usually no longer apparent after 7–10 days. However, opiate drug craving, impaired sleep, and a general feeling of malaise may persist for months (Martin and Jasinski, 1969), again suggesting the occurrence of as yet unidentified disturbances during withdrawal. Symptoms of protracted abstinence may be significant factors in the high incidence of relapse to opiate drug use in subjects who have successfully completed the acute phase of withdrawal.

The opiate-dependent state, like the opiate-tolerant state, is initiated by opiate receptor activation. Thus any drug that can activate the same receptors that are activated by morphine can induce a state of dependence similar to that induced by morphine provided that the drug is administered at a frequency appropriate to its rate of metabolism and excretion. Mu-receptor agonists such as fentanyl, methadone and meperidine can each induce a similar dependent state although there are significant differences in the time-courses of the withdrawal syndrome following discontinuation of administration. Mu-selective agonists are also able to suppress withdrawal symptoms elicited by discontinuation of morphine in morphine-dependent subjects. However, their receptor affinities and efficacies are not identical, and the rates of metabolism and elimination differ substantially. For these reasons, the doses of each drug needed to induce dependence, the time-course for the development of dependence, and the time-course for the withdrawal syndrome are also not identical. The methadone withdrawal syndrome develops more slowly and lasts for substantially longer than the morphine withdrawal syndrome, but its peak severity is lower than that of morphine (Isbell, 1948). These features have led to the clinical use of methadone in the treatment of heroin dependence. Other pharmacological treatments are discussed in Chapter 2.

7.5.3 Behavioural factors in opiate tolerance and dependence

Behavioural factors are important contributors to tolerance to and dependence on opiate drugs in intact animals and man. It is important that investigators evaluating neurochemical and other pharmacological processes induced by chronic opioid administration are aware of behavioural factors that may affect measurements of drug effect in intact animals. Attempts to correlate neurochemical changes measured *in vitro* with changes in a behavioural response measured *in vivo* (e.g. the motor response to a nociceptive stimulus) may be compromised by behavioural factors associated with environmental cues linked to the repeated administration of the drug during the chronic treatment phase of the experiment. It is beyond the scope of this chapter to discuss these factors in detail; readers are referred to recent reviews by Siegal (1989) and Barrett *et al.* (1989) for a more complete consideration of many of the possible situations in which prior experiences of the animals influence their responses to opiates and other drugs.

Siegal has argued for many years that tolerance to the analgesic and some other actions of morphine and related drugs shows many of the features of Pavlovian conditioning. Analgesic tolerance has been shown to be associated with a specific testing environment; animals that are routinely dosed or tested in a particular environment may show no or much less tolerance when dosed or tested in a novel environment (Adams *et al.*, 1969). Environmental cues associated with the location of drug administration or pre-test procedures are assumed to act as conditioning stimuli which evoke a conditioned response in the test environment. Even if environmental cues associated with drug administration can be avoided, the drug itself may induce interoceptive cues that might act as a conditioning stimulus. The ability of opioid agonists to provide discriminative cues is well established (Shannon and Holtzman, 1976). These drug or environmental cues may evoke compensatory conditioned responses which reduce or modify the direct actions of the drug. The phenomenon of state-dependent learning also influences the expression of drug actions; behaviours developed or learned in one drug treatment condition may not be observed under another condition (Overton, 1984). It should also be noted that such behavioural factors are not restricted in their significance to experimental measurements that obviously are behavioural in nature as in analgesic testing, but may also be important in some physiological measures such as drug-induced changes in blood glucose levels and body temperature.

Environmental and interoceptive cues associated with, or induced by, drug administration may not only affect the direct actions of the drug but may also influence withdrawal. Both the induction and suppression of withdrawal symptoms by environmental cues has been demonstrated (Wikler, 1973). As noted above, environmental factors acting as conditioning stimuli may evoke compensatory conditioned responses. When the environmental cues are present in the absence of opiate drug, the evoked compensatory response may be observed as a withdrawal symptom.

These behavioural factors contributing to opiate drug tolerance and dependence clearly are important in the clinical use of opiate drugs for therapeutic purposes, and also in drug effects and withdrawal responses in opiate drug addicts. For the scientist studying the biochemical mechanisms underlying pharmacological tolerance and dependence, it is important to design experiments to avoid as far as possible complications resulting from purely behavioural factors in the measured outcome. This is not to deny the importance of the behavioural factors, but to allow the many mechanisms that contribute to the overall tolerance to opiate drugs to be separately identified and quantified.

7.6 Specific systems regulated by opioids

7.6.1 Spinal and supraspinal sites mediating opioid analgesia

Opiate drugs induce analgesia through actions at multiple levels within the central nervous system. A comment on terminology is necessary here. In man, opiate drugs provide relief from pain, and this action is described as analgesia. In experimental animal studies, it is only possible to infer a relief of pain by observing behaviour in response to the application of a noxious stimulus that is presumed to be painful. In this section, we will continue to use the term analgesia to describe the opiate-induced modification of behavioural responses induced by application of a noxious stimulus although this action is more properly described as antinociception. Electrophysiological studies on neural pathways mediating behavioural responses to noxious stimuli have confirmed that primary sites of opiate action are associated with these pathways, both in laboratory animals and in man.

Sites within the central nervous system mediating opiate analgesia have been defined mainly by localized microinjections of drugs to specific brain regions. The pioneering studies of Tsou and Jang (1964) identified the area surrounding the aqueduct in the midbrain of rabbits as a site at which morphine induced a profound analgesia. These studies have since been extended to other species (Yaksh *et al.*, 1976). Microinjections of morphine into an area lateral to and ventral to the aqueduct known as the periaqueductal grey region (PAG) reliably produce analgesia that can be antagonized by naloxone, either after systemic administration or after co-injection to the same site. Since the PAG is readily accessible to drugs diffusing from the ventricular system, this site is probably a primary mediation site for analgesia induced by intraventricular injections of opiate drugs. Opiate receptors of the μ and κ type are present at moderate density in PAG (Mansour *et al.*, 1988). Many intrinsic neurones containing enkephalin and a smaller number of dynorphin-containing cell soma are present in PAG. The area is also innervated by β-endorphin-containing fibres originating from the arcuate nucleus in the hypothalamus (Khachaturian *et al.*, 1985). Thus this site may participate in the physiological control of transmission in nociceptor pathways. Electrical stimulation of this region in man induces a reduction in pain perception that can be antagonized by naloxone (Hosobuchi *et al.*, 1977).

Analgesia can also be induced by application of opiate drugs or peptides to the ventral surface of the medulla oblongata (Dey and Feldberg, 1976) or to structures located in the ventral medulla. Microinjections into this region have shown that opiates can act within several nuclei in this area, including the nucleus raphe magnus, the nucleus gigantocellularis and the nucleus paragigantocellularis (Takagi *et al.*, 1977) to induce analgesia, at doses even lower than those needed to induce analgesia in the PAG. Mu- and κ-receptors are demonstrable by autoradiographic techniques in the ventral medulla (Mansour *et al.*, 1988). Enkephalin-containing cell soma and fibres, as well as dynorphin-containing and β-endorphin-containing fibres, are scattered throughout the ventral medullary region (Khachaturian *et al.*, 1985). This region may also therefore participate in physiological control of nociceptive transmission.

A third site of opiate analgesic action is the dorsal horn of spinal cord (DHSC). Injection of opioids into the subarachnoid space gives a good analgesic effect limited to regions innervated at or below the level of drug injection. The analgesic action of opiates applied to DHSC is readily antagonized by naloxone administered to the same site, or administered systemically. The neuronal location of opiate action within the dorsal horn remains unclear. Morphine inhibits the release of substance P in sensory pathways (Jessel and Iversen, 1977; Hirota *et al.*, 1985). Since substance P is presumed to be a transmitter in primary afferent neurones, this suggests a possible action of opioids directly on the terminals of the primary sensory neurones. Action of opiates directly on primary afferent neurones is supported in part by observations showing that opiates can act on their peripheral terminals in rat paw to reduce the response to noxious stimuli applied to the same site (Ferreira and Nakamura, 1979). However, opiate inhibition of nociception at the peripheral terminals of primary afferent neurones is enhanced by local inflammatory reactions (Stein *et al.*, 1988) and this site is probably not of major importance for opiate action in non-inflamed tissue. Enkephalins are located in many small interneurones in laminae I and II of the dorsal horn, but there are few enkephalin terminals making axo-axonic synapses with substance P-containing terminals of primary afferent neurones (Bresnahan *et al.*, 1984). Both enkephalin and substance P terminals appear to synapse with dendritic trees of putative transmission neurones in the dorsal horn. Opiates and endogenous opioids may therefore act directly on transmission neurones in the dorsal horn of spinal cord to reduce transmission in nociceptive pathways to the CNS. Mu-, δ- and κ-receptors are present in high concentrations in the doral horn of spinal cord.

The dorsal horn of spinal cord is not only a primary site of opioid analgesic action, but also mediates the analgesic actions of opiates administered supraspinally to the PAG and ventral medulla. When opiates are administered to the PAG or ventral medulla, pathways descending to the dorsal horn of spinal cord are activated, resulting in an inhibitory effect on transmission in nociceptive pathways and a reduction in the response to noxious stimuli (Basbaum *et al.*, 1976; Watkins and Meyer, 1982). The descending pathways are located in the spinal cord in the dorsolateral funiculus. Transection of the dorsolateral funiculus at high cervical sites largely abolishes the analgesic actions of morphine (Basbaum *et al.*, 1976). In the rat, the descending fibres contain 5-hydroxytryptamine (5-HT). Substances preventing the synthesis or action of 5-HT inhibit analgesia induced by brain stimulation (Hayes *et al.*, 1977), suggesting a major role for 5-HT in this system. Noradrenergic systems may also be important, however (Kuraishi *et al.*, 1983). Endogenous opioids within the dorsal horn appear to have a critical role in mediating the inhibitory activity of the descending pathways, since the analgesia induced by activation of the descending pathways is blocked by the intrathecal administration of naloxone (Watkins and Meyer, 1982).

The analgesic action of opiate drugs is potentiated by coincident actions at supraspinal and spinal sites (Yeung and Rudy, 1980). The ED_{50} for morphine, administered intraventricularly in a rat analgesic test, was reduced by 30–40-fold by the simultaneous administration of an equal dose by the intrathecal route (i.e. the total dose required was reduced 15–20-fold). Since the pathways activated by supraspinal morphine ultimately interact at the same or at closely apposed sites to those activated by intrathecally administered drug, an enhanced effect when both systems are activated might be predicted. Repeated systemic administration of morphine results in tolerance to its analgesic action, whether the test dose of drug is administered systemically, intraventricularly or intrathecally. Repeated application of morphine by the intraventricular route, or to spinal cord by intrathecal administration, also induces a degree of tolerance to systemically administered morphine (Yaksh *et al.*, 1977), again suggesting that both spinal and supraspinal sites are significant in the analgesic actions of systemic morphine.

When naloxone is administered intrathecally to rats made tolerant to morphine by repeated intrathecal injection of the drug, a withdrawal syndrome is elicited (Yaksh *et al.*, 1977). This syndrome was particularly characterized by hyperreflexia and extreme sensitivity to handling. In contrast, some other frequent symptoms of systemic naloxone-induced withdrawal in rats made dependent on systemic morphine, including diarrhoea, body weight loss, piloerection, chromodaccryorrhoea and seminal emissions, were much less frequently observed after intrathecal naloxone administration. The significance of the spinal cord in the expression of some opioid withdrawal signs has also been demonstrated by studies in which animals were treated intrathecally with an irreversible antagonist of opioid receptors (β-chlornaltrexamine or β-funaltrexamine) before being implanted with a morphine pellet (de Lander *et al.*, 1984). Escape jumping, wet dog shakes and hypothermia were all reduced in severity after naloxone administration to the morphine-treated animals, but there was no significant change in weight loss.

Direct infusion of opioids into the PAG region in rats also induced a dependent state; subsequent systemic administration of naloxone induced a withdrawal syndrome similar to that observed after morphine pellet implantation (Wei and Loh, 1976; Bozarth and Wise, 1984). Subsequent anatomical and functional studies demonstrating that opioids applied to the PAG activate neurones in the ventral medulla (Watkins and Meyer, 1982), and that the locus coeruleus receives a major excitatory input from a ventral medullary nucleus, the nucleus paragigantocellularis (Ennis and Aston-Jones, 1988), provide support for a neural pathway linking the PAG to the locus coeruleus, a region that has been implicated in the expression of the opioid withdrawal syndrome (see next section).

In summary, opiate agonists, especially those with high efficacy at μ-receptors, induce analgesia through actions at several sites in the CNS. Supraspinal sites include the PAG and the ventral medulla; an action in the dorsal horn of spinal cord is also important. Tolerance to opiate action has been demonstrated to occur at sites at which opioids induce analgesic effects, including the PAG and spinal cord. This is to be anticipated if the primary mechanism of opioid tolerance is an agonist-induced receptor desensitization. Sites at which opioids induce analgesia may also participate in withdrawal reactions in opiate-dependent animals. However, when opiate access during chronic administration is limited to spinal cord, the withdrawal reaction induced by naloxone does not include all of the symptoms associated with opiate withdrawal after systemic application of the opiate.

7.6.2 Locus coeruleus and mechanisms of withdrawal

Numerous studies have linked opiate drug actions with noradrenergic systems. Opiate drugs and peptides inhibit the release of noradrenaline from central (Montel *et al.*, 1974; Werling *et al.*, 1987) and peripheral (Trendelenburg, 1957; Illes *et al.*, 1985) noradrenergic neurones. In recent years interest has focused on the role of the locus coeruleus (LC), a pontine nucleus composed mainly of noradrenergic neurones, in the mediation of opioid withdrawal reactions. The LC receives inputs from a very small number of brain loci, but sends efferents to numerous structures, including the cortex, hippocampus and other forebrain structures, as well as to the cerebellum and spinal cord (Aston-Jones *et al.*, 1986). Agonists with affinity for μ opiate receptors open K^+ channels in LC neurones, induce membrane hyperpolarization, and reduce the firing rate. These effects are antagonized by naloxone. α_2-Adrenergic receptors are coupled to the same K^+ channels; agonists such as clonidine also hyperpolarize LC neurones and can be antagonized by α_2-antagonists such as idazoxan or yohimbine (North and Williams, 1985).

Stimulation of LC neurones produces effects in opiate-naive monkeys that resemble the symptoms of opiate withdrawal in morphine-dependent monkeys (Redmond *et al.*, 1976). Precipitation of withdrawal by naloxone administration to dependent animals induces a marked increase in firing in LC neurones when studied in intact animals (Aghajanian, 1978). The increased firing rate in naloxone-treated dependent animals can be inhibited by the administration of the α_2-agonist clonidine. Several studies have also shown that clonidine treatment suppresses some if not all of the symptoms of opiate withdrawal (Tseng *et al.*, 1975; Laverty and Roth, 1980).

These studies suggest that the LC plays an important role in the expression of opiate withdrawal symptoms. Studies of the properties of LC neurones in slice preparations taken from morphine-dependent rats have shown that these neurones are tolerant to the hyperpolarizing effects of morphine and related opioids (Christie *et al.*, 1987). Similarly, the ability of opioids to inhibit release of noradrenaline from the cortical terminals of the LC neurones is reduced after chronic morphine treatment (Werling *et al.*, 1988b). Nevertheless, in the LC neurone terminals in cortical slices from rats chronically exposed to morphine, there was no evidence of enhanced release of noradrenaline in response to naloxone administration (Cox and Werling, 1988). Thus, the LC neurones in isolated slice preparations from morphine-dependent animals do not demonstrate the enhanced sensitivity to naloxone that is apparent in intact animals. It seems probable that in the intact animal, excitatory inputs to LC are activated during naloxone-precipitated opiate withdrawal. Activation of LC neurones results in the enhanced release of noradrenaline at the many brain and spinal cord structures innervated by the LC, contributing significantly to the opiate withdrawal syndrome. The enhanced release of noradrenaline can be suppressed by agents inhibiting LC neurones, including clonidine and morphine itself, thus reducing the severity of the withdrawal syndrome.

The major excitatory input to the LC is from the nucleus paragiganto-cellularis (PGi) in the ventrolateral medulla. Excitation of the LC from the PGi can be blocked by kynurenic acid, but not by specific antagonists of the NMDA type of glutamate receptor (Ennis and Aston-Jones, 1988), suggesting that kainate-type receptors may mediate the excitation. It has recently been shown that in rats dependent on morphine, kynurenic acid blocks the increased firing of LC neurones induced by naloxone administration (Tung *et al.*, 1990). These results explain the failure to observe withdrawal hyperexcitability in *in vitro* preparations of the LC (Christie *et al.*, 1987), and suggest that opiate withdrawal is in part mediated by activation of excitatory afferents from the PGi to the LC. Excitatory inputs to the LC can also be inhibited by the κ-type opioid agonists U69593 and U50488H (Henderson and McFadzean, 1988), suggesting that modification of opioid withdrawal by κ-agonists may in part occur as a result of inhibition of LC excitation by afferents from the PGi. There are, as yet, no studies on the effects of sustained opiate drug exposure on the activity of PGi neurones. However, it is noteworthy that this nucleus is included in the ventral medullary areas, centred around the nucleus reticularis gigantocellularis, in which microinjections of very small doses of morphine produce a profound analgesic effect in rats not previously treated with opiate drugs (Takagi *et al.*, 1977). Neurones in the PGi are neurochemically heterogeneous (Ennis and Aston-Jones, 1988); it is unclear if opiate drugs can directly modify the activities of neurones forming the excitatory amino acid pathway from the PGi to the LC or whether function of this system is only modified after chronic opiate treatment.

There are recept reports that the activities of adenylate cyclase and cAMP-dependent protein kinase in slices from the LC region of rat brain are increased after chronic opiate treatments (Nestler and Tallman, 1987; Duman *et al.*, 1988). The LC slices contain both the cell soma of the locus noradrenergic neurones and the terminals of inputs to the LC cells, including terminals of afferents from the PGi. It is therefore unclear if the enhanced adenylate cyclase and protein kinase A activity reflect changes associated with opiate tolerance in LC neurones, or are associated with changes in the function of the PGi neurone terminals which might be related to their increased firing during opiate withdrawal.

Collectively, these studies point to an important role for the PGi–LC pathway in the expression of opiate withdrawal symptoms. The extensive efferent network of the LC neurones throughout the CNS (Aston-Jones *et al.*, 1986) provides a system by which significant disturbance of many physiological functions may occur. LC neurones are unusual in that a relatively small number of neurones project to many brain regions. Generally, the effect of LC activation on other systems is to enhance their responsiveness to other synaptic inputs, while reducing target cell basal activity (Foote *et al.*, 1983), perhaps facilitating discrete localization of specific responses in individual systems. Inhibition of this system by opiates in drug-naive animals may contribute to the sedative and depressant effects of acute opiate administration. Excessive and indiscriminate firing of the system during opiate drug withdrawal may lead to the impaired function of many systems and may contribute to the dysphoria associated with withdrawal. It now seems clear, however, that the hyperexcitability associated with opiate withdrawal is not initiated in the LC, but originates in afferent inputs to the LC from the PGi.

Withdrawal symptoms in morphine-dependent rats can also be initiated by administration of naloxone to other brain sites, including the medial thalamus (Wei *et al.*, 1973a) and the PAG region (Bozarth and Wise, 1984). It is possible that antagonist administration at these sites activates pathways independent of the LC in inducing withdrawal reactions, but is seems more likely that antagonists applied to these sites may indirectly activate LC neurones through the PGi. In the case of the PAG, an opioid-regulated excitatory pathways from the PAG to the ventral medulla has been proposed (Watkins and Meyer, 1982).

7.6.3 Opiate reward

The rewarding effects induced by opiate drugs appear to be primary factors in the initiation of addiction to opiates, and in the maintenance of continued drug administration. Some progress has been made in identifying the neural substrates underlying opiate reinforcement of behaviours. Dopamine pathways appear to be important, with most evidence suggesting the involvement of the mesolimbic dopaminergic pathway. This pathway arises from cell bodies in the mesencephalic ventral tegmental area (VTA), and projects anteriorly through the medial forebrain bundle (MFB) to the nucleus accumbens (NAs) and olfactory tubercle (OT). This conclusion is based on experiments in which the effects of microinjections of opiate agonists or antagonists on specific structures in the mesolimbic system, have been studied.

Three experimental approaches to the evaluation of opiate-reinforcing effects have been of particular value in identifying the sites of opiate action. Studies of drug self-administration behaviour have directly evaluated the effects of lesions or the consequences of allowing animals (usually rats) to self-administer drugs directly to the VTA or NAs. However, these studies are technically difficult and are time-consuming and expensive to perform. It is difficult to be certain that the drug does not diffuse from the immediate region surrounding the injection cannula to exert effects at a more distant site. Furthermore, there is always the possibility that repeated self-administrations of drug solutions may damage or perturb the function of local neural elements in close proximity to the injection cannula. Alternative approaches have therefore attempted to evaluate the behaviour-reinforcing properties of opiates while avoiding the need for repeated self-administration of the drug to discrete brain sites.

The technique of intracranial brain self-stimulation (ICSS), in which animals are given access to a lever that when depressed causes an electrical stimulus to be applied through electrodes chronically implanted in the brain (Schaefer, 1988), has also been useful. When the electrodes are implanted in the VTA, the MFB, or the NAs, rats will repeatedly activate the lever to apply electrical stimulation. When the electrodes are located in adjacent areas outside the mesolimbic system, the effect of the stimulus is generally neutral, or at some sites may be aversive. In either case, lever-pressing behaviour is not reinforced and the rats do not continue to activate the lever. By varying the stimulation current intensity, the threshold current for each site that maintains ICSS behaviour can be determined. In general, it has been shown that drugs that support self-administration behaviour will also lower the threshold for ICSS when electrodes are located in the mesolimbic system. Central stimulants like cocaine, and opiate drugs, including morphine, are particularly effective in lowering ICSS thresholds. In each animal, a drug need be administered only once in this procedure, and for drugs that gain access to the CNS after systemic administration there is no requirement for localized microinjections of drug since a degree of anatomical specificity is provided by the placement of the stimulating electrodes. Thus, some of the disadvantages of self-administration procedures are avoided. However, it is possible that drugs might induce reinforcement through other mechanisms or at sites different from those that maintain ICSS behaviour, making it possible that their rewarding properties would not be detected by this technique.

Place preference tests have also been used to examine drug-mediated reward. If drug administration to an animal is uniquely associated with a specific environment (usually a box or enclosure with characteristic shading and texture of the walls and floor or characteristic odour), the animal may choose to enter or to avoid that area if the drug effect was pleasurable or aversive, respectively. Thus, after an initial period of drug training (which may require only one or two trials), during which the drug administration is always paired with one environment while drug vehicle administration is paired with an alternative environment, the animal is tested (while in a drug-free state) by being placed in a neutral area with equal access to the two environments. The amount of time spent by the animal in each environment during the evaluation period is recorded. Opiates, and central stimulants like cocaine and amphetamines, generally cause rats to move to the environment paired with drug administration (Almaric *et al.*, 1987); in the same test paradigm drugs that are aversive will cause the animals to move to the environment paired with drug vehicle. This procedure requires training sessions to establish the association of drug effect with a specific environment. When used to evaluate drug reward, the place preference test makes the assumption that the selection of a specific environment is associated with a rewarding effect of the drug. Other unidentified factors associated with the drug administration and its consequences, however, might also influence the choice of environment during the test procedure.

These experimental approaches to drug-mediated reinforcement of behaviour employ very different techniques with differing sets of advantages and disadvantages, but taken collectively they provide a reasonably reliable evaluation of drug-induced reward. A potential difficulty arises from the fact that each experimental procedure, drug self-administration, ICSS, or place preference, requires some form of motor response by the animal: lever pressing or locomotion to a preferred environment. This is unfortunate, because the mesolimbic system appears to exert a regulatory role in motor function in addition to its involvement in drug reinforcement of behaviour. Therefore, the differentiation of drug-induced facilitation of motor activity and drug-induced reward may be difficult to establish because the neural systems underlying reward are apparently closely associated with pathways regulating motor function.

Several lines of evidence point to the mesolimbic dopaminergic system as a primary site of opiate-mediated reward. Lesions of the VTA (Bozarth and Wise, 1981,1984; Spyraki *et al.*, 1983) or the presumed cellular targets of the mesolimbic dopamine neurones in the NAs (Zito *et al.*, 1985) reduce or extinguish opiate drug self-administration behaviour. Antagonism of dopamine receptors by D_2 receptor antagonists is also reported to reduce opiate reward (Ettenberg *et al.*, 1982; Gerber and Wise, 1989). Rats implanted with indwelling cannulae will self-administer morphine through cannulae located in the VTA but generally do not self-administer opiates when the cannula is located in adjacent areas outside the mesolimbic pathway (Phillips and LePiane, 1980; Bozarth, 1987). Rats also self-administer morphine through cannulae located in the NAs (Olds, 1982), while microinjections of morphine to the NAs have been identified as reinforcing in place preference tests (van der Kooy *et al.*, 1982) and have been shown to facilitate ICSS (Broekamp *et al.*, 1979). In contrast, microinjections of opiate antagonists into the NAs reduce opiate self-administration by the systemic route (Vaccarino *et al.*, 1985). These experiments all indicate the importance of the mesolimbic system in opiate reward. Some studies have suggested that opiates administered to other brain sites might also support self-administration, but in general larger doses of opiates have been injected at each administration, and the extent of spread of drug from the site of administration has not been determined.

The mechanisms of opiate actions in the VTA and the NAs are still uncertain. The evidence for an opioid facilitation of dopamine neurone firing after VTA administration is fairly strong. It is possible that opiates influence the function of inhibitory or excitatory afferent terminals that exert a regulatory control over the firing of VTA neurones. However, it has not been shown that opiates injected into the NAs act on the mesolimbic nerve terminals to increase dopamine release. Lesions of the mesolimbic pathway that usually completely extinguish cocaine self-administration attenuate opiate self-administration but do not extinguish it (Pettit *et al.*, 1984). Thus, the integrity of the dopamine terminals in the NAs is more critical for the self-administration of cocaine than for opiates. It is possible that opiates act on neural elements in the NAs that are postsynaptic to the dopamine terminals and thus facilitate the action of released dopamine. The systems activated and inhibited by dopamine in the NAs also require further study. Uchimura and North (1990) have shown that dopamine acting through D_1 receptors hyperpolarized about 80% of NAs neurones, but also (in the same concentration range) had biphasic effects or depolarized through D_2 receptor activation about 50–60% of NAs neurones from which intracellular recordings were obtained. Presumably these neurones would be destroyed in the kainate lesions demonstrated by Zito *et al.* (1985) to suppress both cocaine and heroin self-administration. Koob *et al.* (1989) have suggested that a major pathway from the NAs to the ventral pallidum is involved in opiate reinforcement. Thus, opiate actions in both the VTA and the NAs are probably important in opiate reward.

Disclaimer: The opinions and assertions contained herein reflect the private views of the authors and are not to be construed as official or reflecting the views of the Uniformed Services University of the Health Sciences or the U.S. Department of Defense.

References

Adams, W.J., Yeh, S.Y., Woods, L.A. & Mitchell, C.L. (1969) *J. Pharmacol. Exp. Ther.* **168**, 252–257.

Aghajanian, G.K. (1978) *Nature (Lond.)* **276**, 186–188.

Aghajanian, G.K. & Wang, Y.Y. (1986) *Brain Res.* **371**, 390–394.

Akil, H., Watson, S.J., Young, E., Lewis, M.E., Khachaturian, H. & Walker, J.M. (1984) *Annu. Rev. Neurosci.* **7**, 223–255.

Almaric, M., Cline, E.J., Martinez, J.L., Jr, Bloom, F.E. & Koob, G.F. (1987) *Psychopharmacology* **91**, 14–19.
Andrews, H.L. & Himmelsbach, C.K. (1944) *J. Pharmacol. Exp. Ther.* **81**, 288–293.
Archer, S. (1986) *Natl Inst. Drug Abuse Res. Monogr. Ser.* **69**, 364–375.
Aston-Jones, G., Ennis, M., Pieribone, V.A., Nickell, W.T. & Shipley, M.T. (1986) *Science* **234**, 734–737.
Barrett, J.E., Glowa, J.R. & Nader, M.A. (1989) In *Psychoactive Drugs: Tolerance and Sensitization* (eds Goudie, A.J. & Emmett-Oglesby, M.W.), pp 181–220. Clifton, New Jersey, Humana Press.
Basbaum, A.I., Clanton, C.H. & Fields, H.L. (1976) *Proc. Natl Acad. Sci. USA* **73**, 4685–4688.
Blasig, J., Meyer, G., Höllt, V., Hengstenberg, J., Dum, J. & Herz, A. (1979) *Neuropharmacology* **18**, 473–481.
Bozarth, M.A. (1987) *Brain Res.* **414**, 77–84.
Bozarth, M.A. & Wise, R.A. (1981) *Life Sci.* **29**, 1881–1886.
Bozarth, M.A. & Wise, R.A. (1984) *Science* **224**, 516–517.
Brase, D.A., Iwamoto, E.T., Loh, H.H. & Way, E.1. (1976) *J. Pharmacol. Exp. Ther.* **197**, 317–325.
Bresnahan, J.C., Ho, R.H. & Beattie, M.S. (1984) *J. Comp. Neurol.* **229**, 497–511.
Broekamp, C.L., Phillips, A.G. & Cools, A.R. (1979) *Pharmacol. Biochem. Behav.* **11**, 289–295.
Cheney, D.L., Judson, B.A. & Goldstein, A. (1972) *J. Pharmacol. Exp. Ther.* **182**, 189–194.
Childers, S.R. (1988) *J. Neurochem.* **50**, 543–553.
Christie, M.J., Williams, J.T. & North, R.A. (1987) *Mol. Pharmacol.* **32**, 633–638.
Cicero, T.J. & Meyer, E.R. (1973) *J. Pharmacol. Exp. Ther.* **184**, 404–408.
Clark, C.R., Birchmore, B., Sharif, N.A., Hunter, J.C., Hill, R.G. & Hughes, J. (1989) *Br. J. Pharmacol.* **93**, 618–626.
Clark, J.C., Liu, L., Price, M., Hersh, B., Edelson, M. & Pasternak, G.W. (1989) *Mol. Pharmacol.* **251**, 461–468.
Cox, B.M. & Werling, L.L. (1988) In *Regulatory Roles of Opioid Peptides* (eds Illes, P. & Farsang, C.), pp 259–267. Weinhein, FRG, VCH.
Cox, B.M., Ginsburg, M. & Willis, J. (1975) *Br, J. Pharmacol.* **53**, 383–391.
de Lander, G.E., Portoghese, P.S. & Takemori, A.E. (1984) *J. Pharmacol. Exp. Ther.* **231**, 91–96.
Dey, P.K. & Feldberg, W. (1976) *Br. J. Pharmacol.* **58**, 383–393.
Douglass, J., Cox, B.M., Quinn, B., Civelli, O. & Herbert, E. (1987) *Endocrinology* **120**, 707–713.
Duman, R.S., Tallman, J.F. & Nestler, E.J. (1988) *J. Pharmacol. Exp. Ther.* **246**, 1033–1039.
Ennis, M. & Aston-Jones, G. (1988) *J. Neurosci.* **8**, 3644–3657.
Ettenberg, A., Pettit, H.O., Bloom, F.E. & Koob, G.F. (1982) *Psychopharmacology* **78**, 204–209.
Evans, C.J., Hammond, D.L. & Frederickson, R.C.A. (1988) In *The Opiate Receptors* (ed. Pasternak, G.W.), pp 23–71. Clifton, NJ, Humana Press.
Fernandes, M., Kluwe, S. & Coper, H. (1977) *Naunyn-Schmiedeberg's Arch. Pharmacol.* **297**, 53–60.
Ferreira, S.H. & Nakamura, M. (1979) *Prostaglandins* **18**, 191–200.
Foote, S.L., Bloom, F.E. & Aston-Jones, G. (1983) *Physiol. Rev.* **63**, 844–914.
Frey, E.A. & Kebabian, J. (1984) *Endocrinology* **115**, 1797–1804.

Gerber, G.J. & Wise, R.A. (1989) *Pharmacol. Biochem. Behav.* **32**, 527–531.
Gilman, A.G. (1986) *Trends Pharmacol. Sci.* **9**, 460–462.
Gouarderes, C., Kopp, N., Cros, J. & Quirion, R. (1986) *Brain Res. Bull.* **16**, 355–361.
Goudie, A.J. & Emmett-Oglesby, N.W. (eds) (1989) *Psychoactive Drugs: Tolerance and Sensitization.* Clifton, New Jersey, Humana Press.
Grevel, J. & Sadee, W. (1983) *Science* **221**, 1198–1201.
Hayes, R.L., Newton, P.G., Rosecrans, J.A. & Mayer, D.J. (1977) *Brain Res.* **122**, 367–372.
Henderson, G. & McFadzean, I. (1988) In *Regulatory Roles of Opioid Peptides* (eds Illes, P. & Farsant, C.), pp 165–174. Weinheim, FRG, VCH.
Hescheler, J., Rosenthal, W., Trautwein, W. & Schulz, G. (1987) *Nature (Lond.)* **325**, 443–447.
Hirota, N., Kuraishi, Y., Hino, Y., Sato, Y., Sato, M. & Takagi, H. (1985) *Neuropharmacology* **24**, 567–570.
Höllt, V., Dum, J., Blasig, J., Schubert, P. & Herz, A. (1975) *Life Sci.* **16**, 1823–1832.
Hosobuchi, Y., Adams, J.E. & Linchitz, R. (1977) *Science* **197**, 183–186.
Hughes, J., Smith, T.H., Kosterlitz, H.W., Fothergill, L.A., Morgan, B.A. & Morris, H.R. (1975) *Nature (Lond.)* **258**, 577–579.
Illes, P., Pfeiffer, N., von Kugelen, I. & Starke, K. (1985) *J. Pharmacol. Exp. Ther.* **232**, 526–533.
Isbell, H. (1948) *Ann. N.Y. Acad. Sci.* **51**, 108–122.
Jessel, T.M. & Iversen, L.L. (1977) *Nature (Lond.)* **268**, 549–551.
Katada, T. & Ui, M. (1982) *J. Biol. Chem.* **257**, 7210–7215.
Khachaturian, H., Lewis, M.E., Schafer, M.K.-H. & Watson, S.J. (1985) *Trends Neurosci.* **8**, 111–119.
Klee, W.L. & Streaty, R.A. (1973) *Nature (Lond.)* **248**, 61–63.
Kolb, L. & Himmelsbach, C.K. (1938) *Am. J. Psychiatry* **94**, 759–795.
Koob, G.F. & Bloom, F.E. (1988) *Science* **242**, 715–723.
Koob, G.F., Stinus, L., Le Moal, M. & Bloom, F.E. (1989) *Neurosci. Biobehav. Rev.* **13**, 135–140.
Kromer, W. (1988) *Pharmacol. Rev.* **40**, 121–162.
Kuraishi, Y., Harada, Y., Aratani, S., Satoh, M. & Takagi, H. (1983) *Brain Res.* **273**, 245–252.
Kurose, H., Katada, T., Amano, T. & Ui, M. (1983) *J. Biol. Chem.* **258**, 4870–4875.
Laverty, R. & Roth, R.H. (1980) *Brain Res.* **182**, 482–485.
Lemaire, S., Magnan, J. & Regnoli, D. (1978) *Br. J. Pharmacol.* **64**, 327–329.
Loh, H.H., Tao, P.-L. & Smith, A.P. (1988) *Synapse* **2**, 457–462.
Lord, J.A.H., Waterfield, A.A., Hughes, J. & Kosterlitz, H.W. (1977) *Nature (Lond.)* **267**, 495–499.
Mansour, A., Khachaturian, H., Lewis, M.E., Akil, H. & Watson, S.J. (1988) *Trends Neurosci.* **11**, 308–314.
Martin, W.R. & Jasinski, D.R. (1969) *J. Psychiatr. Res.* **7**, 9–17.
Martin, W.R., Eades, C.G., Thompson, J.A., Huppler, R.E. & Gilbert, P.E. (1976) *J. Pharmacol. Exp. Ther.* **197**, 517–532.
Misra, A.L., Mule, S.J., Bloch, R. & Vadlamani, N.L. (1973) *J. Pharmacol. Exp. Ther.* **185**, 287–299.
Montel, H., Starke, K. & Weber, F. (1974) *Naunyn-Schmiedeberg's Arch. Pharmacol.* **283**, 357–369.
Morita, K. & North, R.A. (1982) *Brain Res.* **242**, 145–150.
Nestler, E.J. & Tallman, J.F. (1987) *Mol. Pharmacol.* **33**, 127–132.

North, R.A. & Williams, J.T. (1985) *J. Physiol. (Lond.)* **364**, 265–280.
North, R.A., Williams, J.T., Suprenant, A. & Christie, M.J. (1987) *Proc. Natl Acad. Sci. USA* **84**, 5487–5491.
Olds, M.E. (1982) *Brain Res.* **237**, 429–440.
Overton, D.A. (1984) In *Handbook of Psychopharmacology*, vol. 18 (eds Iversen, L.L., Iversen, S.D. & Snyder, S.N.), pp 59–127. New York, Plenum Press.
Pasternak, G.W. & Wood, P.J. (1986) *Life Sci.* **38**, 1889–1898.
Pettit, H.O., Ettenberg, A., Bloom, F.E. & Koob, G.F. (1984) *Psychopharmacology* **84**, 167–173.
Phillips, A. & LePiane, F.G. (1980) *Pharmacol. Biochem. Behav.* **12**, 965–968.
Puttfarcken, P.S., Werling, L.L. & Cox, B.M. (1988) *Mol. Pharmacol.* **33**, 520–527.
Redmond, D.E., Jr, Huang, Y.H., Snyder, D. & Maas, J.W. (1976) *Brain Res.* **116**, 502–510.
Rothman, R.B., Bykov, V., DeCosta, B.R., Jacobson, A.E., Rice, K.C. & Brady, L.S. (1990) *Peptides* **11**, 311–331.
Schaefer, G.J. (1988) *Neurosci. Biobehav. Rev.* **12**, 1–17.
Siegal, S. (1989) In *Psychoactive Drugs: Tolerance and Sensitization* (eds Goudie, A.J. & Emmett-Oglesby, M.W.), pp 115–180. Clifton, New Jersey, Humana Press.
Shannon, H.E. & Holtzman, S.G. (1976) *J. Pharmacol. Exp. Ther.* **198**, 54–65.
Sharma, S.K., Klee, W.A. & Nirenberg, M. (1975) *Proc. Natl Acad. Sci. USA* **72**, 3092–3096.
Sibinga, N.E.S. & Goldstein, A. (1988) *Annu. Rev. Immunol.* **6**, 219–249.
Spyraki, C., Fibiger, H.C. & Phillips, A.G. (1983) *Psychopharmacology* **79**, 278–283.
Stein, C., Millan, M.J., Yassourides, A. & Herz, A. (1988) *Eur. J. Pharmacol.* **155**, 255–264.
Takagi, H., Satoh, M., Akaike, A., Shibata, T. & Kuraishi, Y. (1977) *Eur. J. Pharmacol.* **45**, 91–92.
Tiberi, M. & Magnan, J. (1990) *Mol. Pharmacol.* **37**, 694–703.
Trendelenburg, U. (1957) *Br. J. Pharmacol.* **12**, 79–85.
Tseng, L.-F., Loh, H.H. & Wei, E.T. (1975) *Eur. J. Pharmacol.* **30**, 93–99.
Tsou, K. & Jang, C.S. (1964) *Sci. Sin.* **13**, 1099–1109.
Tung, C.-S., Grenhoff, J. & Svennson, T.H. (1990) *Acta Physiol. Scand.* **138**, 581–582.
Uchimura, N. & North, R.A. (1990) *Br. J. Pharmacol.* **99**, 736–740.
Vaccarino, F.J., Bloom, F.E. & Koob, G.F. (1985) *Psychopharmacology* **85**, 37–42.
Van der Kooy, D., Mucha, R.F., O'Shaughnessy, M. & Bucenicks, P. (1982) *Brain Res.* **243**, 107–117.
Vaupel, D.B. (1983) *Eur. J. Pharmacol.* **92**, 269–274.
Watkins, L.R. & Meyer, D.J. (1982) *Science* **216**, 1185–1192.
Watson, S. & Abbott, A. (1990) *Trends Pharm. Sci.* **13** (Suppl.), 21.
Wei, E. & Loh, H.H. (1976) *Science* **193**, 1262–1263.
Wei, E., Loh, H.H. & Way, E.L. (1973a) *J. Pharmacol. Exp. Ther.* **185**, 108–115.
Wei, E., Loh, H.H. & Way, E.L. (1973b) *J. Pharmacol. Exp. Ther.* **184**, 398–403.
Werling, L.L., Brown, S.R. & Cox, B.M. (1987) *Neuropharmacology* **26**, 987–996.
Werling, L.L., Puttfarcken, P.S. & Cox, B.M. (1988a) *Mol. Pharmacol.* **33**, 423–431.
Werling, L.L., McMahon, P.N. & Cox, B.M. (1988b) *J. Pharmacol. Exp. Ther.* **247**, 1103–1106.
Werling, L.L., McMahon, P.N. & Cox, B.M. (1989) *Proc. Natl Acad. Sci. USA* **86**, 6393–6397.
Werz, M.A. & Macdonald, R.A. (1983) *Neurosci. Lett.* **42**, 173–178.
Werz, M.A. & Macdonald, R.A. (1984) *Neurosci. Lett.* **46**, 185–190.

Werz, M.A. & Macdonald, R.A. (1985) *J. Pharmacol. Exp. Ther.* **234**, 49–56.
Wikler, A. (1973) *Arch. Gen. Psychiatry* **28**, 611.
Wuster, M., Schulz, R. & Herz, A. (1978) *Neurosci. Lett.* **15**, 193–198.
Yaksh, T.L., Yeung, J.C. & Rudy, T.A. (1976) *Brain Res.* **114**, 83–103.
Yaksh, T.L., Kohl, R.L. & Rudy, T.A. (1977) *Eur. J. Pharmacol.* **42**, 275–284.
Yaksh, T.L., Al-Rodhan, N.R.F. & Jensen, T.S. (1988) *Prog. Brain Res.* **77**, 373–396.
Yeung, J.C. & Rudy, T.A. (1980) *J. Pharmacol. Exp. Ther.* **215**, 633–642.
Zito, K.A., Vickers, G. & Roberts, D.C.S. (1985) *Pharmacol. Biochem. Behav.* **25**, 1029–1036.
Zukin, R.S., Eghbali, M., Olive, D., Unterwald, E.M. & Tempel, A. (1988) *Proc. Natl Acad. Sci. USA* **85**, 4061–4065.

CHAPTER 8

TOLERANCE TO AND DEPENDENCE ON PSYCHOTROPIC CANNABINOIDS

R.G. Pertwee

Division of Pharmacology, School of Biomedical Sciences, Marischal College, University of Aberdeen, Aberdeen AB9 1AS, UK

Table of Contents

THE BIOLOGICAL BASES OF DRUG TOLERANCE AND DEPENDENCE
ISBN 0-12-564250-4

8.1 Introduction

Consideration of the tolerance and dependence liabilities of cannabinoids is important not only because cannabis is widely used recreationally but also because there is a continuing interest in the therapeutic potential of naturally occurring and synthetic cannabinoids. Most tolerance and dependence studies have been carried out with cannabis or with its main psychically active constituent, (−)-Δ^9-tetrahydrocannabinol (Δ^9-THC). Other natural constituents of cannabis to have been studied include (−)-Δ^8-tetrahydrocannabinol (Δ^8-THC), which is only slightly less potent than Δ^9-THC, and cannabinol, which is much less active. Experiments have also been performed with several psychically active hydroxy metabolites of Δ^8- or Δ^9-THC and with certain synthetic analogues, for example $\Delta^{6a,10a}$-hexyl-tetrahydrocannabinol (pyrahexyl), $\Delta^{6a,10a}$-dimethylheptyl-tetrahydrocannabinol, levonantradol and nabilone (for chemical formulae and recent reviews of cannabinoid pharmacology see Dewey (1986), Martin (1986) and Pertwee (1990)). There have been relatively few controlled studies with human subjects, and consequently this chapter deals largely with data from animal experiments. Since cannabis itself has often been used in tolerance and dependence studies, it is important to note that this substance contains several pharmacologically active compounds. Not all of these have the same properties and some of them are known to interact pharmacologically with each other. The chemical composition of cannabis can vary from sample to sample and is affected by heat when the material is smoked.

8.2 Signs of tolerance in animals: Δ^9-THC

8.2.1 Effects on unconditioned and conditioned behaviour

Experiments with rats have shown that tolerance can develop to both the stimulant and depressant effects of Δ^9-THC on motor function as measured by changes in locomotor activity (Table 1), rearing activity, grooming and/or co-ordination (Barnes and Fried, 1974; Järbe, 1978; Luthra *et al.*, 1975; Masur *et al.*, 1971; Miczek, 1979; Miczek and Dixit, 1980; Pryor *et al.*, 1977a; Siemens and Doyle, 1979; Sjöden *et al.*, 1973). Tolerance to the depressant effects of Δ^9-THC on motor function has also been observed in other species, including mice (Anderson *et al.*, 1975; Sprague and Craigmill, 1976; Karler *et al.*, 1986), monkeys (Fredericks and Benowitz, 1980; Kaplan, 1979; Sassenrath and Chapman, 1975; Thompson *et al.*, 1974), dogs and rabbits (Dewey *et al.*, 1972b; Kaymakcalan and Deneau, 1972; Martin *et al.*, 1976; Martin and Consroe, 1978). In addition, there are reports that tolerance can develop to the cataleptic effect of Δ^9-THC in mice (Pertwee, 1974; Burstein *et al.*, 1988), to the convulsant effect of the drug in rabbits and mice (Craigmill, 1979; Fish and Consroe, 1981; Karler *et al.*, 1982; Martin and Consroe, 1976) and to the drug's anticonvulsant effect in rats, gerbils and mice (Colasanti *et al.*, 1982; Corcoran *et al.*, 1978; Fried and McIntyre, 1973; Karler and Turkanis, 1980; Karler *et al.*, 1974a,b, 1982; Ten Ham *et al.*, 1975).

Experiments with monkeys, pigeons and rats have shown that repeated treatment with Δ^9-THC can produce tolerance to the drug's effects on several types of conditioned behaviour (Table 1). Since food reinforcement was often used in these studies, it is important to note that tolerance can also develop to the depressant effect of Δ^9-THC on food consumption, at least in rats (Miczek, 1979; Verberne *et al.*, 1980).

Results obtained by Magour *et al.* (1977) point to the importance of measuring the time-course of drug-induced effects in tolerance studies. Rats given Δ^9-THC twice daily appeared completely tolerant to the drug's depressant effect on locomotor activity when tested on day 9, 4 hours after an injection of the drug, but only marginally tolerant when tested 2 hours earlier. This was because the pretreatment reduced the duration of the drug's effect but had only a small effect on intensity.

8.2.2 Body temperature, blood pressure and heart rate

Tolerance to the hypothermic effect of Δ^9-THC has been reported to develop rapidly in monkeys (Thompson *et al.*, 1974), chicks (Abel, 1972; Abel *et al.*, 1973), rats and mice (Table 1). It can also develop to the ability

Table 1 Signs of tolerance to certain effects of Δ^9-THC in monkeys, pigeons, rats and mice.

Species	Pretreatment	Effect to which tolerance developed	Time taken for tolerance to develop	References
Monkey	2 mg/kg i.v. or 1 or 2 mg/kg i.m. or 1 to 16 mg/kg p.o. every 24 h	Effects of Δ^9-THC on conditioned behaviour (usually inhibitory)	2 to 15 days	1 to 5
Pigeon	0.3 or 10 mg/kg i.v. or 0.5 to 20 mg/kg i.m. or 10 mg/kg p.o. every 24, 48 or 72 h (or only one pretreatment)	Effects of Δ^9-THC on conditioned behaviour (inhibitory)	2 to 21 days	6 to 12
Rat	4 to 100 mg/kg i.p. or 8 to 32 mg/kg s.c. or 10 to 60 mg/kg p.o. every 24 or 48 h	Effects of Δ^9-THC on conditioned behaviour (usually inhibitory)	2 to 50 days	12 to 28
Rat	10 to 40 mg/kg i.p. or 2 to 6 mg/kg i.v. or 25 mg/kg s.c. or 10 mg/kg p.o. every 24 h or twice daily	Effect of Δ^9-THC on spontaneous locomotor activity (usually inhibitory)	2 to 42 days	24, 25, 29 to 37

Rat	2 to 6 mg/kg i.v. or 0.3 to 40 mg/kg i.p. or 10 or 20 mg/kg s.c. or 10 to 25 mg/kg p.o. every 24 h or twice daily	Hypothermic effect of Δ^9-THC	2 to 15 days	23 to 25, 27, 32 to 35, 38 to 46
Mouse	5 to 80 mg/kg i.p. or 20 to 200 mg/kg s.c. or 10 mg/kg p.o. every 24 h	Hypothermic effect of Δ^9-THC	2 to 9 days	47 to 52

References: 1, Branch *et al.* (1980); 2, Elsmore (1972); 3, Elsmore (1976); 4, Ferraro and Grisham (1972); 5, Harris *et al.* (1972); 6, Abel *et al.* (1974); 7, Chait *et al.* (1981); 8, Cherek *et al.* (1980); 9, Dewey *et al.* (1973); 10, Kosersky *et al.* (1974); 11, McMillan *et al.* (1970); 12, McMillan *et al.* (1973); 13, Bailey and Pradhan (1972); 14, Becker and Reid (1977); 15, Carlini *et al.* (1970); 16, Davis and Borgen (1975); 17, Hirschhorn and Rosecrans (1974); 18, Larsen and Pryor (1977); 19, Manning (1976b); 20, McMillan *et al.* (1972); 21, Newman *et al.* (1972); 22, Newman *et al.* (1974); 23, Pryor *et al.* (1977a); 24, Pryor *et al.* (1977b); 25, Pryor *et al.* (1978); 26, Silva *et al.* (1968); 27, Ten Ham (1977); 28, Webster *et al.* (1973); 29, Aulakh *et al.* (1980); 30, Davis *et al.* (1972); 31, Magour *et al.* (1977); 32, Miczek (1979); 33, Miczek and Dixit (1980); 34, Taylor and Fennessy (1978a); 35, Taylor and Fennessy (1982); 36, Tulunay *et al.* (1982); 37, Verberne *et al.* (1980); 38, Adams *et al.* (1976); 39, Carder and Deikel (1976); 40, Järbe (1978); 41, Kaymakcalan and Deneau (1972); 42, Kaymakcalan *et al.* (1977); 43, Kosersky (1978); 44, Tulunay *et al.* (1981); 45, Uran *et al.* (1980); 46, Verberne *et al.* (1985); 47, Anderson *et al.* (1975); 48, Bloom and Dewey (1978); 49, Fitton and Pertwee (1982); 50, Liu (1974); 51, Spaulding *et al.* (1972); 52, Ten Ham and De Jong (1974).

of Δ^9-THC to produce hypotension in unanaesthetized hypertensive rats (Birmingham, 1973; Kosersky, 1978; Nahas *et al.*, 1973a,b), bradycardia in unanaesthetized normotensive rats (Hine, 1985; Kawasaki *et al.*, 1980; Kaymakcalan and Sivil, 1974; Pryor *et al.*, 1977a,b, 1978) and hypotension or bradycardia in anaesthetized rats (Adams *et al.*, 1976; Li, 1981). In other experiments with anaesthetized rats it was found that tolerance developed to the ability of Δ^9-THC to potentiate the pressor response to noradrenaline (Li, 1981) and that it did not develop to an initial, transient pressor effect of Δ^9-THC (Adams *et al.*, 1976). Fredericks *et al.* (1981) studied the effect of repeated administration of Δ^9-THC on heart rate and blood pressure in four unanaesthetized rhesus monkeys. Single administration of the drug produced tachycardia and hypotension, preceded in two of the animals by a transient rise in blood pressure. With repeated drug administration, tolerance developed rapidly to the drug-induced tachycardia and hypertension but not to the hypotensive effect.

8.2.3 Endocrine effects

Tolerance has been reported to develop to the ability of Δ^9-THC to stimulate the release of corticosteroids into the circulation of rats and mice (Pertwee, 1974; Miczek and Dixit, 1980), to block surges in serum luteinizing hormone and prolactin levels at first pro-oestrus in rats (Field and Tyrey, 1986), to depress thyroid function in rats (Kaymakcalan and Deneau, 1972; Nazar *et al.*, 1977) and to reduce plasma levels of growth hormone and prolactin in mice (Dalterio *et al.*, 1981).

8.2.4 Antinociceptive effect

Tolerance has been demonstrated in a number of experiments with rats or mice using the tail-flick test (Bloom and Dewey, 1978; Dewey *et al.*, 1972a; Hine, 1985; Martin, 1985), the hot plate test (Kaymakcalan, 1979; Kaymakcalan and Deneau, 1972) or abdominal stretching tests (Chesher, 1980; Kaymakcalan and Deneau, 1972). Kaymakcalan *et al.* (1974) found that daily administration of Δ^9-THC produced tolerance to its depressant effect on the response of dogs to electrical stimulation of the tooth. Tolerance to Δ^9-THC-induced antinociception has also been reported to occur in neonatal chicks (Abel, 1972).

8.2.5 EEG activity

Tolerance has been observed in several rat studies (Fried, 1976; Moreton and Davis, 1973; Stadnicki *et al.*, 1974a). For example, Fried (1976) reported that rats became tolerant to Δ^9-THC-induced suppression of hippocampal theta I activity (4 to 6 c.p.s.). Moreton and Davis (1973) studied the effects of Δ^9-THC on EEG patterns in rats during sleep. Tolerance to the drug's ability to reduce the incidence of EEG signs of paradoxical sleep developed within 4 days and was still present 13 days after drug withdrawal. Tolerance to effects of Δ^9-THC or cannabis on EEG patterns has also been reported to occur in monkeys (Stadnicki *et al.*, 1974b) and rabbits (Martin and Consroe, 1978, 1981).

8.2.6 Neuropharmacological effects

8.2.6.1 Neurotransmitters

Results from studies with rats suggest that repeated administration of Δ^9-THC can reduce its ability to alter brain levels of dopamine (DA), 5-hydroxytryptamine (5-HT) and noradrenaline (NA) (Aulakh *et al.*, 1980; Bensemana and Gascon, 1974; Poddar and Ghosh, 1976a; Sofia *et al.*, 1977), to modify catecholamine turnover in the brain as measured by the rate of fall in NA or DA concentration after pretreatment with α-methyl-*p*-tyrosine (Poddar and Ghosh, 1976a), to elevate tryptophan levels in blood and brain (Filipovic and Trkovnik, 1980) and to depress tyrosine levels in blood (Poddar and Ghosh, 1976a). The pretreatment used in the study by Aulakh *et al.* (1980) also induced tolerance to effects of the drug on spontaneous activity.

Taylor and Fennessy (1978a) found that daily administration of Δ^9-THC to rats led to the development of tolerance to effects of the drug on motor activity and body temperature (hypothermia). This was associated with a progressive reduction in the drug's ability to elevate brain levels of 5-hydroxyindole acetic acid (5-HIAA). Towards the end of the treatment period, the drug elicited hyperthermic responses and falls in brain levels of 5-HIAA. That onset of tolerance (and hence a rightward shift in the dose–response curve) should lead to reversals in the direction of these Δ^9-THC-induced changes is not unexpected, there being evidence that sub-hypothermic doses of the drug can elevate body temperature and depress brain levels of 5-HIAA (Taylor and Fennessy, 1977). Brain levels of 5-HT were unaffected by single administration of Δ^9-THC but decreased after six or more injections. It was suggested by Taylor and Fennessy (1978a) that the changes in 5-HIAA levels observed following Δ^9-THC administration reflected drug-induced alterations in 5-HT release, that Δ^9-THC-induced hypothermia is mediated by 5-HT-releasing pathways and that tolerance to the hypothermic response develops because the stimulant effect of the cannabinoid on 5-HT release disappears when the drug is given repeatedly. Experiments carried out more recently (Verberne *et al.*, 1985) have yielded results which suggest that onset of tolerance to the hypothermic effect of Δ^9-THC in rats is also associated with reduced release of histamine in the cerebral cortex, hypothalamus, midbrain and cerebellum/pons/medulla oblongata.

In other experiments with rats, Miczec and Dixit (1980) investigated whether development of tolerance to effects of Δ^9-THC on body temperature, food intake, motor activity and plasma levels of corticosterone was associated with changes in brain levels of NA, DA or 5-HT. Single injection of the drug did not alter the concentration of any of these putative transmitters whereas changes did occur when the same dose was given repeatedly. In contrast to the results obtained by Taylor and Fennessy (1978a), only rises in 5-HT levels were seen to occur (in telencephalon, diencephalon, mesencephalon, cerebellum and striatum). In addition, there were falls in striatal NA levels and rises in striatal DA levels. Increases in brain levels of 5-HT following the repeated administration of Δ^9-THC have also been noted in experiments with mice (Anton *et al.*, 1974). The same pretreatment had no effect on brain levels of 5-HIAA.

Hershkowitz and Szechtman (1979) studied the effect of *in vivo* treatment of mice with Δ^9-THC on uptake of [^{3}H]DA into cerebral cortical synaptosomes. Whereas the cannabinoid produced increases in uptake when given to mice which had not been exposed to the drug before, it had no effect in mice which had been repeatedly pretreated with Δ^9-THC. Friedman *et al.* (1976) found that repeated *in vivo* administration of Δ^9-THC (or Δ^8-THC) to rats reduced the ability of these drugs to inhibit the formation of [^{3}H]acetylcholine ([^{3}H]ACh) in striatal slices preloaded with [^{3}H]choline. Δ^8-THC (but not Δ^9-THC) was also shown to induce tolerance to its inhibitory effect on [^{3}H]ACh formation by cerebral cortical slices. Tolerance to the inhibitory effect of the two cannabinoids on [^{3}H]ACh formation in hypothalamic slices did not develop.

8.2.6.2 Enzymes

Poddar and Ghosh (1976b) found that when rats were repeatedly injected with Δ^9-THC they became tolerant to both stimulatory and inhibitory effects of this drug on brain adenosine triphosphatase (ATPase) activity. The inhibitory effect of Δ^9-THC on synaptosomal Na^+/K^+-ATPase was reduced and its stimulatory effect on microsomal Na^+/K^+-ATPase and Mg^{2+}-ATPase abolished.

8.2.6.3 Binding studies

Hillard and Bloom (1982) studied the effects of Δ^9-THC on specific binding of the β-adrenoceptor antagonist dihydroalprenolol to cerebral cortical tissue obtained from mice. Twice-daily *in vivo* administration of the cannabinoid over 6 days was found to decrease the number of binding sites for [^{3}H]dihydroalprenolol without affecting the affinity of these sites. The effect of single *in vivo* administration of Δ^9-THC was not reported. It is noteworthy, therefore, that single *in vitro* addition of the drug (3 and 10 μM) to cerebral cortical tissue taken from unpretreated animals was found to produce an increase in binding. It did this by increasing the affinity of the binding sites for [^{3}H]dihydroalprenolol and not by altering the number of these sites. More recently, Evans *et al.* (1987) investigated the effect of repeated *in vivo* treatment with Δ^9-THC on specific binding of [^{3}H]dihydroalprenolol to ventricular plasma membranes prepared from the rat heart. It was found that administration of the drug once every week day for 90 days produced no detectable change in binding site density or affinity. Again, the effect of a single *in vivo* drug treatment was not reported.

8.3 Signs of tolerance in animals: cannabis and psychotropic cannabinoids other than Δ^9-THC

Tolerance of the sort produced by Δ^9-THC has also been observed in experiments with other psychoactive constituents of cannabis (Δ^8-THC and cannabinol), with cannabinoid metabolites such as the 11-hydroxy metabolites of Δ^8- and Δ^9-THC, with synthetic analogues of tetrahydrocannabinol such as $\Delta^{6a,10a}$-dimethylheptyl-THC, nantradol, levonantradol and nabilone, and with cannabis itself (e.g. Delini-Stula, 1973; Dykstra, 1983; Edery and Gottesfeld, 1975; Fish and Consroe, 1981; Frankenheim, 1974; Hine *et al.*, 1977; Johansson *et al.*, 1975; Kosersky *et al.*, 1974; Lomax, 1971; Luthra *et al.*, 1976; Page and West, 1977; Poddar and Ghosh, 1976b; Rating *et al.*, 1972; Smith, 1991; Watanabe *et al.*, 1982, 1983; Young *et al.*, 1981). In addition, there is evidence that tolerance can develop to the ability of cannabis and of Δ^8-THC and several of its metabolites to prolong sleep induced by barbiturates or ethanol in mice or rats (Rating *et al.*, 1972; Friedman and Gershon, 1974; Narimatsu *et al.*, 1983; Siemens and Kalant, 1974; Watanabe *et al.*, 1982, 1987). Tolerance to the effects of Δ^8-THC on the duration of sleep induced by hexobarbitone or ethanol does not seem to be associated with any change in the metabolism or disposition of these drugs (Friedman and Gershon, 1974; Rating *et al.*, 1972).

There is also evidence that tolerance can develop to the effect of cannabis on specific binding of the DA D_2 receptor antagonist, spiroperidol, to a crude synaptic membrane preparation derived from mouse corpus striatum (Agrawal *et al.*, 1985). Single administration of cannabis (50 or 100 mg/kg i.p.)

augmented the affinity of binding sites for [^{3}H]spiroperidol but had no effect on the number of these sites. Daily administration of cannabis for 14 days either abolished this effect (50 mg/kg per day i.p.) or led to a reduction in binding (100 mg/kg per day i.p.). More recently, Agrawal *et al.* (1989) reported that repeated cannabis administration (50 or 100 mg/kg per day i.p. for 14 days) produced tolerance to the ability of the drug (injected *in vivo*) to increase the affinity of mouse striatal muscarinic binding sites for [^{3}H]quinuclidinyl benzylate. Interestingly, pretreatment with the higher dose also produced tolerance to the ability of cannabis to enhance oxotremorine-induced tremor in mice and to increase the permeability of the blood–brain barrier, as measured by entry of sodium fluorescein into mouse brain. In other experiments, repeated oral administration of cannabis (100 mg/kg per day for 28 days) was shown to enhance the specific binding of [^{3}H]diazepam to a crude membrane fraction prepared from mouse frontal cortex (Sethi *et al.*, 1986). This occurred through an increase in binding site affinity. Single administration of the same dose had no detectable effect on [^{3}H]diazepam binding.

Finally, Tayal *et al.* (1974) reported that rats subjected to a 6-day pretreatment with cannabis became tolerant not only to the effect of the drug on a conditioned avoidance response but also to its inhibitory effect on brain monoamine oxidase activity.

8.4 Signs of tolerance in cultured cells

Burstein *et al.* (1985) found that a single prior exposure of WI-38 human lung fibroblasts to Δ^9-THC (0.08–1.6 μM for 30 min) reduced its ability to stimulate prostaglandin E_2 production by the same (washed) cells 24 hours later. The degree of tolerance increased with the number of prior exposures to Δ^9-THC, the drug's effect disappearing completely after three successive 30-min pretreatments, applied at 24-hour intervals. Similar results were obtained in experiments with cannabidiol and cannabicyclol. Additional experiments demonstrated that tolerance to the effect of Δ^9-THC on prostaglandin production was reversible, that cells rendered completely tolerant to Δ^9-THC could still increase their production of prostaglandin E_2 (in response to a calcium ionophore) and that the Δ^9-THC pretreatments used did not affect cell number. Tolerance was also shown to develop to the ability of Δ^9-THC to increase [^{14}C]arachidonate release from preloaded cells.

Dill and Howlett (1988) investigated the effect of cannabinoid pretreatment on the ability of two cannabinoids to inhibit secretin-induced production of cyclic adenosine 3′,5′-monophosphate (cyclic AMP) by a cloned neuroblastoma cell line (N18TG2). It was found that the degree of inhibition produced by 1 μM Δ^9-THC or desacetyllevonantradol (DALN) could be decreased by prior exposure of the cells to the same cannabinoid (1 μM) for 24 hours. It is noteworthy, however, that in the experiments with Δ^9-THC, even though the cells were washed after their first (24-hour) drug treatment, the cannabinoid's inhibitory effect on the secretin response carried over to the second part of the experiment. As a result, although the percentage inhibition produced by the second Δ^9-THC treatment was less in Δ^9-THC-pretreated cells (17%) than in control cells (35%), the absolute amount of cyclic AMP produced following the administration of secretin in the presence of the cannabinoid (about 300 pmol/mg protein in 4 min) was little affected by the Δ^9-THC pretreatment. Additional results obtained in the same study showed that pretreatment with one cannabinoid (Δ^9-THC or DALN) produced tolerance to the other's inhibitory effect (percentage inhibition of the secretin response). However, prior exposure to either cannabinoid did not render cells tolerant to carbachol-induced inhibition of the secretin response. There was good evidence that none of the treatments used produced changes in cell growth rate, cell protein content or cell morphology.

8.5 Signs of tolerance in man

Present knowledge about cannabinoid tolerance in man comes largely from work carried out before 1981 (for reviews see Hollister, 1986; Jones, 1983). There have been a number of laboratory studies. These were performed with experienced cannabis users and fall essentially into two categories. The first consists of experiments which have examined the relationship between subjects' self-reported rates of cannabis consumption (outside the laboratory) and responsiveness to cannabis/cannabinoids measured in the laboratory. The second category is made up of studies which have investigated the extent to which tolerance can be induced by Δ^9-THC, pyrahexyl or cannabis when these are repeatedly administered in a controlled environment. The results from both types of study provide good evidence that tolerance can develop in man to many of the effects of cannabis and Δ^9-THC. These include effects on mood, memory, EEG, sleep, heart rate, blood pressure, intraocular pressure, body temperature, salivary flow and performance in psychomotor tasks (Jones *et al.*, 1976; see also Jones, 1983). Tolerance may also occur to the antiemetic effect of Δ^9-THC (Chang *et al.*, 1979). Human experiments, like those with animals (Sections 8.2 to 8.4, 8.7 and 8.9.1), have yielded data which suggest that tolerance to cannabinoids can develop rapidly, that the rate of onset of cannabinoid tolerance is affected by the treatment dose and by the frequency with which this is administered and that cross-tolerance can occur between cannabis and ethanol (for review see Jones, 1983).

As pointed out by Jones (1983), most tolerance studies with human subjects have been conducted without double-blind or placebo treatments. This is an important limitation since there is evidence that certain responses to cannabis can be markedly influenced by the subjects 'expectations' (Jones, 1971). An additional interpretational difficulty associated with many of those studies in which the development of tolerance has been followed in the laboratory arises from the practice of allowing dose levels and frequency of administration to be decided by the subjects themselves. It is noteworthy, therefore, that the production of tolerance by cannabis and Δ^9-THC has been clearly demonstrated in experiments with human subjects in which drug administrations were made double-blind and in which placebo treatments and predetermined drug regimens were used (Jones *et al.*, 1976; see also Jones. 1983).

8.6 Mechanisms of tolerance

Mechanisms of drug-induced tolerance can be divided into two main types, dispositional (pharmacokinetic) and non-dispositional (broadly equivalent to pharmacodynamic). Dispositional tolerance arises from any change in drug absorption, distribution, metabolism or excretion which leads to a reduction in the concentration of the active form of the drug at its site of action. In contrast, non-dispositional tolerance arises from some change that reduces the ability of a given drug concentration to elicit a response (see also Chapter 1).

8.6.1 Dispositional tolerance

8.6.1.1 Metabolic tolerance

Cannabinoids are known to undergo extensive metabolism (for review see Agurell *et al.*, 1986) and the notion that they produce tolerance by inducing some change in their own metabolism is, therefore, well worth exploring. Evidence that cannabinoid metabolism can be enhanced by cannabinoid pretreatment already exists. Magour *et al.* (1977) reported that the conversion of Δ^9-THC and its 11-hydroxy metabolite to 'highly polar metabolites' could be increased in rats by pretreating the animals with Δ^9-THC for 4 days. The same pretreatment was found to decrease the duration of the drug's depressant effect on locomotor activity. Mantilla-Plata and Harbison (1975) pretreated mice with $[^{14}C]\Delta^9$-THC intravenously for 5 days and observed that radioactivity levels in the brain were markedly less after the fifth injection than after the first. They also noted that plasma levels of radioactivity fell more quickly at the end of the pretreatment period than at the beginning. Ho *et al.* (1973) found that Δ^9-THC was metabolized more rapidly by microsomes prepared from the livers of rats which had been given the drug repeatedly for 4 weeks than it was by microsomes prepared from saline-pretreated animals. Similar results were obtained by Watanabe *et al.* (1986) in experiments with mice pretreated with Δ^8-THC or 11-hydroxy-Δ^8-THC for 7 days. Lemberger *et al.* (1971) investigated the effect of repeated exposure to cannabis on the disposition and metabolism of intravenously injected [^{14}C]Δ^9-THC in man. It was found that the rate of disappearance of radioactivity from plasma during the second, slower elimination phase was markedly greater in chronic cannabis smokers than in subjects professing no prior exposure to the drug. Signs of increased Δ^9-THC metabolism following cannabinoid pretreatment have also been detected in other experiments with human subjects (Hunt and Jones, 1980) as well as in experiments with dogs (Martin *et al.*, 1976).

Although it is generally accepted that repeated pretreatment with cannabinoids can increase the rate at which these drugs are metabolized, there are several reasons for believing that such increases play, at most, only a minor role in the production of cannabinoid tolerance. These reasons can be summarized as follows.

(i) There is evidence that the production of tolerance to Δ^9-THC is not always associated with increases in the rate of its removal from the body. More specifically, there are reports that onset of tolerance to its convulsant/anticonvulsant or hypothermic effects in mice, to its inhibitory effect on rotarod performance in rats and mice, to its depressant effect on key pecking for food in pigeons and to its ability to depress respiration in mouse brain homogenates after *in vivo* administration is not accompanied by any detectable increase in the rate of its metabolism or elimination (Dewey *et al.*, 1973; Karler *et al.*, 1982; Lawrence and Pertwee, 1973; McMillan *et al.*, 1973; Nazar *et al.*, 1974; Siemens and Doyle, 1979; Sprague and Craigmill, 1976). Indeed, in some of these studies onset of tolerance has been shown to be associated with signs of a decrease in the rate of metabolism of Δ^9-THC or with signs of an accumulation of cannabinoids in blood, brain and other tissues (Dewey *et al.*, 1973; McMillan *et al.*, 1973; Siemens and Doyle, 1979). It has also been found that development of tolerance to the effect of cannabis on the duration of ethanol-induced sleep in rats is not accompanied by any change in ability to metabolize or excrete Δ^9-THC (Siemens and Kalant, 1974). Perez-Reyes *et al.* (1974), Lindgren *et al.* (1981) and Ohlsson *et al.* (1982) compared the elimination rates of Δ^9-THC in frequent users of cannabis with those in less frequent users and found little difference between the two groups. However, data from two of these studies (Lindgren *et al.*, 1981; Perez-Reyes *et al.*, 1974) suggest that there was also little difference in the sensitivity of the two groups to Δ^9-THC.

(ii) In some of the experiments in which an enhancement of cannabinoid metabolism has been found to parallel onset of tolerance, the changes in metabolism appear to be far too small to account for the degree of the tolerance produced. In these experiments, conducted with human subjects (Hunt and Jones, 1980) or dogs (Martin *et al.*, 1976), a comparison was made between Δ^9-THC metabolism and disposition in tolerant and non-tolerant groups by injecting both groups with [^{14}C]- or [^{3}H]Δ^9-THC and then measuring radioactivity levels in plasma, urine and/or faeces. In the dog experiments, levels of radioactivity were also monitored in peripheral tissues, in various areas of the brain and in subcellular fractions of brain tissue. Tolerance was defined, in man, as a diminution in Δ^9-THC-induced tachycardia and skin hypothermia and in the intensity of the drug's psychological effects and, in dogs, as a reduction in Δ^9-THC-induced impairment of spontaneous motor activity.

(iii) In two of the studies in which pretreatment with cannabinoids was found to hasten cannabinoid metabolism (Δ^8-THC or Δ^9-THC) (Ho *et al.*, 1973; Watanabe *et al.*, 1986), there was seen to be an increase in the production of pharmacologically active metabolites. These metabolites, 11-hydroxy-Δ^8-THC and 11-hydroxy-Δ^9-THC, are known to be even more potent than their parent compounds (for review see Razdan, 1986).

(iv) Pretreatment of mice with Δ^9-THC by a peripheral route (s.c.) has been shown to produce tolerance to the hypothermic effect of a low dose of the drug (10 μg) administered directly into the IVth cerebral ventricle (Fitton and Pertwee, 1982). This finding constitutes evidence against dispositional tolerance only if Δ^9-THC is not metabolized within the brain to less active metabolites. Some experiments with mouse or rat brain microsomal preparations (Christensen *et al.*, 1971; Ho *et al.*, 1973; Jones *et al.*, 1974) have yielded results which suggest that Δ^9-THC is not metabolized by brain tissue at all. However, results from other experiments with brain microsomes (Watanabe *et al.*, 1988) suggest that some metabolism does occur, albeit mainly to 4′-hydroxy- (mice, rats and rabbits) or 5′-hydroxy-Δ^9-THC (guinea-pigs), both of which probably possess marked pharmacological activity (4′-hydroxy- and 5′-hydroxy-Δ^8-THC are at least as potent as their parent compound, Δ^8-THC (for review see Razdan, 1986)).

8.6.1.2 Other types of dispositional tolerance

The role of 'non-metabolic' dispositional mechanisms has yet to be explored. One hypothesis still to be fully tested is that tolerance to cannabinoids is mediated by the immune system (Nahas *et al.*, 1973b). Thus it could be that cannabinoids (bound to plasma proteins) raise antibodies and that these can produce tolerance by removing cannabinoid molecules from free solution.

8.6.2 Non-dispositional tolerance

Mechanisms for non-dispositional drug tolerance can be thought of as being either 'direct' or 'indirect'. The former operate by reducing sensitivity at the site of action itself whereas the latter act beyond the site of action, for example to reduce transmission along some neuronal pathway mediating a drug effect. The evidence that cannabinoid tolerance is non-dispositional comes mainly from data suggesting that it cannot be accounted for by changes in cannabinoid metabolism or disposition (Section 8.6.1). For psychoactive cannabinoids, there is little other information and hence it is only possible to speculate about the nature of the underlying 'direct' or 'indirect' mechanisms.

8.6.2.1 Possible 'direct' mechanisms of tolerance to psychotropic cannabinoids

Psychotropic cannabinoids are thought to owe many of their pharmacological properties to an ability to produce functional changes in neuronal membranes and there is good evidence that this ability depends on the molecular shape and structure of the cannabinoids rather than on their marked lipophilicity (Thomas *et al.*, 1990; see also Pertwee, 1990). Whilst some cannabinoid-induced changes in membrane function may be brought about by non-receptor-mediated processes involving, for example, the induction of conformational changes in membrane phospholipids (Hillard *et al.*, 1990; see also Pertwee, 1990), it is now clear that changes in membrane function can also be produced by the activation of a specific cannabinoid receptor. Thus (i) cannabinoids show chemical and stereochemical selectivity, biological selectivity and high potency in certain preparations (for review see Pertwee, 1990), (ii) high-affinity, specific cannabinoid binding sites have been demonstrated in the membranes of cultured cells and rat brain synaptosomes (Bidaut-Russell *et al.*, 1990; Devane *et al.*, 1988; Herkenham *et al.*, 1990; Howlett *et al.*, 1990), and (iii) a cannabinoid receptor has been cloned (Matsuda *et al.*, 1990). There is also evidence that cannabinoid receptors are linked to adenylate cyclase through a guanine nucleotide regulatory protein (Devane *et al.*, 1988; Howlett *et al.*, 1990; see also Pertwee, 1990).

The binding studies were carried out using a tritium-labelled, synthetic cannabinoid, CP-55,940. Experiments with unlabelled cannabinoids have shown that their ability to displace [^{3}H]CP-55,940 correlates reasonably well with their psychopharmacological potency (Bidaut-Russell *et al.*, 1990; Devane *et al.*, 1988; Herkenham *et al.*, 1990; Howlett *et al.*, 1990). It has also been shown that the binding of [^{3}H]CP-55,940 to brain tissue is unaffected by a wide range of non-cannabinoids. These include ligands known to bind to receptors for noradrenaline, dopamine, acetylcholine, GABA or opioid peptides. The experiments with [^{3}H]CP-55,940 have also demonstrated that cannabinoid binding sites are not uniformly distributed throughout the brain. Instead, they are localized, in high density, in areas of the brain (substantia nigra, globus pallidus, entopeduncular nucleus, corpus striatum, cerebral cortex, hippocampus and cerebellum) at which cannabinoids might be expected to produce their characteristic effects on cognition and memory and at which they are already known to affect motor function (Pertwee and Wickens, 1991; see also Pertwee, 1990). Some cannabinoid-sensitive brain areas such as the hypothalamus and brain stem appear to be relatively sparsely populated with [^{3}H]CP-55,940 binding sites. Although this might well be because the actions of cannabinoids in these parts of the brain (e.g. those responsible for hypothermia; see Pertwee (1985)) are mediated by mechanisms that do not involve a cannabinoid receptor, it might equally well be because cannabinoid receptors are concentrated at only a limited number of critical sites within the hypothalamus and brain stem or because these brain areas contain other type(s) of cannabinoid receptor with a low affinity for [^{3}H]CP-55,940.

It follows from what is now known about their mode(s) of action that 'direct' tolerance to psychoactive cannabinoids could arise from a reduction in the affinity and/or density and/or efficacy of a population of cannabinoid receptors. It could also arise from some other change in membrane composition or organization and, indeed, there is already evidence that changes in membrane composition can modify the effects of cannabinoids on membrane 'fluidity' and that *in vivo* administration of Δ^9-THC can change the phospholipid composition of central neuronal membranes (for review see Pertwee, 1990).

8.6.2.2 Possible 'indirect' mechanisms of tolerance to psychotropic cannabinoids

There is evidence that psychotropic cannabinoids can affect many areas of the brain and that the changes produced are mediated by numerous pathways through the release of a wide range of different transmitters (for further details see Pertwee (1990)). It follows that tolerance to at least some effects of the cannabinoids could arise indirectly from some change in one or more of the pathways mediating these effects, for example a change in sensitivity to a neurotransmitter. In line with this notion are reports that the development of tolerance to cannabinoids is associated with changes in transmitter synthesis, concentration and turnover and that repeated administration of cannabis or Δ^9-THC can alter the affinity or density of central adrenergic, dopaminergic and cholinergic binding sites (Sections 8.2.6 and 8.3). The same kind of mechanism could also explain the development of non-dispositional cross-tolerance between psychoactive cannabinoids and other types of centrally active drug (Section 8.7). This is because some of the neuronal pathways responsible for the expression of a particular drug response are likely to be the same no matter whether the response is elicited by a cannabinoid or by some other drug. It is through a functional change in one of these common pathways that 'indirect' cross-tolerance might arise.

Although the changes underlying the production of 'indirect' non-dispositional tolerance to a drug may be at the level of an individual transmitter or neuronal pathway, more complex mechanisms are also possible. For example, animal or human subjects may become tolerant by learning to cope with the effects of a drug ('learned' tolerance). Whilst there is evidence from certain conditioned behavioural studies that such a learning process can give rise to cannabinoid tolerance (Carder and Olson, 1973; Larsen and Pryor, 1977; Manning, 1976a; Smith, 1991), there is also evidence, from other conditioned behavioural studies with cannabinoids, that a process of this kind is not always involved (Johansson *et al.*, 1974; Ten Ham, 1977; Webster *et al.*, 1973). The role of 'learned' tolerance in the development of tolerance to other effects of cannabinoids has yet to be explored.

8.7 Cross-tolerance studies

Cross-tolerance, either symmetrical or asymmetrical, can develop amongst certain psychoactive cannabinoids (Dill and Howlett, 1988; Fish and Consroe, 1981; McMillan *et al.*, 1972; Narimatsu *et al.*, 1983; Page and West, 1977; Watanabe *et al.*, 1987; Yamamoto *et al.*, 1985). It can also develop between cannabinoids and morphine, certain barbiturates, phenytoin, ethanol, chlorpromazine, reserpine, tetrabenazine, prostaglandin E_2, oxotremorine and 5-HT (e.g. Burstein *et al.*, 1988; Carder and Deikel, 1976; Chait *et al.*, 1981; Englert *et al.*, 1973; Hedley *et al.*, 1984; Hine, 1985; Karler *et al.*, 1974b; McMillan *et al.*, 1980, 1983; Narimatsu *et al.*, 1983; Newman *et al.*, 1972, 1974; Siemens and Doyle, 1979; Singh *et al.*, 1978; Sprague and Craigmill, 1976; Tulunay *et al.*, 1982; Watanabe *et al.*, 1984; Yamamoto *et al.*, 1985). For two effects (antinociception and hypothermia) the data are conflicting, there being some reports that cross-tolerance between cannabinoids and morphine does develop (Bloom and Dewey, 1978; Chesher, 1980; Hine, 1985; Kaymakcalan and Deneau, 1972; Narimatsu *et al.*, 1983, 1987) and others that it does not (Yamamoto *et al.*, 1985; Martin, 1985). Burstein *et al.* (1989) reported that Δ^9-THC-induced catalepsy could be attenuated in mice by triggering the production of anti-prostaglandin E_2 antibodies. This was achieved by pretreating the animals with a thyroglobulin–prostaglandin E_2 conjugate.

There is evidence, at least for ethanol and barbiturates (barbitone), that dispositional or metabolic changes do not play a major role in the development of cross-tolerance with cannabinoids (Chait *et al.*, 1981; Siemens and Doyle, 1979; Sprague and Craigmill, 1976). It is also unlikely that rats or mice pretreated with Δ^9-THC become tolerant to certain behavioural effects of ethanol because they learn to compensate for some drug-induced change in brain function (Newman *et al.*, 1972; Siemens and Doyle, 1979; Sprague and Craigmill, 1976).

8.8 Dependence studies

8.8.1 Withdrawal signs in animals

8.8.1.1 Behavioural changes

There are only a few reports that abrupt withdrawal from treatment with cannabis or one of its constituents (Δ^8- or Δ^9-THC) can trigger behaviour different from that observed in drug-treated or control animals. Examples include increased motor activity and grooming behaviour in rats (Kaymakcalan *et al.*, 1977; Sjöden *et al.*, 1973; see also Section 8.8.5.1), altered susceptibility to convulsions induced by electroshock in mice (Karler and Turkanis, 1980; Karler *et al.*, 1986), increased aggressiveness in monkeys (Beardsley *et al.*, 1986; Kaymakcalan, 1972; Stadnicki *et al.*, 1974b) and in dominant male mice (Cutler *et al.*, 1975) and changed operant performance in monkeys (Beardsley *et al.*, 1986; Branch *et al.*, 1980).

Kaymakcalan (1972) reported that as well as increasing aggressiveness and irritability, withdrawal of Δ^9-THC from six rhesus monkeys which had been injected with the drug four times a day for 36 days (0.1–0.4 mg/kg i.v.) caused muscle tremor and twitching, yawning, photophobia, piloerection, penile erection, anorexia, sitting in 'propped-up positions', the consumption of faeces, biting and licking of fingers, hair pulling, staring 'in circles', grasping as if catching flies and cage wall slapping. These changes appeared within 12 hours of withdrawal and lasted for about 5 days. Fredericks and Benowitz (1980) repeatedly injected four rhesus monkeys with Δ^9-THC, 0.5 mg/kg i.v. every 6 hours for 3 weeks. During this period tolerance developed to behavioural effects of the drug which included suppression of gross movement and of eye contact/tooth baring. Withdrawal of the drug treatment caused the frequency or duration of these types of behaviour to increase well beyond that which had been observed in the same animals before any exposure to Δ^9-THC. This 'rebound' effect was first detected 3 days after drug withdrawal. It was a transient phenomenon, disappearing within 12 days of withdrawal.

Rats subjected to Δ^9-THC treatments known to induce tolerance to the drug's effects on motor activity, food consumption and body temperature (see Sections 8.2.1 and 8.2.2) have been reported to show marked changes in behaviour when injected with clomipramine, imipramine or fluoxetine on the day after Δ^9-THC withdrawal (Taylor and Fennessy, 1978b, 1982; Verberne *et al.*, 1980). Among the most prominent of these responses were writhing and backward kicking of the hind legs. Other behavioural responses were wet dog shakes, jumping, tremor, ptosis, chewing movements, excessive grooming, yawning, squealing and ataxia. Body temperature changes and diarrhoea were not observed. The behavioural 'syndrome' was not induced by Δ^9-THC withdrawal *per se*. Nor, indeed, was it induced by naloxone (Verberne *et al.*, 1980) (cf. Section 8.8.5.1). Since it could be partially suppressed by giving Δ^9-THC shortly before clomipramine (Verberne *et al.*, 1981, 1985) and since it was only observed in Δ^9-THC-pretreated animals, the syndrome most probably results from an unmasking of changes triggered by Δ^9-THC withdrawal. The three drugs found to provoke the behavioural syndrome are all inhibitors of the neuronal uptake of 5-HT and it has therefore been proposed that the syndrome may be mediated by 5-HT (Taylor and Fennessy, 1978b; Verberne *et al.*, 1980). There is also evidence for an involvement of histamine (Verberne *et al.*, 1985).

8.8.1.2 EEG changes

Stadnicki *et al.* (1974b) reported that cannabis withdrawal could trigger an increase in the incidence of EEG desynchronization in one of two rhesus monkeys that had been rendered tolerant to the drug's effects on EEG. In experiments with rats, Pirch *et al.* (1972, 1973) showed that withdrawal from a daily pretreatment with cannabis known to produce tolerance to the drug's depressant effect on EEG voltage gave rise to a transient 'rebound' voltage increase. Moreton and Davis (1973) found that withdrawal from rats of a Δ^9-THC treatment producing tolerance to the drug's inhibitory effect on paradoxical sleep led to a slight increase in the proportion of time spent in this sleep state.

8.8.2 Withdrawal signs in man

Much of the important literature in this area was published before 1981 and has been extensively reviewed by Jones (1983). In essence, signs of withdrawal have been demonstrated in experiments with cannabis, Δ^9-THC and pyrahexyl although not in experiments with cannabidiol. They have been produced in the laboratory either by depriving regular cannabis users of cannabis or by abruptly terminating cannabis or cannabinoid treatments administered under controlled conditions. In at least some of these experiments, double-blind procedures were used and placebo treatments included (cf. Section 8.5). The signs of cannabis/cannabinoid withdrawal detected in such experiments have been relatively mild. They have been likened to the changes observed following withdrawal of short, low-dose treatments with opioids or ethanol (for review see Jones, 1983) and include changes in mood, sleep, heart rate, body temperature, salivary flow, body weight, caloric intake and appetite. Restlessness, tremor, mild nausea, hot flushes and sweating have also been noted. There is evidence that the cannabinoid withdrawal syndrome is transient and that it can be attenuated by re-administration of cannabis or Δ^9-THC or, indeed, by treatment with ethanol or hexobarbitone. There is also evidence that the intensity of the syndrome in man is governed by the pretreatment dose and by the frequency with which this has been administered.

8.8.3 Effects on electrical intracranial self-stimulation

When given at doses ranging from 1 to 20 mg/kg i.p., Δ^9-THC has been found to decrease the rates at which rats press a lever to receive electrical stimulation through electrodes implanted in the ventral tegmentum (A10 area, dorsal to the interpenduncular nucleus) or lateral or posterior hypothalamus (Bailey and Pradhan, 1972; Bhattacharyya *et al.*, 1980; Pradhan *et al.*, 1972; Wayner *et al.*, 1973). This finding does not necessarily support the idea that Δ^9-THC has a depressant effect on central reward mechanisms since the same dose range has also been found to inhibit certain other types of conditioned behavioural response (Pradhan *et al.*, 1972; Wayner *et al.*, 1973). Other studies, also with rats, have been directed at investigating the effect of cannabinoids on rewarding brain stimulation thresholds. Kucharski *et al.* (1983) found that levonantradol increased the current required to maintain electrical self-stimulation of the medial forebrain bundle–lateral hypothalamic area. The response was abolished by doses above 0.3 mg/kg. In contrast, Δ^9-THC has been found to decrease the threshold for self-stimulation (Gardner *et al.*, 1988). Again, the electrodes were implanted in the medial forebrain bundle, albeit at sites posterior to the hypothalamus. There is evidence that this effect of Δ^9-THC depends on the drug's ability to enhance dopamine release from nerve terminals in the nucleus accumbens and medial prefrontal cortex and that the effect of Δ^9-THC on dopamine release (at least in the nucleus accumbens) depends on the presence of endogenous opioid peptides (Chen *et al.*, 1990a,b). These findings have prompted the suggestion that cannabis may 'resemble other drugs of abuse in producing as a final common neuropharmacological action, acute facilitation of the mesocorticolimbic dopamine reward-relevant circuitry' (Chen *et al.*, 1990a,b).

8.8.4 Intravenous self-administration of cannabinoids

Several studies have been directed at investigating the extent to which animals will self-administer cannabinoids intravenously, the overall aim being to assess the reinforcing properties of this drug group. Some of these studies have been made with animals which have never before received a drug ('naive' animals). The others have been performed with animals previously exposed to a series of cannabinoid injections ('forced' injections) or already trained to self-administer cocaine or codeine. Kaymakcalan (1972) was unable to train six naive rhesus monkeys to self-administer Δ^9-THC. However, two of the monkeys did self-administer the drug after having first been subjected to forced Δ^9-THC injections four times a day for 36 days. Three other rhesus monkeys were similarly pretreated with Δ^9-THC and then provided with cocaine for intravenous self-administration. Only one of these animals could be trained to self-administer this drug. The same animal also self-administered Δ^9-THC when this was substituted for the cocaine. Harris *et al.* (1974), like Kaymakcalan (1972), failed to induce any significant degree of self-administration of Δ^9-THC in naive rhesus monkeys. They were also unable to demonstrate self-administration of the drug by rhesus monkeys first trained to self-administer cocaine or subjected over a 30-day period to forced injections of Δ^9-THC. Similarly, Young *et al.* (1981) found that three rhesus monkeys conditioned to press a lever in order to self-administer codeine did not continue to press the lever when the codeine was replaced by nantradol or levonantradol.

Van Ree *et al.* (1978) were able to demonstrate self-administration of Δ^9-THC by rats first subjected for 4 days to hourly forced intravenous injections of the drug. The results obtained suggest that Δ^9-THC, taken intravenously, has relatively weak reinforcing properties. Thus significant levels of self-administration were not observed in all of the rats studied and the drug intake of those animals that did show this type of behaviour was markedly less than that observed in parallel experiments with opioids or amphetamine. Takahashi and Singer (1979, 1980) conditioned fasted rats to bar press for food and found that the response rates of trained animals increased markedly when bar pressing was allowed to trigger intravenous injections of

Δ^9-THC as well as food reinforcement. However, such increases in responding did not occur if there was no food reinforcement or if the animals were not sufficiently fasted.

8.8.5 Cross-dependence studies

8.8.5.1 Experiments with morphine and naloxone

There are reports from two laboratories that several opioid-like withdrawal signs can be induced in Δ^9-THC-pretreated rats either by drug withdrawal or by naloxone (Hirschhorn and Rosecrans, 1974; Kaymakcalan *et al.*, 1977; Tulunay *et al.*, 1980). In addition there is evidence that cannabinoids can suppress certain signs precipitated by opioid withdrawal or by naloxone in morphine- or methadone-pretreated rats, mice, guinea-pigs and chronic spinal dogs (Bhargava, 1976a,b, 1978; Frederickson *et al.*, 1976; Gilbert, 1981; Hine *et al.*, 1975a,b,c; Jacob *et al.*, 1981; Lal *et al.*, 1981; Young *et al.*, 1981). Not all of the many changes precipitated by naloxone after morphine pretreatment appear to be equally susceptible to this inhibitory effect. For example, experiments directed at studying the effect of Δ^9-THC on a selected range of responses elicited by naloxone in morphine-pretreated rats showed that, at certain doses, the cannabinoid reduced the incidence of naloxone-induced defaecation, diarrhoea and wet dog shakes/escapes without significantly affecting the incidence of naloxone-induced vocalization, ear blanching, ptosis, chewing movements, abnormal posture or teeth chattering (Hine *et al.*, 1975a).

Zaluzny *et al.* (1979) studied the effect of Δ^9-THC on the 'quasi-morphine withdrawal syndrome' (QMWS). This is induced by phosphodiesterase inhibitors and resembles the withdrawal syndrome precipitated by naloxone in morphine-dependent animals. It was found that Δ^9-THC shared the ability of morphine to suppress the QMWS in rats (agitation and grooming, wet dog shakes, head shakes and ptosis). Only the effect of morphine was naloxone reversible. Further studies showed that the QMWS could also be suppressed by cannabinol but not by cannabidiol (Chesher and Jackson, 1985).

8.8.5.2 Experiments with phenobarbitone and ethanol

Gildea and Bourn (1977) found that Δ^9-THC could reduce the incidence and severity of audiogenic seizures in rats which had been withdrawal from phenobarbitone after a 4-week period of repeated phenobarbitone administration. On the other hand, Δ^9-THC and nabilone were found to increase the severity of convulsions induced by handling mice which had been continuously exposed to ethanol vapour (and repeatedly injected with pyrazole) over the preceding 3 days (Kralik *et al.*, 1976; Sprague and Craigmill, 1978). However, handling-induced convulsions were also observed in Δ^9-THC- and nabilone-injected mice which had not been pretreated with ethanol.

8.8.6 Mechanisms of dependence

Little is known about the mechanisms underlying cannabinoid dependence. However, many of the data that are available can be readily explained in terms of classical theories which postulate an involvement of non-dispositional tolerance in the production of drug dependence and can provide plausible explanations for most signs of dependence other than drug-seeking behaviour. According to these theories, tolerance may develop because, in the continued presence of a drug, counteractive processes arise which produce effects opposite in direction to the acute effects of the drug. As long as the drug remains at its site of action, the presence of such counteractive processes is indicated by a suppression of these acute effects (tolerance). However, if the drug disappears from its site of action with sufficient rapidity or if an antagonist is given, the now unopposed counteractive processes precipitate a withdrawal syndrome made up of effects opposite in direction to the drug's acute effects ('rebound' effects). In the continued absence of the drug, the counteractive processes gradually disappear.

The evidence that cannabinoid dependence may develop through such a mechanism is circumstantial. It can be summarized as follows.

(i) Cannabinoid tolerance appears to be largely non-dispositional in nature (Section 8.6).

(ii) There are several reports that withdrawal of cannabis or Δ^9-THC can give rise to 'rebound' effects (Section 8.8.1).

(iii) Effects precipitated by cannabinoid withdrawal are transient. They are detected within 12–24 hours of withdrawal and disappear within 2–12 days (Section 8.8.1).

(iv) In the few cannabinoid studies in which both tolerance and dependence have been investigated, it has been found that animals showing signs of dependence were also tolerant (Branch *et al.*, 1980; Fredericks and Benowitz, 1980; Taylor and Fennessy, 1982; Verberne *et al.*, 1980, 1985; see also Section 8.8.1.2). This finding is at least consistent with the notion that cannabinoid tolerance is a prerequisite for cannabinoid dependence.

(v) Cannabis and Δ^9-THC can suppress their own withdrawal signs when re-administered after withdrawal (Beardsley *et al.*, 1986; Section 8.8.2).

The involvement of counteractive processes in the production of cannabinoid tolerance and dependence could well account for the observation that 5-HT uptake inhibitors can elicit novel responses in Δ^9-THC-pretreated rats showing signs of tolerance but not of dependence (no withdrawal syndrome) (Section 8.8.1.1). One possibility is that Δ^9-THC administration can lead to a fall in the activity of certain 5-HT-releasing neurones and that tolerance can develop through a compensatory change in transmission along these pathways, for example an increase in the sensitivity of postsynaptic 5-HT receptors (counteractive process). The finding that there was no withdrawal syndrome could indicate that sufficient amounts of Δ^9-THC remained at the site of action in the post-withdrawal period to prevent expression of the counteractive process. An uptake inhibitor would be expected to upset such a balance between drug and counteractive process in favour of the latter by causing an accumulation of 5-HT at its receptors.

8.9 General discussion and summary

8.9.1 Tolerance

There is strong evidence that tolerance can develop to many of the effects of cannabinoids and that it can occur in a wide range of species. These include man, monkey, dog, rabbit, rat, mouse, gerbil, pigeon and the domestic hen. Although usually demonstrated *in vivo*, cell culture experiments have shown that cannabinoid tolerance can also develop *in vitro*. The main characteristics of cannabinoid tolerance may be summarized as follows:

(i) Tolerance can develop to many of the effects of cannabis and of its main psychically active constituent, Δ^9-THC. Tolerance also develops to other psychoactive constituents of cannabis (e.g. Δ^8-THC and cannabinol), to certain psychoactive cannabinoid metabolites, for example the 11-hydroxy metabolites of Δ^8- and Δ^9-THC, and to synthetic analogues of tetrahydrocannabinol such as levonantradol and nabilone (Sections 8.2 to 8.5).

(ii) Cannabinoid tolerance can be rapid in its onset (it can take 24 hours or less to develop) and intense in its degree. Examples of effects to which tolerance has been shown to develop particularly rapidly are hypothermia (Ten Ham and De Jong, 1974; Anderson *et al.*, 1975), depression of locomotor activity (e.g. Tulunay *et al.*, 1982; Verberne *et al.*, 1980) and elevation of plasma corticosterone levels (Pertwee, 1974). To date, the greatest degree of tolerance to have been observed has been a reduction in sensitivity of at least 100-fold to an effect of Δ^9-THC on conditioned behaviour in pigeons (Chait *et al.*, 1981; McMillan *et al.*, 1972).

(iii) There is evidence that the rate of onset and degree of tolerance produced by cannabinoids is governed by the treatment dose (Abel *et al.*, 1973; Uran *et al.*, 1980; see also Jones, 1983) and by the frequency with which this dose is administered (Davis and Borgen, 1975; Liu, 1974; Pirch *et al.*, 1972; see also Jones, 1983).

(iv) Tolerance seems to develop more readily to some effects than others. For example, it has been shown that monkeys can become tolerant to Δ^9-THC-induced tachycardia without also becoming tolerant to the drug's hypotensive effect (Fredericks *et al.*, 1981). In mice, tolerance has been shown to develop more rapidly to the depressant effects of Δ^9-THC on body temperature and locomotor activity than to its depressant effect on intestinal motility (Anderson *et al.*, 1975). There is also evidence that rats exhibiting marked tolerance to some behavioural effects of Δ^9-THC or cannabis can still distinguish clearly between these drugs and their vehicles in operant discrimination tasks (Bueno and Carlini, 1972; Greenberg *et al.*, 1975). Further examples are to be found in studies involving the anticonvulsant effects of cannabinoids or their effects on motor activity, conditioned behaviour or EEG (Branch *et al.*, 1980; Colasanti *et al.*, 1982; Ferraro and Grilly, 1973; Harris *et al.*, 1972; Karler *et al.*, 1982; Miczek, 1979; Miczek and Dixit, 1980; Pirch *et al.*, 1972, 1973; Singh and Das, 1977; Ten Ham *et al.*, 1975).

(v) Although reversible, cannabinoid tolerance can persist long after drug withdrawal. Reports that it can last 2, 3 or 4 weeks after withdrawal are not uncommon (Harris *et al.*, 1972; Karler *et al.*, 1982; Larsen and Pryor, 1977; Singh and Das, 1977) and there is one report that signs of tolerance to an effect of Δ^9-THC on conditioned behaviour were still detectable 3 months after withdrawal (Chait *et al.*, 1981).

(vi) Whereas some cannabinoid dose–response relationships are monophasic, others are biphasic or bell-shaped (for review see Pertwee, 1990). Consequently, although tolerance (i.e. a rightward shift of the dose–response curve) can lead to an attenuation of the drug's acute effect (monophasic, biphasic or bell-shaped response) it may also lead to its reversal (biphasic response) or enhancement (bell-shaped response). One example of the reversal of a response is the replacement of hypothermia by hyperthermia (Lomax, 1971; Miczek, 1979; Miczek and Dixit, 1980; Singh and Das, 1976, 1977, 1978; Singh *et al.*, 1978; Taylor and Fennessy, 1978a; Verberne *et al.*, 1985; see also Section 8.2.6.1). Another example is the replacement of a depressant effect on motor activity by a stimulant effect (Luthra *et al.*, 1975). The diminution or disappearance of an effect with a biphasic or bell-shaped dose–response curve as a result of repeated cannabinoid administration (e.g. Poddar and Ghosh, 1976a) could be due to either a rightward or a leftward movement in the dose–response curve, one possible cause of the latter being an accumulation of the drug at its site of action.

8.9.2 Dependence

Cannabinoid dependence has been the subject of far fewer studies than cannabinoid tolerance. Even so, there is no doubt that it can occur, experiments with monkeys, rats, mice and humans having demonstrated that abrupt withdrawal from treatments with cannabis or Δ^9-THC can be followed within a day or two by the onset of behavioural and EEG effects which differ markedly both from those produced by cannabinoid administration and from those observable in drug-free human subjects or animals (Sections 8.8.1 and 8.8.2). The effects are transient and can be suppressed by cannabinoid re-administration. Experiments with monkeys and rats have also shown that withdrawal of Δ^9-THC can induce cannabinoid-seeking behaviour (Section 8.8.4). The data suggest that cannabinoids possess much weaker reinforcing properties than opioids or amphetamine. There is also evidence from experiments with rats that cannabinoids share the ability of other drugs of abuse to enhance transmission in certain putative reward pathways (Section 8.8.3). There is no evidence that dependence develops to psychically inactive cannabinoids such as cannabidiol (Karler and Turkanis, 1980; Sections 8.8.2 and 8.8.5.1).

8.9.3 Mechanisms of tolerance and dependence

Although there is little doubt that tolerance to psychoactive cannabinoids is mainly non-dispositional in nature (Section 8.6), the detailed mechanisms remain to be elucidated. Those underlying the development of cannabinoid dependence and of cross-tolerance and cross-dependence between cannabinoids and other centrally active drugs are also little understood. Two observations, that tolerance to cannabinoids can be long-lasting and that the cannabinoid withdrawal syndrome is relatively mild, could both well reflect a tendency for these highly lipophilic substances to disappear only slowly from their sites of action after withdrawal.

An important reason for the present paucity of knowledge about the basis of tolerance and dependence to cannabinoids is the shortage of information about the mechanisms underlying acute effects. Results from tolerance and dependence studies could themselves contribute to the elucidation of these mechanisms. There are already data from such studies which support an involvement of acetylcholine, dopamine, 5-hydroxytryptamine, opioids and prostaglandins in responses elicited by Δ^9-THC (Sections 8.2.6, 8.3, 8.7 and 8.8.6).

Future studies should be directed at investigating the role of the putative cannabinoid receptor in the development of cannabinoid tolerance or dependence (Section 8.6.2.1). It is worth bearing in mind that there may be an endogenous ligand for this receptor and that this too might have a part to play in the development of tolerance to or dependence upon cannabinoids. The role, in the production of tolerance, of the neurochemical changes that occur in the brain during repeated cannabinoid administration also requires further investigation. Other experiments should be directed at developing cannabinoid antagonists as the expected ability of such drugs to precipitate withdrawal signs in cannabinoid-pretreated animals could well form the basis of an improved experimental model for the study of cannabinoid dependence.

8.9.4 Clinical implications

Since cannabis is widely taken for recreational purposes and since certain cannabinoids may come to have a place in modern medicine or are already used therapeutically, the existence of cannabinoid tolerance and dependence has important clinical implications. In particular, the ease with which quite marked degrees of tolerance can develop to cannabinoids must be borne in mind when clinical trials are performed. Cross-tolerance with other classes of drug arising either from the recreational or therapeutic use of cannabinoids could also be of clinical significance. Although cannabinoid withdrawal alone does not give rise to a particularly intense syndrome, experiments with rats have shown that quite severe changes can be precipitated if certain other drugs (tricyclic antidepressants or fluoxetine) are given shortly after withdrawal (Section 8.8.1.1). Interactions of this sort have not yet been reported to occur in man.

References

Abel, E.L. (1972) *Experientia* **28**, 1188–1189.

Abel, E.L., McMillan, D.E. & Harris, L.S. (1973) *Br. J. Pharmacol.* **47**, 452–456.

Abel, E.L., McMillan, D.E. & Harris, L.S. (1974) *Psychopharmacologia* **35**, 29–38.

Adams, M.D., Chait, L.D. & Earnardt, J.T. (1976) *Br. J. Pharmacol.* **56**, 43–48.

Agrawal, A.K., Kumar, P., Singh, N., Seth, P.K. & Bhargava, K.P. (1985) *Res. Commun. Subst. Abuse* **6**, 11–22.

Agrawal, A.K., Kumar, P., Gulati, A. & Seth, P.K. (1989) *Res. Commun. Subst. Abuse* **10**, 155–168.

Agurell, S., Halldin, M., Lindgren, J.-E., Ohlsson, A., Widman, M., Gillespie, H. & Hollister, L. (1986) *Pharmacol. Rev.* **38**, 21–43.

Anderson, P.F., Jackson, D.M., Chesher, G.B. & Malor, R. (1975) *Psychopharmacology* **43**, 31–36.
Anton, A.H., Serrano, A., Beyer, R.D. & Lavappa, K.S. (1974) *Life Sci.* **14**, 1741–1746.
Aulakh, C.S., Bhattacharyya, A.K., Hossain, M.A. & Pradhan, S.N. (1980) *Neuropharmacology* **19**, 97–102.
Bailey, P.T. & Pradhan, S.N. (1972) *Neuropharmacology* **11**, 831–838.
Barnes, C. & Fried, P.A. (1974) *Psychopharmacologia* **34**, 181–190.
Beardsley, P.M., Balster, R.L. & Harris, L.S. (1986) *J. Pharmacol. Exp. Ther.* **239**, 311–319.
Becker, B.M. & Reid, L.D. (1977) *Bull. Psychon. Soc.* **10**, 325–327.
Bensemana, D. & Gascon, A.L. (1974) *Rev. Can. Biol.* **33**, 269–278.
Bhargava, H.N. (1976a) *Eur. J. Pharmacol.* **36**, 259–262.
Bhargava, H.N. (1976b) *Psychopharmacology* **49**, 267–270.
Bhargava, H.N. (1978) *Pharmacol. Biochem. Behav.* **8**, 7–11.
Bhattacharyya, S.K., Aulakh, C.S., Pradhan, S., Ghosh, P. & Pradhan, S.N. (1980) *Neuropharmacology* **19**, 87–95.
Bidaut-Russell, M., Devane, W.A. & Howlett, A.C. (1990) *J. Neurochem.* **55**, 21–26.
Birmingham, M.K. (1973) *Br. J. Pharmacol.* **48**, 169–171.
Bloom, A.S. & Dewey, W.L. (1978) *Psychopharmacology* **57**, 243–248.
Branch, M.N., Dearing, M.E. & Lee, D.M. (1980) *Psychopharmacology* **71**, 247–256.
Bueno, O.F.A. & Carlini, E.A. (1972) *Psychopharmacologia* **25**, 49–56.
Burstein, S., Hunter, S.A. & Renzulli, L. (1985) *J. Pharmacol. Exp. Ther.* **235**, 87–91.
Burstein, S., Hunter, S.A., Latham, V. & Renzulli, L. (1988) In *Marijuana: An International Research Report* (eds Chesher, G., Consroe, P. & Musty, R.), pp 371–376. Canberra, Australian Government Publishing Service.
Burstein, S.H., Hull, K., Hunter, S.A. & Shilstone, J. (1989) *Mol. Pharmacol.* **35**, 6–9.
Carder, B. & Deikel, S.M. (1976) *Behav. Biol.* **17**, 313–332.
Carder, B. & Olson, J. (1973) *Pharmacol. Biochem. Behav.* **1**, 73–76.
Carlini, E.A., Hamaoui, A., Bieniek, D. & Korte, F. (1970) *Pharmacology* **4**, 359–368.
Chait, L.D., Brocco, M.J. & McMillan, D.E. (1981) *Psychopharmacology* **75**, 1–4.
Chang, A.E., Shiling, D.J., Stillman, R.C., Goldberg, N.H., Seipp, C.A., Barofsky, I., Simon, R.M. & Rosenberg, S.A. (1979) *Annals Int. Med.* **91**, 819–824.
Chen, J.P., Paredes, W., Li, J., Smith, D., Lowinson, J. & Gardner, E.L. (1990a) *Psychopharmacology* **102**, 156–162.
Chen, J.P., Paredes, W., Lowinson, J.H. & Gardner, E.L. (1990b) *Eur. J. Pharmacol.* **190**, 259–262.
Cherek, D.R., Thompson, T. & Kelly, T. (1980) *Pharmacol. Biochem. Behav.* **12**, 305–309.
Chesher, G.B. (1980) *Proc. Australian Physiol. Pharmacol. Soc.* **11**, 24–28.
Chesher, G.B. & Jackson, D.M. (1985) *Pharmacol. Biochem. Behav.* **23**, 13–15.
Christensen, H.D., Freudenthal, R.I., Gidley, J.T., Rosenfeld, R., Boegli, G., Testino, L., Brine, D.R., Pitt, C.G. & Wall, M.E. (1971) *Science* **172**, 165–167.
Colasanti, B.K., Lindamood, C. & Craig, C.R. (1982) *Pharmocol. Biochem. Behav.* **16**, 573–578.
Corcoran, M.E., McCaughran, J.A. & Wada, J.A. (1978) *Epilepsia* **19**, 47–55.
Craigmill, A.L. (1979) *Res. Commun. Psychol. Psychiat. Behav.* **4**, 51–63.
Cutler, M.G., Mackintosh, J.H. & Chance, M.R.A. (1975) *Psychopharmacologia* **44**, 173–177.
Dalterio, S.L., Michael, S.D., MacMillan, B.T. & Bartke, A. (1981) *Life Sci.* **28**, 761–766.
Davis, W.M. & Borgen, L.A. (1975) *Arch. Int. Pharmacodyn.* **213**, 97–112.

Davis, W.M., Moreton, J.E., King, W.T. & Pace, H.B. (1972) *Res. Commun. Chem. Path. Pharmacol.* **3**, 29–35.

Delini-Stula, A. (1973) *Pharmakopsychiatrie* **6**, 189–197.

Devane, W.A., Dysarz, F.A., Johnson, M.R., Melvin, L.S. & Howlett, A.C. (1988) *Mol. Pharmacol.* **34**, 605–613.

Dewey, W.L. (1986) *Pharmacol. Rev.* **38**, 151–178.

Dewey, W.L., Harris, L.S. & Kennedy, J.S. (1972a) *Arch. Int. Pharmacodyn.* **196**, 133–145.

Dewey, W.L., Jenkins, J., O'Rourke, T. & Harris, L.S. (1972b) *Arch. Int. Pharmacodyn.* **198**, 118–131.

Dewey, W.L., McMillan, D.E., Harris, L.S. & Turk, R.F. (1973) *Biochem. Pharmacol.* **22**, 399–405.

Dill, J.A. & Howlett, A.C. (1988) *J. Pharmacol. Exp. Ther.* **244**, 1157–1163.

Dykstra, L.A. (1983) *Psychopharmacology* **79**, 322–324.

Edery, H. & Gottesfeld, Z. (1975) *Br. J. Pharmacol.* **54**, 406–408.

Elsmore, T.F. (1972) *Psychopharmacologia* **26**, 62–72.

Elsmore, T.F. (1976) *Pharmacol. Biochem. Behav.* **5**, 123–128.

Englert, L.F., Ho, B.T. & Taylor, D. (1973) *Br. J. Pharmacol.* **49**, 243–252.

Evans, E.B., Seifen, E., Kennedy, R.H., Kafiluddi, R., Paule, M.G., Scallet, A.C., Ali, S.F.& Slikker, W. (1987) *Pharmacol. Biochem. Behav.* **28**, 171–174.

Ferraro, D.P. & Grilly, D.M. (1973) *Science* **179**, 490–492.

Ferraro, D.P. & Grisham, M.G. (1972) *Physiol. Behav.* **9**, 49–54.

Field, E. & Tyrey, L. (1986) *J. Pharmacol. Exp. Ther.* **238**, 1034–1038.

Filipovic, N. & Trkovnik, M. (1980) *Arch. Hig. Rada. Toksikol.* **31**, 293–297.

Fish, B.S. & Consroe, P. (1981) *Experientia* **37**, 295–296.

Fitton, A.G. & Pertwee, R.G. (1982) *Br. J. Pharmacol.* **75**, 409–414.

Frankenheim, J.M. (1974) *Psychopharmacologia* **38**, 125–144.

Fredericks, A.B. & Benowitz, N.L. (1980) *Psychopharmacology* **71**, 201–202.

Fredericks, A.B., Benowitz, N.L. & Savanapridi, C.Y. (1981) *J. Pharmacol. Exp. Ther.* **216**, 247–253.

Frederickson, R.C.A., Hewes, C.R. & Aiken, J.W. (1976) *J. Pharmacol. Exp. Ther.* **199**, 375–384.

Fried, P.A. (1976) *Psychopharmacology* **50**, 285–291.

Fried, P.A. & McIntyre, D.C. (1973) *Psychopharmacologia* **31**, 215–227.

Friedman, E. & Gershon, S. (1974) *Psychopharmacologia* **39**, 193–198.

Friedman, E., Hanin, I. & Gershon, S. (1976) *J. Pharmacol. Exp. Ther.* **196**, 339–345.

Gardner, E.L., Paredes, W., Smith, D., Donner, A., Milling, C., Cohen, D. & Morrison, D. (1988) *Psychopharmacology* **96**, 142–144.

Gilbert, P.E. (1981) *J. Clin. Pharmacol. (Suppl.)* **21**, 311s–319s.

Gildea, M.L. & Bourn, W.M. (1977) *Life Sci.* **21**, 829–832.

Greenberg, I., Kuhn, D. & Appel, J.B. (1975) *Pharmacol. Biochem. Behav.* **3**, 931–934.

Harris, R.T., Waters, W. & McLendon, D. (1972) *Psychopharmacologia* **26**, 297–306.

Harris, R.T., Waters, W. & McLendon, D. (1974) *Psychopharmacologia* **37**, 23–29.

Hedley, D., Pertwee, R.G. & Sutherland, J.F. (1984) *Br. J. Pharmacol.* **83**, 423P.

Herkenham, M., Lynn, A.B., Little, M.D., Johnson, M.R., Melvin, L.S., de Costa, B.R. & Rice, K.C. (1990) *Proc. Natl Acad. Sci. USA* **87**, 1932–1936.

Hershkowitz, M. & Szechtman, H. (1979) *Eur. J. Pharmacol.* **59**, 267–276.

Hillard, C.J. & Bloom, A.S. (1982) *Brain Res.* **235**, 370–377.

Hillard, C.J., Pounds, J.J., Boyer, D.R. & Bloom, A.S. (1990) *J. Pharmacol. Exp. Ther.* **252**, 1075–1082.

Hine, B. (1985) *Psychopharmacology* **87**, 34–38.

Hine, B., Friedman, E., Torrelio, M. & Gershon, S. (1975a) *Science* **187**, 443–445.
Hine, B., Friedman, E., Torrelio, M. & Gershon, S. (1975b) *Neuropharmacology* **14**, 607–610.
Hine, B., Torrelio, M. & Gershon, S. (1975c) *Psychopharmacol. Commun.* **1**, 275–283.
Hine, B., Torrelio, M. & Gershon, S. (1977) *Pharmacology* **15**, 65–72.
Hirschhorn, I.D. & Rosecrans, J.A. (1974) *Psychopharmacologia* **36**, 243–253.
Ho, B.T., Estevez, V.S. & Englert, L.F. (1973) *Res. Commun. Chem. Path. Pharmacol.* **5**, 215–218.
Hollister, L.E. (1986) *Pharmacol. Rev.* **38**, 1–20.
Howlett, A.C., Champion, T.M., Wilken, G.H. & Mechoulam, R. (1990) *Neuropharmacology* **29**, 161–165.
Hunt, C.A. & Jones, R.T. (1980) *J. Pharmacol. Exp. Ther.* **315**, 35–44.
Jacob, J.J., Ramabadran, K. & Campos-Madeiros, M. (1981) *J. Clin. Pharmacol. (Suppl.)* **21**, 327s–333s.
Järbe, T.U.C. (1978) *Arch. Int. Pharmacodyn.* **231**, 49–56.
Johansson, J.O., Henriksson, B.G. & Järbe, T.U.C. (1974) *Physiol. Psychol.* **2**, 431–432.
Johansson, J.O., Järbe, T.U.C. & Henriksson, B.G. (1975) *T.-I.-T. J. Life Sci.* **5**, 17–28.
Jones, G., Widman, M., Agurell, S. & Lindgren, J.-E. (1974) *Acta. Pharm. Suecica* **11**, 283–294.
Jones, R.T. (1971) *Pharmacol. Rev.* **23**, 359–369.
Jones, R.T. (1983) In *Cannabis and Health Hazards* (eds Fehr, K. & Kalant, H.), pp 617–689. Toronto, Addiction Research Foundation.
Jones, R.T., Benowitz, N. & Bachman, J. (1976) *Annals N.Y. Acad. Sci.* **282**, 221–239.
Kaplan, J.N. (1979) *Pharmacol. Biochem. Behav.* **11**, 539–543.
Karler, R. & Turkanis, S.A. (1980) *Br. J. Pharmacol.* **68**, 479–484.
Karler, R., Cely, W. & Turkanis, S.A. (1974a) *Life Sci.* **15**, 931–947.
Karler, R., Cely, W. & Turkanis, S.A. (1974b) *Res. Commun. Chem. Pathol. Pharmacol.* **9**, 23–39.
Karler, R., Borys, H.K. & Turkanis, S.A. (1982) *Naunyn-Schmiedeberg's Arch. Pharmacol.* **320**, 105–109.
Karler, R., Calder, L.D. & Turkanis, S.A. (1986) *Neuropharmacology* **25**, 441–446.
Kawasaki, H., Watanabe, S. & Ueki, S. (1980) *Eur. J. Pharmacol.* **65**, 63–69.
Kaymakcalan, S. (1972) In *Cannabis and its Derivatives* (eds Paton, W.D.M. & Crown, J.), pp 142–149. London, Oxford University Press.
Kaymakcalan, S. (1979) In *Marihuana: Biological Effects* (eds Nahas, G.G. & Paton, W.D.M.), pp 591–604. Oxford, Pergamon Press.
Kaymakcalan, S. & Deneau, G.A. (1972) *Acta Med. Turcica (Suppl. 1)* 5–27.
Kaymakcalan, S. & Sivil, S. (1974) *Pharmacology* **12**, 290–295.
Kaymakcalan, S., Turker, R.K. & Turker, M.N. (1974) *Psychopharmacologia* **35**, 123–128.
Kaymakcalan, S., Ayhan, I.H. & Tulunay, F.C. (1977) *Psychopharmacology* **55**, 243–249.
Kosersky, D.S. (1978) *Arch. Int. Pharmacodyn.* **233**, 76–81.
Kosersky, D.S., McMillan, D.E. & Harris, L.S. (1974) *J. Pharmacol. Exp. Ther.* **189**, 61–65.
Kralik, P.M., Ho, B.T. & Matthews, H.R. (1976) *Experientia* **32**, 723–725.
Kucharski, L.T., Williams, J.E.G. & Kornetsky, C. (1983) *Pharmacol. Biochem. Behav.* **19**, 149–151.
Lal, H., Bennett, D.A., Shearman, G.T., McCarten, M.D., Murphy, R. & Angeja, A. (1981) *J. Clin. Pharmacol. (Suppl.)* **21**, 361s–366s.
Larsen, F.F. & Pryor, G.T. (1977) *Pharmacol. Biochem. Behav.* **7**, 323–329.
Lawrence, D.K. & Pertwee, R.G. (1973) *Br. J. Pharmacol.* **49**, 373–374.

Lemberger, L., Tamarkin, N.R., Axelrod, J. & Kopin, I.J. (1971) *Science* **173**, 72–74.
Li, D.M.F. (1981) *Clin. Exp. Pharmacol. Physiol.* **8**, 101–108.
Lindgren, J.-E., Ohlsson, A., Agurell, S., Hollister, L. & Gillespie, H. (1981) *Psychopharmacology* **74**, 208–212.
Liu, R.K. (1974) *Res. Commun. Chem. Pathol. Pharmacol.* **9**, 215–228.
Lomax, P. (1971) *Res. Commun. Chem. Pathol. Pharmacol.* **2**, 159–167.
Luthra, Y.K., Rosenkrantz, H., Heyman, I.A. & Braude, M.C. (1975) *Toxicol. Appl. Pharmacol.* **32**, 418–431.
Luthra, Y.K., Rosenkrantz, H. & Braude, M.C. (1976) *Toxicol. Appl. Pharmacol.* **35**, 455–465.
Magour, S., Coper, H. & Fahndrich, C. (1977) *Psychopharmacology* **51**, 141–145.
Manning, F.J. (1976a) *Pharmacol. Biochem. Behav.* **5**, 269–273.
Manning, F.J. (1976b) *Pharmacol. Biochem. Behav.* **4**, 17–21.
Mantilla-Plata, B. & Harbison, R.D. (1975) *Toxicol. Appl. Pharmacol.* **34**, 292–300.
Martin, B.R. (1985) In *Marihuana '84* (ed. Harvey, D.J.), pp 685–692. Oxford, IRL Press.
Martin, B.R. (1986) *Pharmacol. Rev.* **38**, 45–74.
Martin, B.R., Dewey, W.L., Harris, L.S. & Beckner, J.S. (1976) *J. Pharmacol. Exp. Ther.* **196**, 128–144.
Martin, P. & Consroe, P. (1976) *Science* **194**, 965–967.
Martin, P. & Consroe, P. (1978) *Pharmacol. Biochem. Behav.* **9**, 753–758.
Martin, P. & Consroe, P. (1981) *Physiol. Psychol.* **9**, 219–222.
Masur, J., Martz, R.M.W. & Carlini, E.A. (1971) *Psychopharmacologia* **19**, 388–397.
Matsuda, L.A., Lolait, S.J., Brownstein, M.J., Young, A.C. & Bonner, T.I. (1990) *Nature* **346**, 561–564.
McMillan, D.E., Ford, R.D., Frankenheim, J.M., Harris, R.A. & Harris, L.S. (1972) *Arch. Int. Pharmacodyn.* **198**, 132–144.
McMillan, D.E., Dewey, W.L., Turk, R.F., Harris, L.S. & McNeil, J.H. (1973) *Biochem. Pharmacol.* **22**, 383–397.
McMillan, D.E., Harris, L.S., Frankenheim, J.M. & Kennedy, J.S. (1970) *Science* **169**, 501–503.
McMillan, D.E., Leander, J.D. & Dudley, K.H. (1980) *J. Pharmacol. Exp. Ther.* **212**, 85–90.
McMillan, D.E., Hardwick, W.C. & Wells, J.D. (1983) *Arch. Int. Pharmacodyn.* **264**, 4–14.
Miczek, K.A. (1979) *Psychopharmacology* **60**, 137–146.
Miczek, K.A. & Dixit, B.N. (1980) *Psychopharmacology* **67**, 195–202.
Moreton, J.E. & Davis, W.M. (1973) *Neuropharmacology* **12**, 897–907.
Nahas, G.G., Schwartz, I.W., Adamec, J. & Manger, W.M. (1973a) *Proc. Soc. Exp. Biol. Med.* **142**, 58–60.
Nahas, G.G., Zagury, D., Schwartz, I.W. & Nagel, M.-D. (1973b) *Nature* **243**, 407–408.
Narimatsu, S., Watanabe, K., Yamamoto, I. & Yoshimura, H. (1983) *Res. Commun. Subst. Abuse* **4**, 301–314.
Narimatsu, S., Yamamoto, I., Watanabe, K. & Yoshimura, H. (1987) *Eur. J. Pharmacol.* **141**, 437–443.
Nazar, B.L., Harclerode, J., Roth, R.I. & Butler, R.C. (1974) *Life Sci.* **14**, 2513–2520.
Nazar, B., Kairys, D.J., Fowler, R. & Harclerode, J. (1977) *J. Pharm. Pharmacol.* **29**, 778–779.
Newman, L.M., Lutz, M.P., Gould, M.H. & Domino, E.F. (1972) *Science* **175**, 1022–1023.

Newman, L.M., Lutz, M.P. & Domino, E.F. (1974) *Arch. Int. Pharmacodyn.* **207**, 254–259.
Ohlsson, A., Lindgren, J.-E., Wahlen, A., Agurell, S., Hollister, L.E. & Gillespie, H.K. (1982) *Biomed. Mass Spec.* **9**, 6–10.
Page, J.G. & West, L.E. (1977) *Pharmacology* **15**, 233–241.
Perez-Reyes, M., Timmons, M.C. & Wall, M.E. (1974) *Arch. Gen. Psychiatry* **31**, 89–91.
Pertwee, R.G. (1974) *Br. J. Pharmacol.* **51**, 391–397.
Pertwee, R.G. (1985) In *Marihuana '84* (ed. Harvey, D.J.), pp 263–277. Oxford, IRL Press.
Pertwee, R.G. (1990) In *Psychotropic Drugs of Abuse* (ed. Balfour, D.J.K.), pp 355–429. New York, Pergamon Press.
Pertwee, R.G. & Wickens, A.P. (1991) *Neuropharmacology* **30**, 237–244.
Pirch, J.H., Cohn, R.A., Barnes, P.R. & Barratt, E.S. (1972) *Neuropharmacology* **11**, 231–240.
Pirch, J.H., Osterholm, K.C., Cohn, R.A. & Barratt, E.S. (1973) *Arch. Int. Pharmacodyn.* **203**, 213–220.
Poddar, M.K. & Ghosh, J.J. (1976a) *Ind. J. Biochem. Biophys.* **13**, 273–277.
Poddar, M.K. & Ghosh, J.J. (1976b) *Ind. J. Biochem. Biophys.* **13**, 267–272.
Pradhan, S.N., Bailey, P.T. & Ghosh, B. (1972) *Res. Commun. Chem. Pathol. Pharmacol.* **3**, 197–204.
Pryor, G.T., Husain, S., Larsen, F., McKenzie, C.E., Carr, J.D. & Braude, M.C. (1977a) *Pharmacol. Biochem. Behav.* **6**, 123–136.
Pryor, G.T., Larsen, F.F., Carr, J.D. & Braude, M.C. (1977b) *Pharmacol. Biochem. Behav.* **7**, 331–345.
Pryor, G.T., Larsen, F.F., Husain, S. & Braude, M.C. (1978) *Pharmacol. Biochem. Behav.* **8**, 295–318.
Rating, D., Broermann, I., Honecker, H., Kluwe, S. & Coper, H. (1972) *Psychopharmacologia* **27**, 349–357.
Razdan, R.K. (1986) *Pharmacol. Rev.* **38**, 75–149.
Sassenrath, E.N. & Chapman, L.F. (1975) *Fed. Proc.* **34**, 1666–1670.
Sethi, B.B., Trivedi, J.K., Kumar, P., Gulati, A., Agarwal, A.K. & Sethi, N. (1986) *Biol. Psychiatry* **21**, 3–10.
Siemens, A.J. & Doyle, O.L. (1979) *Pharmacol. Biochem. Behav.* **10**, 49–55.
Siemens, A.J. & Kalant, H. (1974) *Can. J. Physiol. Pharmacol.* **52**, 1154–1166.
Silva, M.T.A., Carlini, E.A., Claussen, U. & Korte, F. (1968) *Psychopharmacologia* **13**, 332–340.
Singh, P.P. & Das, P.K. (1976) *Psychopharmacology* **50**, 199–204.
Singh, P.P. & Das, P.K. (1977) *Ind. J. Exp. Biol.* **15**, 280–284.
Singh, P.P. & Das, P.K. (1978) *Psychopharmacology* **56**, 309–316.
Singh, P.P., Bhattacharya, S.K. & Das, P.K. (1978) *Ind. J. Exp. Biol.* **16**, 326–329.
Sjöden, P.-O., Järbe, T.U.C. & Henriksson, B.G. (1973) *Pharmacol. Biochem. Behav.* **1**, 243–249.
Smith, J.B. (1991) *Psychopharmacology* **103**, 115–120.
Sofia, R.D., Dixit, B.N. & Barry, H. (1977) *Arch. Int. Pharmacodyn.* **229**, 52–58.
Spaulding, T.C., Ford, R.D., Dewey, W.L., McMillan, D.E. & Harris, L.S. (1972) *Eur. J. Pharmacol.* **19**, 310–317.
Sprague, G.L. & Craigmill, A.L. (1976) *Pharmacol. Biochem. Behav.* **5**, 409–415.
Sprague, G.L. & Craigmill, A.L. (1978) *Pharmacol. Biochem. Behav.* **9**, 11–15.
Stadnicki, S.W., Schaeppi, U., Rosenkrantz, H. & Braude, M.C. (1974a) *Life Sci.* **14**, 463–472.

Stadnicki, S.W., Schaeppi, U., Rosenkrantz, H. & Braude, M.C. (1974b) *Psychopharmacologia* **37**, 225–233.
Takahashi, R.N. & Singer, G. (1979) *Pharmacol. Biochem. Behav.* **11**, 737–740.
Takahashi, R.N. & Singer, G. (1980) *Pharmacol. Biochem. Behav.* **13**, 877–881.
Tayal, G., Gupta, L., Agarwal, S.S. & Arora, R.B. (1974) *Ind. J. Exp. Biol.* **12**, 375–376.
Taylor, D.A. & Fennessy, M.R. (1977) *Eur. J. Pharmacol.* **46**, 93–99.
Taylor, D.A. & Fennessy, M.R. (1978a) *Psychopharmacology* **56**, 279–285.
Taylor, D.A. & Fennessy, M.R. (1978b) *J. Pharm. Pharmacol.* **30**, 654–656.
Taylor, D.A. & Fennessy, M.R. (1982) *J. Pharm. Pharmacol.* **34**, 240–245.
Ten Ham, M. (1977) *Pharmacol. Biochem. Behav.* **6**, 183–185.
Ten Ham, M. & De Jong, Y. (1974) *Eur. J. Pharmacol.* **28**, 144–148.
Ten Ham, M., Loskota, W.J. & Lomax, P. (1975) *Eur. J. Pharmacol.* **31**, 148–152.
Thomas, B.F., Compton, D.R. & Martin, B.R. (1990) *J. Pharmacol. Exp. Ther.* **255**, 624–630.
Thompson, G.R., Fleischman, R.W., Rosenkrantz, H. & Braude, M.C. (1974) *Toxicol. Appl. Pharmacol.* **27**, 648–665.
Tulunay, F.C., Uran, B., Ayhan, I.H., Ulku, E. & Kaymakcalan, S. (1980) *Res. Commun. Subst. Abuse* **1**, 151–157.
Tulunay, F.C., Ayhan, I.H., Portoghese, P.S. & Takemori, E.A. (1981) *Eur. J. Pharmacol.* **70**, 219–224.
Tulunay, F.C., Ayhan, I.H. & Sparber, S.B. (1982) *Psychopharmacology* **78**, 358–360.
Uran, B., Tulunay, F.C., Ayhan, I.H., Ulku, E. & Kaymakcalan, S. (1980) *Pharmacology* **21**, 391–395.
Van Ree, J.M., Slangen, J.L. & De Wied, D. (1978) *J. Pharmacol. Exp. Ther.* **204**, 547–557.
Verberne, A.J.M., Taylor, D.A. & Fennessy, M.R. (1980) *Psychopharmacology* **68**, 261–267.
Verberne, A.J.M., Taylor, D.A. & Fennessy, M.R. (1981) *Psychopharmacology* **73**, 97–98.
Verberne, A.J.M., Fennessy, M.R., Lewis, S.J. & Taylor, D.A. (1985) *Pharmacol. Biochem. Behav.* **23**, 153–159.
Watanabe, K., Narimatsu, S., Yamamoto, I. & Yoshimura, H. (1982) *Eur. J. Pharmacol.* **77**, 53–56.
Watanabe, K., Yamamoto, I. & Yoshimura, H. (1983) *Eur. J. Pharmacol.* **94**, 349–351.
Watanabe, K., Yamamoto, I., Narimatsu, S. & Yoshimura, H. (1984) *Res. Commun. Subst. Abuse* **5**, 89–101.
Watanabe, K., Arai, M., Narimatsu, S., Yamamoto, I. & Yoshimura, H. (1986) *Biochem. Pharmacol.* **35**, 1861–1865.
Watanabe, K., Narimatsu, S., Yamamoto, I. & Yoshimura, H. (1987) *J. Pharm. Pharmacol.* **39**, 945–947.
Watanabe, K., Tanaka, T., Yamamoto, I. & Yoshimura, H. (1988) *Biochem. Biophys. Res. Commun.* **157**, 75–80.
Wayner, M.J., Greenberg, I., Fraley, S. & Fisher, S. (1973) *Physiol. Behav.* **10**, 109–132.
Webster, C.D., LeBlanc, A.E., Marshman, J.A. & Beaton, J.M. (1973) *Psychopharmacologia* **30**, 217–226.
Yamamoto, I., Watanabe, K., Narimatsu, S., Hamajima, K. & Yoshimura, H. (1985) *Eur. J. Pharmacol.* **111**, 159–166.
Young, A.M., Katz, J.L. & Woods, J.H. (1981) *J. Clin. Pharmacol. (Suppl.)* **21**, 348s–360s.
Zaluzny, S.G., Chesher, G.B., Jackson, D.M. & Malor, R. (1979) *Psychopharmacology* **61**, 207–216.

CHAPTER 9

THE ROLE OF GENETICS IN VULNERABILITY TO DRUG DEPENDENCE

Frank R. George[1], Mary C. Ritz[2] and Gregory I. Elmer[2]

[1] *Department of Psychology & Center on Alcoholism, Substance Abuse and Addiction, University of New Mexico, North East Albuquerque, New Mexico 871 31-1161, USA*

[2] *National Institute on Drug Abuse, Addiction Research Center, Box 5180, Baltimore, Maryland 21224, USA*

Table of Contents

THE BIOLOGICAL BASES OF DRUG TOLERANCE AND DEPENDENCE
ISBN 0-12-564250-4

9.1 Introduction

Drug dependence and its resultant adverse medical and social consequences have increased dramatically in recent years, leading to serious economic and political challenges worldwide as well as psychological, physiological and social problems for individuals and their families. In response to strong appeals, increased research efforts have been applied to understanding the biological mechanisms and determinants of drug abuse. Current major research efforts include the elucidation of specific biochemical mechanisms of action of abused substances and the contribution of specific biological or genetic risk factors which may contribute towards dependence. In this chapter, we introduce the methods and concepts of behavioural genetic studies as they apply to drug abuse, we review the current state of knowledge concerning genetic contributions to drug dependence, and we present a review of animal pharmacogenetic models of drug abuse, particularly ethanol, opiates and psychostimulants.

9.1.1 Introduction to behavioural genetics

The study of variation in behaviour among individuals, its genetic and environmental bases, and its implications for society comprise the field of behavioural genetics. A related field involving genetic factors related to drug effects is known as pharmacogenetics. Both of these areas represent the integration of genetics with the behavioural and neural sciences, incorporating work from physiological, molecular, population and whole animal levels of analysis.

9.1.2 Interactions between genes and their environments

Members of a population commonly show large differences in the expression of traits. This variation in traits is referred to as phenotypic variability, or V_P, and can routinely be seen for many morphological traits, such as height and hair colour, as well as for behavioural traits, such as activity level. The sources of variation of traits can be mathematically expressed as follows:

$$V_p = V_g + V_e + (V_g \times V_e)$$

While this equation is an abbreviated version of the true expression, the major components are present and it serves to illustrate the point being made, which is that phenotypic variability (V_p), which for the purposes of this discussion would typically be variability in some drug-related behaviour across non-identical individuals, is the result of genetic variability (V_g) among those individuals studied, plus the differential effects of the different environments in which they each currently exist and have previously existed (V_e), plus the sum of the interactions between these specific genotypes and their specific environments ($V_g \times V_e$). In real life, the last (and most complex) component, the genotype by environment interaction (commonly expressed as $G \times E$), is usually the most critical. Genes cannot exist without an environment, and the environment modifies the final expression of specific genetic combinations.

It is primarily this last point that the reader should keep in mind throughout the discussions in this chapter. It is possible that some behavioural effects may be determined to such an extent by genetic makeup that no environmental factor can noticeably alter that effect, or that some environmental effects are so strong that they affect virtually all genotypes. However, for the most part it appears that behavioural responses, in particular responses to drugs, lie somewhere in between these two extremes, so that both genetic and environmental influences, and thus interactions between the two, are critical.

The importance of $G \times E$ interactions is illustrated through the classic medical genetics example of phenylketonuria (PKU), a biochemical disorder resulting in severe behavioural deficits. PKU is a genetically determined deficiency in the enzyme phenylalanine hydroxylase, which converts phenylalanine, an amino acid found in many foods, to tyrosine. As a result PKU individuals build up high levels of phenylalanine, which is responsible for the behavioural deficits in PKU patients.

A critical point here is that phenylalanine is a dietary constituent, and thus an environmental factor. An important clinical question then becomes whether an individual's behaviour can be changed by altering levels of phenylalanine. The answer is that it can. Early detection and intervention through dietary reduction of phenylalanine can dramatically improve the abilities of PKU patients. Therefore, even though PKU individuals differ genetically from non-PKU persons in their ability to metabolize phenylalanine, the behavioural expression of PKU is dependent upon a $G \times E$ interaction, namely the existence of the PKU genotype within a high-phenylalanine environment.

This example also illustrates that behavioural genetics is the study of both genetic and environmental influences upon behaviour. This results from the fact that genotype can not only be manipulated as an independent variable, such as through the use of multiple inbred rodent strains or multiple sets of identical twins, but can also be controlled, as in the use of a single inbred rat strain. When genotype is completely controlled or held constant, then the resulting variability among subjects is due to environmental factors. When specific environmental variables are being systematically varied, as in many studies on substance abuse, genetic control through the use of genetically defined subjects can provide a very powerful approach for testing the significance of specific environmental factors on behaviour.

9.1.2.1 Applications to drug dependence

It is possible to apply this line of reasoning to the study of addiction processes. The use of genetic models is a powerful tool for examining the biological substrates of drug-mediated behaviours, but can also aid in determining the mechanisms of environmental influences on drug-related behaviours. For example, genes may contribute to the mediation of cocaine self-administration by determining the amount of neurotransmitter release or reuptake in response to neural stimulation. Similarly, genes control numbers of neurones, receptors and specific neural connections. Thus, individuals may be differentially affected by environmental stressors. If this stress is affecting catecholamine production, then these subjects could have responses to cocaine which differ from those of other individuals. These responses could be related to peripherally mediated effects, differential toxic effects or alterations in the reinforcing effects of cocaine.

Before further discussing how behavioural genetic concepts and methods can be applied to the experimental analysis of drug dependence, it is important to briefly describe some of the ideas and terms which are the foundation of this field.

9.1.3 Genotype as an independent variable

A unifying concept in behavioural genetics is that genes may be utilized as independent variables, and can be either controlled or manipulated like other experimental variables. Control results from the ability to produce offspring from specified matings, and manipulation derives from the ability to chose which, and how many, specific genotypes are to be included in a particular study. Importantly, when genotype is held constant, then any variability among subjects is due to environmental factors. Behavioural genetic paradigms can be complex, but most studies employ simple but elegant mating paradigms based upon Mendelian principles (McClearn and DeFries, 1973). Much information concerning the extent of genetic contributions to a trait, its mode of transmission (e.g. dominant or recessive), and an estimate of the number of genes which mediate the trait, can be ascertained within only a few generations of specified matings.

While the production of specified offspring is an important aspect of behavioural genetic analysis, in most studies related to dependence it is not necessary for the experimenter to actually perform genetic manipulations. Instead, the experimenter is only required to select currently existing genetically defined animals from stocks maintained at commercial or university breeding facilities. The choice of animals is typically based upon some morphological or behavioural aspect of a specific genetic stock which makes that stock most suitable for the experiment being designed. For example, it may be advantageous in alcohol self-administration studies to choose animals which show low levels of emotionality when placed in novel situations so that they are more readily trained to lever press in an operant chamber.

9.1.4 Techniques and terms

9.1.4.1 Inbreeding

Inbreeding is a reduction in genetic variance within a population so that individuals become more genetically alike with subsequent generations. Inbreeding results from the mating of individuals which are closely related, such as siblings. A strain maintained by brother–sister matings for at least 20 generations is considered to be inbred, and use of the word 'strain' denotes a history of inbreeding.

In the laboratory, it is extremely difficult to maintain a truly non-inbred, or heterogeneous, population free of the effects of inbreeding. As a result, 'randomly bred' or 'representative' animals are usually neither. Instead, these animals are highly but indeterminately inbred, resulting in poorly defined, genetically distinct populations which vary within and across breeders. An example in research is 'Sprague-Dawley' rats.

Inbreeding can, however, be of significant value. Because members of an inbred strain are genetically identical, use of a single strain controls for genetic variation, resulting in controlled populations over time and across laboratories. This eliminates much of the need for repeated replications of basic findings. Thus, inbred strains provide a powerful and economical approach to research.

9.1.4.2 Selective breeding

Selective breeding is the intermating of particular individuals in order to change a particular trait. Selection is often conducted bidirectionally to produce maximally distinct populations, for example high versus low ethanol drinking. Measures then shown to covary with the selected trait are proposed to be causally related. Thus, in addition to producing animals which are characterized by significantly different values for a given trait, selected lines serve as powerful research tools to test hypotheses regarding the mechanisms of action of drugs.

Most selective breeding studies of interest to pharmacologists have used some response to ethanol as the selected trait. The most characterized selected lines are the Long Sleep and Short Sleep mice (McClearn and Kakihana, 1981), bred respectively for long versus short duration of loss of the righting reflex (i.e. 'sleeping time') following ethanol administration. These lines currently differ in their CNS sensitivity to ethanol by approximately 20-fold. Selected lines relevant to the study of drug dependence include the Alcohol Accepting and Alcohol Non-Accepting rats (Eriksson, 1968) and the alcohol preferring and Non-Preferring rats (Li *et al.*, 1979).

9.1.4.3 Genetic correlation

Correlating potency of effect with potency of binding at a specific site is often used in pharmacology to determine the site of action of a drug. However, the molecular binding site may be only one component in a sequence of events culminating in a behavioural response. A powerful behavioural genetic tool which enables pharmacogeneticists to study multiple factors responsible for drug actions is genetic correlation.

Genotypes which differ for a given behavioural trait can be used to test hypotheses concerning causal relationships with other independent variables. A lack of correlation indicates that the measures studied are not mechanistically related. A strong positive correlation, especially a perfect rank order correlation across genotypes, enables one to reasonably conclude that the measures are causally related.

9.2 Human genetic studies on dependence

Most reliable human studies on substance abuse can be divided into two groups based on methodology. These are twin studies and adoption studies. The best studies incorporate the use of both methods, using twins which have been split apart by circumstance and adopted by different families, thus being raised in different environments. These methodological factors are extremely important in being able to distinguish genetic from environmental effects, but contribute to the lack of studies in this area. Not only are twins and adoptees relatively rare, but individuals must also have substance abuse disorders, and substance abuse information must also be available for co-twins, and adoptive and biological parents.

A number of studies have examined possible genetic contributions to human drug abuse. Most of these studies have examined frequency of alcohol drinking, while fewer have studied genetic factors in clinically diagnosed alcoholism or alcohol abuse. There are very few human genetic studies on opiates or psychostimulants.

The first adoption study on alcoholism failed to find differences between adopted biological offspring of alcoholics and non-alcoholics (Roe, 1944). Since then, however several studies have shown that adopted biological sons of alcoholics have higher rates of alcoholism than do adopted biological sons of non-alcoholics (Goodwin *et al.*, 1973; Cloninger *et al.*, 1981; Cadoret and Gath, 1978). Interestingly, studies with adopted females have been less consistent (Cadoret and Gath, 1978; Bohman *et al.*, 1981). Twin studies are also more consistent for males, and again suggest a significant genetic component in terms of developing alcohol abuse disorders (Hrubec and Omenn, 1981; Gurling *et al.*, 1981; Pickens and Svikus, 1991).

The only other drug for which there exists a body of human genetic data, albeit small, is nicotine. Most of these studies have reported significant genetic contributions to incidence of smoking among twins (Shields, 1962; Pedersen, 1981).

The database for possible genetic influences in the determinants of human opiate-reinforced behaviour is virtually non-existent, in part because methods used to determine genetic contributions in alcoholism are not as readily applied to opiate dependence, due to restrictions in sample populations and established databases. What little information exists on genetic predisposition to opiate dependence in humans is embedded in studies of alcoholism and the covariance of multiple drugs of abuse. For example, Cadoret *et al.* (1986) investigated the correlation between the degree of drug dependence in adopted adults with that of alcohol abuse in the parents. The results suggest that alcohol problems in biological relatives appear to be associated with the abuse of a number of drugs, including opiates.

For cocaine, individual differences in human response to particular treatment regimens have been reported, but these differences have not been studied systematically. In addition, since the problem of cocaine dependence has only recently increased to catastrophic proportions, studies of the genetic and environmental antecedents of human cocaine abuse are currently in their infancy. To date, few studies of genetic influences on human predispositions for the effects of psychostimulants have been performed. In one study, the effects of amphetamine on the responses of six pairs of male monozygotic twins for several cognitive, psychomotor, personality and mood variables were assessed (Crabbe *et al.*, 1983). In general, both baseline and drug-induced responses to amphetamine were similar in twin pairs. However, shared environmental effects could not be ruled out by this study. Another study has shown that cocaine metabolism was significantly inhibited in patients with histories of succinylcholine sensitivity and low dibucaine numbers (phenotype A) relative to normal controls (phenotype U). Intermediate metabolism was observed in heterozygote offspring of phenotype A patients. Thus, the authors recommended caution in using cocaine for topical anaesthesia in patients with succinylcholine sensitivity or low dibucaine numbers (Jatlow *et al.*, 1979).

9.3 Animal models of drug dependence

Most animal drug-taking studies can be divided into two groups based on methodology. One group consists of studies using preference procedures; the other consists of studies using operant conditioning methods.

9.3.1 Preference or choice procedures

The two-bottle water–drug preference procedure was developed by Richter and Campbell (1940), and has been used in hundreds of studies, most involving ethanol. However, the relevance of most of this work to human drug dependence is unclear. Despite limitations, however, the use of inbred strains in many preference studies has provided valuable information about the contribution of genetic factors to drug taking (McClearn and Rodgers, 1959, 1961). For example, C57BL/6 mice prefer ethanol whereas DBA/2 mice are strong ethanol-avoiders. Such large variability in preference served as the basis for two major selection programmes, the ALKO AA (alcohol-accepting) and ANA (alcohol non-accepting) lines (Eriksson, 1968, 1972; Eriksson and Rusi, 1981; Hilakivi *et al.*, 1984) and the P (preferring) and NP (non-preferring) rat lines (Li *et al.*, 1981). The success of these selection programmes indicates that ethanol consumption is strongly influenced by genetic factors. The preferring lines characteristically drink most of their daily liquid intake in the form of 10% ethanol solutions, and consume almost as much ethanol in a free choice situation as they can metabolize. In contrast, the non-preferring animals drink very small amounts of ethanol daily. Ethanol intake (g/kg per day) for AA and P males averages 5.8 ± 1.8 and 6.3 ± 1.7 respectively, while intake for the ANA and NP males averages 1.8 ± 1.2 and 1.0 ± 0.7 respectively (Hilakivi *et al.*, 1984; Li *et al.*, 1981). These values lie at the extremes of those found in heterogeneous rats or across several inbred strains (Li and Lumeng, 1984). This suggests that these selective breeding programmes have produced lines of rats in which ethanol-drinking behaviour, as described by the preference model, is maximized in one line and minimized in the other (see also Chapter 4).

Preference studies have also shown large genetic differences in intake of non-alcohol drugs. There are several reports of genetic differences in intake of opioids (Nichols and Hsaio, 1967; Suzuki *et al.*, 1988; Broadhurst, 1979; Carroll *et al.*, 1986), and more recently cocaine (George and Goldberg, 1988, 1989). These findings provide foundation evidence that genetic factors play an important role in determining the persistence of non-alcohol drug-taking behaviours, and are discussed in greater detail below. A different type of preference procedure which has been applied to study drug dependence is the conditioned place preference model (see Chapters 5 and 7). The contribution of genetic factors to drug responses in this model is discussed in Section 9.5.2.

9.3.2 Operant studies of drug-reinforced behaviour

The operant approach to studying drug-taking behaviour grew out of operant behaviour studies initiated by Skinner. In the 1960s it was demonstrated that chronically catheterized laboratory animals would intravenously self-inject drugs by pressing a lever which activated a syringe pump (Weeks, 1962). We now know that animals from a number of non-human species will self-administer most of the drugs that humans abuse. In most self-administration studies the intravenous route has been used; however, behaviour reinforced with drugs has been demonstrated via several other routes of administration, including intramuscular (Goldberg *et al.*, 1976), intragastric (Altshuler *et al.*, 1975; Waller *et al.*, 1984), inhalation (Yanagita *et al.*, 1970) and oral (Meisch, 1984). The oral route, in particular, is important in genetic studies because of the relative ease of the oral methodology, which does not involve surgery. Thus, large numbers of animals can be tested over sustained periods of time (Elmer *et al.*, 1986; Ritz *et al.*, 1986; George, 1987, 1988). These operant drug-taking studies provide a good animal model for studying the processes that initiate and maintain drug dependence.

It is important to integrate findings from preference studies with findings from operant studies on drug-reinforced behaviour in order to determine the degree to which home cage preference paradigms and operant chamber studies on drug taking are measuring the same or similar phenomena, both behaviourally and biochemically. In addition, these studies should be useful in determining the relationship between drug-reinforced behaviour and other drug-related behaviours, such as neuronal sensitivity. The issue of commonality of self-administration behaviour or reinforcement across drugs, i.e. the extent to which reinforcement in an individual, or genotype, from one drug is predictive of reinforcement from other drugs, can also be effectively addressed by using genetically defined animals in drug-taking studies using several different methods of self-administration, including operant and preference paradigms.

9.4 Genetic studies on alcohol reinforcement in animals

9.4.1 Operant alcohol self-administration studies

Over the past several years, our laboratories have investigated the relationship between genetic factors and the conditions under which ethanol comes to serve as a positive reinforcer. Genetic correlations between variables have been ascertained in an attempt to determine the degree of commonality between ethanol preference in a two-bottle choice paradigm, neuronal sensitivity to ethanol and ethanol self-administration under operant conditions.

The rodent stocks used in these experiments included the ALKO Alcohol-Accepting (AA) and Alcohol Non-Accepting (ANA) rats, LEWIS/CRLBL (LEW) and Fischer 344/CRLBL (F344) inbred rat strains, C57BL/6J (C57) and BALB/cJ (BALB) inbred mouse strains, and LS/Ibg (LS) and SS/Ibg (SS) selectively bred mice. The AA and ANA rat lines were derived from a heterogeneous foundation stock in a two-way selection for high and low ethanol drinking. The AA rats consume almost as much ethanol in a free-choice situation as they can metabolize, while the non-preferring animals drink very small amounts of ethanol (Eriksson, 1968). AA rats are also less sensitive to ethanol than their ANA counterparts, as determined by a number of tasks (Eriksson, 1972). The LEW and F344 rat strains were selected because they have a long history of genetic divergence and are readily available from commercial vendors. The F344 are a low ethanol preferring line (Li and Lumeng, 1984), and are more sensitive to ethanol than the LEW rats (Suzuki *et al.*, 1989; unpublished results from our laboratories). Similarly, the C57 and BALB mouse strains have a genetically divergent history as well as documented differences in ethanol preference and sensitivity. C57 mice are high preferring and are less sensitive to ethanol than the low preferring BALB mice (McClearn and Rodgers, 1961; Crabbe and Belknap, 1980). Finally, LS mice show approximately a 20-fold greater sensitivity to ethanol relative to SS mice (McClearn and Kakihana, 1981; Crabbe and Belknap, 1980). Both of these latter two lines show very low preference for ethanol (Chan, 1976; Fuller, 1980; Collins, 1981).

In studies with AA and ANA rats, ethanol served as a reinforcer only for AA rats, and was neither reinforcing nor aversive for ANA rats (Ritz *et al.*,

1986, 1989a, b). Ethanol deliveries were consistently greater than water (vehicle) deliveries for the AA rats and varied as an orderly function of ethanol concentration. Conversely, in non-preferring ANA animals, ethanol did not serve as a reinforcer. Since ethanol-drinking behaviour, as described by the preference model, is maximized in the AAs and minimized in the ANAs, then, if ethanol preference and ethanol-reinforced behaviour are equivalent measures of ethanol drinking, more heterogeneous Sprague-Dawley (SD) rats should exhibit ethanol-reinforced responding which could be described as intermediate between that of the AA and ANA animals. Findings obtained with the AA rats have been compared with those obtained with SD rats (Ritz *et al.*, 1989a, b). SD rats maintained higher levels of responding and greater ethanol intake, relative to AA rats, at all concentrations of ethanol tested. Thus, ethanol-reinforced behaviour appears to be partially, but not completely, analogous to ethanol preference. These data are consistent with the suggestion that ethanol self-administration is a polygenic trait, determined by a combination of multiple genes, each of which may differentially interact with various environmental conditions.

The next series of experiments systematically investigated oral ethanol self-administration in two inbred strains of rats, F344 and LEW (Suzuki *et al.*, 1988). In this case, ethanol maintained higher response rates and was consumed in larger volumes than the water vehicle, and blood ethanol levels increased with increases in ethanol concentration for both strains, but to different degrees. LEW rats drank substantially more ethanol than F344 rats. An orderly function between ethanol concentration and number of deliveries was observed for the LEW rats, whereas for the F344 rats much smaller differences were seen between ethanol- and water-maintained responding. For the LEW strain, as the fixed-ratio size was increased, the number of responses increased almost in direct proportion to the fixed-ratio size increase. Similar results were obtained in F344 rats, but the amount of responding was lower and less consistent. LEW rats showed significantly higher response rates, numbers of ethanol deliveries, and blood ethanol levels than F344 rats. Ethanol-induced behavioural activation was also observed in LEW rats, but not in F344 rats. These results support the conclusion that ethanol serves as a strong positive reinforcer for LEW rats and as a weak positive reinforcer for F344 rats. The results here indicate that genotype is important in determining not only whether, but also to what extent, ethanol functions as a reinforcer.

In operant self-administration studies using C57 and BALB mice (Elmer *et al.*, 1986, 1987a, b, 1988), lever pressing for and consumption of ethanol (8% w/v) in C57 mice markedly exceeded that for water and resulted in blood ethanol levels of 199 ± 27 mg/dl. These levels significantly exceeded the ethanol intake of the BALB mice while intake of water was low and not significantly different between strains. The 8% ethanol drinking of the BALB/cJ mice did not differ from their water drinking. Thus, ethanol was established as a positive reinforcer for C57 mice but not for BALB mice. Next, ethanol-reinforced behaviour was studied over ethanol concentrations ranging from 1% to 32%. The purpose was to determine if differences between strains varied as a function of ethanol concentration. Ethanol served as a reinforcer for the C57 mice at concentrations of 4%, 8% and 16%. Results with the BALB mice were very different from those with the C57BL/6J mice. The level of responding of the BALB mice did not increase above baseline levels at any of the concentrations tested, and levels of responding decreased below baseline at 32%. Thus, ethanol did not serve as a reinforcer for the BALB mice at any of the concentrations tested. We then tested whether and to what extent ethanol would maintain responding under increasing fixed ratio size, i.e. increased work requirements to obtain the drug. As fixed-ratio size increased, there were proportional increases in response rates only in C57 mice.

In studies conducted using the LS and SS mice, there were significant line differences in the number of lever presses for ethanol, intake of ethanol and post-session blood ethanol levels (Elmer *et al.*, 1990). LS mice were significantly higher in all measures than SS mice. LS mice made approximately 135 responses per 30-minute session, resulting in average post-session blood ethanol levels of 166 ± 30 mg/dl. Responding in the SS mice was sporadic, with a mean of approximately 25 responses per session. When the ethanol solution was replaced by water, responding declined over days for the LS mice, and remained low for the SS mice. These results, plus other findings (Elmer *et al.*, 1990), demonstrate that ethanol serves as an effective reinforcer for LS mice but not SS mice over a broad range of conditions.

In summary, these studies suggest that the preference model of animal ethanol drinking provides some information, within theoretical limits, about the reinforcing effects of ethanol. However, it appears that the preference model may describe ethanol drinking behaviour only under somewhat specific environmental conditions, and may not be analogous to or highly predictive of the reinforcing effects of ethanol under other situations or in humans.

9.4.2 Relationship between reinforcement, preference and neuronal sensitivity

There exists a substantial body of ethanol preference and neuronal sensitivity data for the genotypes which we have studied in operant self-administration studies (Belknap, 1980; Crabbe and Belknap, 1980; Erwin *et al.*, 1976, 1980; Eriksson, 1972; Eriksson and Rusi, 1981; Fuller, 1980; George, 1987, 1988; Hilakivi *et al.*, 1984; Li *et al.*, 1979; Li and Lumeng, 1984; McClearn and Rodgers, 1959, 1961; Melchior and Meyers, 1976; Rodgers and McClearn,

1962; Spuhler and Deitrich, 1984). These data can be combined to estimate the degree of commonality between ethanol preference, neuronal sensitivity to ethanol and ethanol-reinforced behaviour. These data are summarized in Table 1.

The relationship between reinforcement from ethanol and either ethanol preference or sensitivity to ethanol as determined by sleep time has been estimated by rank ordering the available data on these measures. The relationship between reinforcement from ethanol and ethanol preference is shown in Figure 1. The results of this analysis suggest that there exists a moderate but not significant positive relationship between these two measures of ethanol drinking (Kendall's Tau = 0.39). The most notable exception to a general positive relationship are the LS mice, which show a high degree of reinforcement from ethanol but very low ethanol preference. For some genotypes, measures of ethanol self-administration and preference were inversely related to sleep time.

The relationship between reinforcement from ethanol and loss of righting reflex (neuronal sensitivity) to ethanol is quite different. There is virtually no relationship between propensity to self-administer ethanol and this measure of neuronal sensitivity to ethanol (Kendall's Tau = 0.12). Whether ethanol serves as a positive reinforcer in the LS and SS mice is also an important test of the relationship between sensitivity to ethanol and reinforcement from

Table 1 Rank order relationships between ethanol self-administration, ethanol preference, and ethanol sleep time.

Genotype	Self-administration	Preference	Sleep Time
Rats			
LEW	+ + +	NA	−
P	+ + +	+ + +	−
AA	+ +	+ + +	−
F344	+ −	−	+ +
ANA	− − −	− − −	+
NP	− − −	− − −	+
Mice			
C57BL/6J	+ + +	+ + +	−
LS	+ +	− −	+ + +
BALB/cJ	− − −	− −	+
SS	− − −	− −	− − −

From George (1987).

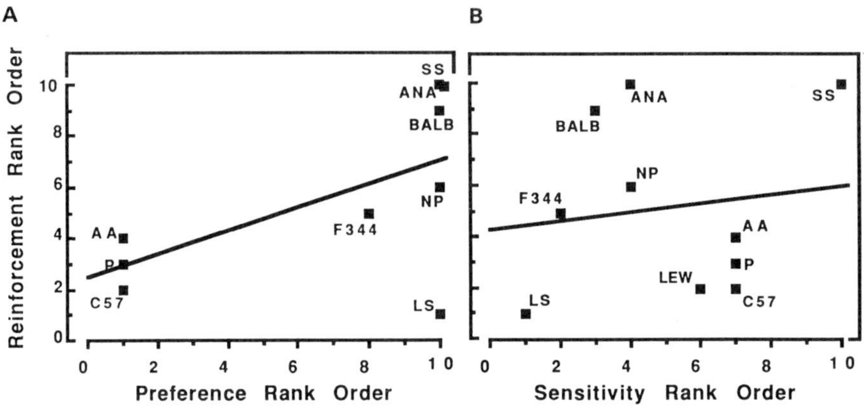

Figure 1 Comparison of rank order for ethanol reinforcement versus ethanol preference (1A) and ethanol reinforcement versus neurosensitivity to ethanol defined by duration of loss of the righting reflex (1B) for several rat and mouse genotypes. Linear regression lines are included for illustrative purposes. Actual concordance between measures is based upon determination of Kendall's Tau coefficient for rank order correlations. From George (1990).

ethanol, since these animals represent extreme values on the continuum of sensitivity to ethanol across genotype. The fact that ethanol was established as a reinforcer in LS mice but not in SS mice is the opposite of what would be expected if reduced sensitivity to ethanol was a primary factor in the establishment of this drug as a reinforcer. Thus, sensitivity to ethanol may be a limiting factor with regard to absolute intake, but sensitivity does not apparently influence the ability of ethanol to function as a reinforcer.

The inclusion of data from the LS and SS lines, in conjunction with data from the other genotypes, shows that acute responses to ethanol, as measured by duration of loss of the righting reflex, is not related to the ability of this drug to function as a positive reinforcer.

9.5 Genetic studies on opiates

Despite the absence of data directly demonstrating genotypic influences on opiate-reinforced behaviour in humans, it is possible to hypothesize that genetic influences exist in humans by examining the literature on animal models. For example, opiate-related physiological and behavioural effects demonstrate a high degree of genetic influence (Nichols and Hsiao, 1967; Oliverio *et al.*, 1975; Belknap *et al.*, 1989). In addition, genotypic variance in response to opioids has been demonstrated across a number of species including mice (Judson and Goldstein, 1978; Belknap *et al.*, 1982, 1989), rats (Satinder, 1977; Dymshitz and Lieblich, 1987) and monkeys (Ternes *et al.*, 1983).

9.5.1 Behavioural genetic studies of opiate preference

Nichols and Hsiao (1967) selectively bred rats for high and low morphine consumption in a two-bottle choice procedure. These experiments utilized a method that involved chronic i.p. morphine administration, cyclic choice exposure, an abstinence period and a final choice test between the drug and vehicle solution in a two-bottle preference test. A choice test between 0.5 mg/ml morphine in tap water versus tap water was given before and after chronic morphine administration in order to establish baseline rates of drug intake. The rats were then exposed to a 3-day cycle of complete liquid deprivation, morphine as the sole liquid, then tap water as the sole liquid. This 'cyclic-reinforcing' stage consisted of ten 3-day cycles with intermittent choice test days. A final choice test is given after an abstinence period of 2 weeks. This protocol was based upon the assumption that opiates would have greater reinforcement efficacy if taken during opiate withdrawal and took advantage of the repeated withdrawal periods to condition opiate-reinforced drinking. From a population of Sprague-Dawley rats that were exposed to these procedures, rats displaying high opiate drinking were randomly inbred as were the low opiate drinking rats. This breeding produced a bidirectional shift in opiate preference following the training procedures without changing the initial baseline preference scores in either line.

Eriksson and Kianmaa (1971) performed a genetic analysis of morphine preference in CBA/Ca, a non-preferring strain, and C57BL/6J mice, a preferring strain, along with their F1, F2, and backcross generations using a similar cyclic-reinforcing technique to that of Nichols and Hsiao (1967). Their analysis of a 5-day preference measure between morphine in tap water and tap water following these techniques demonstrated high heritability and dominance in the direction of morphine preference. These early studies clearly demonstrate the ability of genetic factors to influence opiate preference.

The majority of subsequent studies investigating genotype-dependent opiate self-administration have incorporated saccharin in the morphine solution to enhance morphine intake (Eidelberg *et al.*, 1975; Horowitz, 1976, 1981; Horowitz *et al.*, 1977; Whitney and Horowitz, 1978; Hadaway *et al.*, 1979). Consistently, C57BL/6J mice prefer morphine/saccharin (M/S) solutions to tap water and DBA/2J mice avoid M/S solutions. In a study that compared

M/S versus water intake across nine inbred strains, DBA/2J, AKR/J and SJL/J avoided the M/S solution, BALB/cJ mice showed no preference, I^s/Bl and C3HeB/FeJ showed a modest preference for the M/S solution, and three sublines of the C57BL mice (10J, 6J and 6A) showed almost complete preference for the M/S solution. Interestingly, when the drug was presented unadulterated, C57BL/6J and 10J mice did not show a preference for morphine; only the C57BL/6A mice demonstrated a morphine preference. However, while saccharin-adulterated solutions may be a valid method for the induction of large opiate intake, unless the opposing choice solution is the vehicle used for morphine administration the results will not be effectively related to opiate-reinforced behaviour. In studies of genetic differences in drug-reinforced behaviour, the possibility of confounding drug × vehicle × genotype interactions must either be kept to a minimum or explored thoroughly.

Recently, Carney *et al.* (1991) have demonstrated clear opioid preference differences between C57BL/6J and DBA/2J mice. Initially, saccharin was added to etonitazene in order to ensure adequate experience with the pharmacological effects of the drug. When the saccharin concentration was gradually reduced to 0%, only the C57BL/6J mice preferred etonitazene to the vehicle. This study demonstrates a distinct difference between two inbred strains in their preference for etonitazene following adequate exposure to the pharmacological effects of the drug and in the absence of confounding drug × vehicle interactions.

In a study by Forgie *et al.* (1988), the contribution of taste factors involved in morphine and etonitazene preference was investigated. Initial comparisons of morphine or etonitazene in water versus a presumed equally bitter solution of quinine in water demonstrated opiate preference in the C57 mice and not in the DBA mice. Interestingly, in a separate group of DBA and C57 mice, the C57 but not the DBA mice preferred saccharin to a saccharin/quinine solution.

In addition to possible vehicle and drug history effects across genotype, food deprivation has been shown to be an important environmental variable in etonitazene preference. Although food deprivation has been shown to significantly increase drug intake across a wide range of conditions and drug classes (Carroll and Meisch, 1984), it appears that food deprivation will enhance intake only in those animals genetically predisposed to accept a particular drug as a reinforcer (George, 1987, 1988). George and Meisch (1984) and Carroll *et al.* (1986) demonstrated significant effects of food deprivation in C57BL/6J and DBA/2J mice and in Sprague-Dawley and Wistar rats, respectively. Food-satiated C57BL/6J mice showed a slight preference for etonitazene in water versus water and DBA/2J mice showed an aversion. Reduction to 80% of free-feeding weight greatly increased preference in the C57 mice and slightly decreased preference in the DBA/2J mice. Similarly, food deprivation doubled etonitazene intake in Wistar rats and decreased etonitazene intake in SD rats by approximately 50%. It appears that food deprivation significantly enhances the reinforcement efficacy of a drug that is serving as a positive reinforcer and may enhance the aversive properties of the drug.

Satinder (1977) investigated morphine intake in selectively bred rats: the MNR/Har/Lu and MR/Har/Lu bred for low and high open-field emotional reactivity, respectively; RLA/Lu and RHA/Lu, bred for low and high rates of avoidance learning, respectively; and RCA/Lu rats which were used as the control line. It was possible to induce all five lines to consume morphine in distilled water in a forced choice procedure that included a sucrose fading period along with forced drinking at increasing concentrations of morphine. A choice test comparing each respective increase in morphine concentration between the morphine solution and vehicle followed each increase in concentration. All lines except the MNR and RLA lines demonstrated significant changes in preference ratios as a function of increasing concentration (0.2–0.9 mg/ml). However, only the RLA/Lu, RHA/Lu and MR/Har/Lu rats had preference ratios greater than 0.5. Withdrawal of morphine resulted in a significant decrease in the body weights of all the genetic lines, demonstrating that pharmacologically active quantities of morphine were taken in all lines.

When using preference as a measure of opiate-reinforced behaviour a number of pitfalls must be avoided. For example, genetic differences in the development of conditioned taste aversion may confound differences seen in drug self-administration (Stolerman and D'Mello, 1984). It is important to compare intake of the drug versus that of the vehicle across time. If drug consumption decreases below that of the original levels, conditioned taste aversion may have developed either to the olfactory/gustatory or pharmacological effects of the drug. In addition, it is important that each genotype be exposed to the pharmacological effects of the drug prior to assessment of drug reinforcement. If the genotype under investigation never consumed enough of the drug to experience the interoceptive effects it is possible that the strain is avoiding the drug for reasons other than the post-ingestional effects. Further, the amount of drug intake during tests of self-administration behaviour should be pharmacologically relevant, especially since many opiate compounds display limited absorption following oral administration. The temporal pattern of drug self-administration should reflect adequate levels of drug intake given the specific genotype under investigation and interpretations should take into account pharmacokinetic differences in absorption and distribution that exist across strains (Eidelberg *et al.*, 1975; Belknap *et al.*, 1989).

9.5.2 Genetic studies of opiate-reinforced behaviour

One method used for determination of genetic differences in drug reinforcement has been conditioned place preference. This method is based upon the classical conditioning of a discriminative environment upon single or repeated drug administration. If the subject is reinforced by the test drug then a greater amount of time should be spent in the environment associated with the drug effect (cf. Swerdlow *et al.*, 1989). Dymshitz and Lieblich (1987) used a conditioned place preference paradigm to investigate differences in the ability of morphine and heroin to enter the preferred chamber in two strains of rats, LC2-Hi and LC2-Lo, selectively bred for high and low self-stimulation rates, respectively. Only the LC2-Hi rats demonstrated a significant change in place preference upon conditioning with either morphine (5 mg/kg) or heroin (1 mg/kg). Carney *et al.* (1991), in addition to demonstrating significant differences in etonitazene preference between C57BL/6J and DBA/2J mice, also demonstrated similar dose-dependent differences in etonitazene conditioned place preference. C57BL/6J mice spent significantly more time in the etonitazene-paired compartment following a single trial pairing while DBA/2J mice spent an equivalent amount of time in both the saline- and drug-paired chambers. Interestingly, unlike the preference studies (see Section 9.5.1), conditioned place preference does not indicate a role for aversive stimulus properties in DBA/2J avoidance of opiates since a greater amount of time was not spent in the saline-paired chamber versus the drug-paired chamber.

Very few studies have utilized classical operant paradigms to investigate genetic differences in opiate-reinforced behaviour. The use of schedule-controlled behaviour in determining the extent or degree of drug-reinforced behaviour is a powerful tool that effectively manipulates environmental conditions that may differentiate genetic predispositions to opiate-reinforced behaviour. Suzuki *et al.* (submitted) studied operant self-administration of the potent, orally active opiate agonist etonitazine in LEW and F344 rats. The same strategies used previously to establish oral intake of drugs were effective in establishing etonitazine as a reinforcer, but only for the LEW rats. Responding for etonitazine significantly exceeded responding for vehicle in LEW rats; however, etonitazine intake was actually lower than vehicle intake for F344 rats (George and Goldberg, 1989).

In two studies of Y-maze activity, the operant response was entrance into the drug-appropriate arm of the maze in order to receive drug or vehicle injections. In the first study, Y-maze choice behaviour was investigated in two outbred mouse stocks, ICR and Swiss-Webster, and in C57BL/6J and BALB/cJ inbred strains (Eidelberg *et al.*, 1975). Mice were first made dependent upon morphine (40 mg/kg per day for 6 days) prior to establishing individual side preferences in a Y-maze. Following the determination of side preferences, the mice were given saline when they entered their preferred side and morphine (40 mg/kg) when they entered the opposite side. This training protocol effectively reversed the original arm choice in every group except for the BALB/cJ strain. Interestingly, under similar Y-maze conditions, when BALB/cJ mice were implanted with a chronic indwelling cannula to the lateral hypothalamus without prior dependence induction, this strain showed classical acquisition curves upon morphine (0.1 μg/injection) injection availability and classical extinction curves when saline was substituted (Cazala *et al.*, 1987). When 4.0 mg/kg naloxone was given prior to the session, extinction behaviour was once again demonstrated. These studies demonstrate the importance of environment, i.e. drug history and route of administration, in susceptibility to the reinforcing properties of morphine.

9.5.3 Relationship between reinforcement and other opiate effects

Opiate-reinforced behaviour is one of the many opiate-related phenotypes that demonstrate genetic influence. Genetic differences in many other opioid-related phenotypes such as analgesia, activity, hypothermia, muscle rigidity and opiate receptor affinity have been shown (Broadhurst, 1979). In general, the rank orders of genotypes for sensitivity among these measures are not consistent (Table 2). Genetic independence of opiate-related behaviours is not surprising since the effects of opiates are influenced by a number of neurochemical mediators. Even within a particular measure such as analgesia, the neuronal systems mediating this phenotype are dependent upon the type of stimulus applied, the measured response, and the environmental context (Franklin and Abbott, 1989). For example, thermal pain is thought to be mediated primarily by μ-receptor agonists that are enhanced by 5-HTergic

Table 2 Genetic relationships between opiate-related phenotypes.

Strain	Open field activity	Hot plate analgesia	Preference	Reinforcement
C57BL/6J	+++	−	+++	++++
BALB/cJ	++	++	−	+
DBA/2J	−−	+++	−−	−

Open field activity: Oliverio and Castellano (1974).
Analgesia: Oliverio and Castellano (1974).
Preference: Horowitz (1981).
Reinforcement: Eidelberg *et al.* (1975); Cazala *et al.* (1987); Carney *et al.* (1991).

systems (Tyers, 1980; Abbott *et al.*, 1986; Basbaum and Fields, 1984) whereas chemical irritants are thought to act via μ- and κ-receptors that are dampened by 5-HTergic systems (Abbott *et al.*, 1982, 1986). Thus, genetic contributions to opiate-related phenotypes is dependent upon both the measure employed and the environmental context under which it is studied.

9.6 Genetic studies on cocaine

9.6.1 Mechanisms of psychostimulant-reinforced behaviour

Cocaine is a powerfully addicting drug which also has serious toxic and lethal effects. It produces these and a variety of other pharmacological effects through its interactions with several CNS binding sites. It is well established that cocaine inhibits neuronal reuptake of dopamine, noradrenaline and 5-HT, and that the transporters for these neurotransmitters appear to be labelled by [^{3}H]cocaine (Reith *et al.*, 1980; Kennedy and Hanbauer, 1983; Shoemaker *et al.*, 1985; Calligaro and Eldefrawi, 1987). In addition, receptor binding studies have shown that (−)cocaine interacts with both σ and muscarinic cholinergic receptors in brain (Sharkey *et al.*, 1988a, b).

The goal of recent biological investigations in our laboratories and others has been to determine which cocaine binding sites might be associated with the reinforcing effects of cocaine and other pharmacologically and chemically related compounds. Using one strategy, a fundamental requirement for the identification of the receptors related to cocaine self-administration is a significant relationship between the potency of cocaine and related compounds in producing reinforcing effects in operant self-administration studies and the potency of these compounds at particular binding sites in brain. Multiple regression analyses of the potencies of cocaine-related drugs in operant self-administration studies on their potencies at monoamine transporters indicated that cocaine inhibition of [^{3}H]mazindol binding to dopamine transporters is significantly positively correlated with the reinforcing effects of cocaine-related drugs (Ritz *et al.*, 1987). Thus, cocaine inhibition of dopamine uptake has been shown to be the primary biochemical influence on the reinforcing effects of cocaine.

The results from these biochemical studies are consistent with and confirmed by many behavioural studies which have utilized lesioning techniques and pharmacological manipulations to elucidate the biochemical mechanisms associated with the reinforcing effects of cocaine. Dopaminergic neuronal systems, especially in brain mesolimbic pathways, have been implicated in the reinforcing effects of both cocaine and amphetamine (Goeders and Smith,

1983; Martin-Iverson *et al.*, 1986, Chapter 6). Selective dopaminergic receptor blockade attentuates the reinforcing properties of both (−)cocaine and (+)amphetamine in animals (deWit and Wise, 1977; Ettenberg *et al.*, 1982; de La Garza and Johanson, 1982; Wilson and Schuster, 1972; Goeders *et al.*, 1986; Yokel and Wise, 1975, 1976; Risner and Jones, 1976; Davis and Smith, 1975). Dopaminergic agonists, in contrast, substitute for intravenous self-administration of cocaine and *d*-amphetamine (Woolverton *et al.*, 1984; Yokel and Wise, 1978), and affect operant responding for cocaine (Koob *et al.*,1987; Wilson and Schuster, 1972; Woolverton, 1986; Kleven *et al.*, 1988; Woolverton and Virus, 1989).

Data suggest that 5-HTergic neuronal systems may attenuate the reinforcing potencies of amphetamine, but not cocaine. Lesions of 5-HTergic neurones with the neurotoxin 5, 7-dihydroxytryptamine increase rates of responding for intravenous administrations of *d*-amphetamine under commonly used fixed-ratio operant schedules of reinforcement (Lecesse and Lyness, 1984). In contrast, pretreatments with the 5-HT precursor L-tryptophan or with 5-HT uptake blockers decrease amphetamine-reinforced self-injections under similar operant conditions (Lyness, 1983; Smith *et al.*, 1986; Yu *et al.*, 1986). Consistent with biochemical results (Ritz and Kuhar, 1989), a similar study has shown that the potent 5-HT reuptake inhibitor fluoxetine does not appear to attenuate rates of responding for cocaine, while it does decrease responding associated with amphetamine (Porrino *et al.*, 1989). However, some evidence suggests that 5-HTergic systems may modulate cocaine-reinforced responding under quite different operant conditions, specifically those involving continuous access to the drug over extended periods of time and those requiring the completion of increasingly greater numbers of operant responses prior to administration of cocaine (Carroll *et al.*, 1990).

9.6.2 Genetic studies of psychostimulant actions

Data concerning the influences of genetic variables on cocaine effects in animal models are relatively sparse. Goudie *et al.* (1989) have described individual differences between rats in ability to discriminate cocaine in an operant paradigm. Furthermore, conditioned taste aversion tests of the animals in the study suggest that animals sensitive to the dysphoric effects of cocaine were less sensitive to its discriminative cues. Using a different approach, the recent integration of behavioural genetic research designs and animal models of drug self-administration has begun to suggest that the reinforcing effects of cocaine, like those of alcohol and opiate-related compounds, are mediated by at least some inherited traits. Recent operant studies have shown that cocaine, self-administered orally, serves as a strong reinforcer in Lewis rats, serves as a marginal reinforcer in NBR rats and does not serve as a reinforcer in ACI or F344 rats (George and Goldberg, 1988, 1989). Another study utilizing a limited access two-bottle choice procedure has also shown that cocaine serves as a positive reinforcer for Lewis (LEW) rats, but not F344 rats (George and Goldberg, 1988). Intake of 0.57 mg/ml (−)cocaine base versus water was measured during one-hour home cage preference testing, and during one-hour operant self-administration sessions, as described in detail elsewhere (George and Goldberg, 1988, 1989). Except for the test period, all rats had *ad libitum* access to food and water. Using adjunctive procedures, all rats showed large amounts of cocaine intake during training and thus had been exposed to the CNS effects of this drug. Thus, low intake could not be solely attributed either to a lack of association between consuming cocaine and the resultant effects of the drug nor to aversive taste factors. After training, and in the absence of presession food, liquid intake of cocaine solutions was higher in LEW than in F344 rats in both the home cage and operant chamber test groups, and exceeded intake of water only in LEW rats. Thus, orally delivered cocaine may readily function as a reinforcer for LEW but not F344 rats.

Since previous receptor binding studies indicated that the dopamine transporter is the primary cocaine binding site in the brain associated with its reinforcing effects, accounting for over 90% of the variance in the reinforcing potency of cocaine and related drugs (Ritz *et al.*, 1987), it was hypothesized that differences between strains with respect to cocaine self-administration might be associated with differences in this brain binding site. However, receptor binding studies using the same rat strains shown to differ in cocaine self-administration indicated that there were no differences in either affinity or number for striatal [^{3}H]GBR 12935 binding to dopamine transporters, [^{3}H]SCH 23390 binding to striatal dopaminergic D_1 receptors or [^{3}H]spiperone binding to striatal dopaminergic D_2 receptors (George *et al.*, 1991). In addition, there were no differences observed between these strains in the affinity of (−)cocaine at [^{3}H]GBR 12935 sites. These results suggest that although the dopamine transporter plays a primary role in determining the reinforcing potency of cocaine in animals for which cocaine serves as a reinforcer, differences in cocaine binding to this site may not account for individual or strain differences in whether or not cocaine will serve as a reinforcer. Alternatively, other experiments designed to assess localized receptor density will be necessary to elucidate the influence of specific dopaminergic neuronal systems on genetic differences in the reinforcing properties of cocaine.

Another report describes differences between eight inbred strains of mice using conditioned place preference (Seale and Carney, 1991). This research indicates clear differences between strains in place preference associated with 32 mg/kg cocaine (i.p.), with C57BL/6J, A/J, SWR/J and BALB/cByJ strains exhibiting a strongly positive response, DBA/2J, C57BL/6ByJ and AKR/J strains exhibiting moderate responses, and C3H/HeJ mice exhibiting a strongly negative response. In addition, similar patterns of conditioned place preference for these strains associated with amphetamine were also observed with the potent dopamine inhibitor GBR 12909, and etonitazene, suggesting that strains which exhibit conditioned place preference following pretreatments with one of these drugs will tend to exhibit the same behaviour after pretreatment with another drug.

Several studies have also shown that genetic differences strongly influence cocaine- and amphetamine-induced locomotor activation. Dose–response curves for cocaine and amphetamine illustrated clear differences between ACI, NBR, Lewis and F344 inbred rat strains with respect to both potencies and efficacies of these drugs (George *et al.*, 1991). Similar differences in locomotor activation have been shown across several strains of inbred mice. BALB/cByJ exhibit very small increases in activity compared with C57BL/6J, C57BL/6ByJ, DBA/2J or A/J strains of mice (Seale and Carney, 1991; Schuster *et al.*, 1977; Ruth *et al.*, 1988). However, cocaine apparently does not produce locomotor activation in LS mice (George and Ritz, 1990). Interestingly, there are no differences in striatal dopamine transporters or dopaminergic receptors associated with these observed strain differences in locomotor activity (George *et al.*, 1991; George and Ritz, 1990). Cocaine also readily produces locomotor depressant effects at low doses in C57BL/6J, DBA/2J and LS mice, but only marginally in SS mice (George, 1989; George and Ritz, 1990). Studies also suggest that the stimulant, reinforcing and lethal effects of cocaine are not genetically correlated (George and Goldberg, 1989). This may explain the sudden death syndrome associated with cocaine use: some individuals may be more sensitive to the lethal effects of cocaine and so succumb to cardiovascular toxicity at doses that, for them, produce marginal euphoric effects.

Two studies indicate that genotype influences sensitization to cocaine effects. Schuster *et al.* (1977) reported that greater sensitization to the locomotor effects of cocaine were observed in A/J mice relative to C57BL/6J mice. Furthermore, studies of recombinant inbreds derived from C57BL/6J and BALB/cBy mice suggest that initial locomotion scores and sensitization scores are mediated by separate genetic determinants. A more recent study has shown that sensitization to cocaine-induced hyperactivity and stereotypy is significantly inhibited in Brattleboro homozygotes which lack vasopressin compared to their heterozygote, littermate controls (Post *et al.*, 1982).

Other studies show genetic differences in physiological and metabolic responses to cocaine. Cerebral glucose utilization studies indicate that Lewis rats are more affected by acutely administered cocaine than are F344 rats across several brain regions (London *et al.*, 1991). Interestingly, glucose utilization began to be significantly affected in each strain near the ED_{50}

value for each strain in terms of cocaine's locomotor stimulant effects. Both sex and strain differences have been reported for hepatotoxicity in response to acute doses of cocaine. Specifically, measurements of serum glutamic-pyruvic transaminase (SGPT) levels from a single injection of cocaine (20–100 mg/kg) indicated 100–150-fold increases in male C57Bl/6Ibg, DBA/2Ibg, C3h/2Ibg and BALB/cJ mice, with BALB and C57BL mice being most and least sensitive, respectively (Boyer *et al.*, 1988). In contrast, SGPT levels increased only 2–10-fold in females in response to cocaine. In females, C3H and C57BL mice were most sensitive while BALB and DBA mice were more resistant to the hepatotoxic effects of cocaine. The P-450 inducer phenobarbitone resulted in enhanced cocaine-induced hepatotoxicity in C57BL and BALB, but not C3H and DBA mice. Similar sex and strain differences in measurements of serum glutamic oxaloacetic transaminase (SGOT) levels and periportal necrosis resulting from single injections of cocaine in $B6AF_1$ and BALB/cBy mice have been shown to be influenced by specific inducing agents such as phenobarbitone and pine bedding (Thompson *et al.*, 1984).

9.7 Biological vulnerability to drug abuse

9.7.1 Are there 'addiction-prone' populations?

Many studies indicate that alcoholism has a significant predisposing genetic component. In addition to the many studies showing genetic differences in alcohol-seeking behaviour in experimental animals, and twin and adoption studies showing a significant genetic component for alcohol abuse, we also know that humans who are Family History Positive (FHP) for alcoholism are at substantially greater risk for developing the disorder. FHP individuals also show different electroencephalographic patterns in response to alcohol than do FH-negative persons. Importantly, the twin studies show that identical twins are more concordant for alcoholism than fraternal twins, and the more severe the cases of alcoholism, the greater the difference between the identical and the fraternal concordance rates, strongly suggesting a genetic component. Thus, while any individual may become dependent upon alcohol, there appear to be significant biological differences in the degree of risk for alcoholism. This information, when combined with animal studies on non-alcohol drug taking, suggests that there are human populations at high risk for developing other types of drug dependence.

9.7.2 Genetic commonalities in animal drug-reinforced behaviours

Taken together, recent pharmacogenetic studies provide preliminary data concerning the degree of commonality of self-administration behaviour across multiple drugs and genotypes. Findings supporting the commonality of ethanol, cocaine and opioid self-administration across several genotypes are summarized in Table 3. Overall, a high degree of qualitative commonality exists across these genotypes and drugs. Genotypes which showed strong reinforcement from ethanol also showed similar levels of reinforcement from cocaine and etonitazene. Conversely, genotypes which showed weak or no reinforcement from ethanol showed similarly low levels of responding for either cocaine or etonitazene.

These initial results from operant studies of self-administration across different drugs and genotypes are intriguing as they suggest that genotypic patterns of reinforcement from ethanol may correlate highly with patterns of reinforcement from cocaine and opiates. Thus, drug-seeking behaviours maintained by ethanol, cocaine and opiates may have at least some common biological determinants.

9.7.3 Are there 'addiction' genes?

It is unlikely that specific 'addiction' genes exist, in the way that there are specific genes which regulate the production of the PKU-related enzyme

Table 3 Commonality of self-administration behaviour across drugs and genotypes.

Genotype	Alcohol	Opiates	Cocaine
Rats			
LEW	+++	+++	++
F344	+−	−−−	−
Mice			
C57BL/6J	+++	+++	+++
DBA/2J	−−−	−−−	NA
BALB/cJ	−−−	−−−	NA

Note: Plus symbols indicate relative degree of positive reinforcement. Negative symbols indicate degree of non-reinforcement or avoidance. Three symbols is maximum response relative to all genotypes tested. NA, data not available. Based on George (1990).

tyrosine hydroxylase. Rather, it seems more probable that the biological contributions to drug addiction result from the interactions among several genes, each of which regulates a common and necessary biological system. However, in the case of persons who would be at high risk for drug abuse, the specific versions of these genes are present in a combination which is most conducive to making a drug an effective reinforcer. One important area where several genes could act in concert to produce an organism highly responsive to drugs is in the mesolimbic region, where dopaminergic and other neurotransmitter pathways interact in ways important to the reinforcing effects of drugs. Normal variations in receptor numbers, metabolic enzymes, and second messenger systems could, in the high-risk individuals, be combined in a manner which maximizes the reinforcing drug effect. Importantly, however, particular genotypes susceptible to these positive reinforcing effects must be existing in an environment conducive to addictive behaviour, e.g. high stress, ready drug availability, etc., in order for the addictive phenotype to become fully expressed.

9.7.4 Prevention and treatment applications

Realizing that individuals may differ in the risk of becoming dependent, as well as understanding the biological factors related to risk, can aid in the prevention and treatment of drug abuse. Resources for addiction intervention can be scarce, making a targeting of high-risk persons for the most intensive education and counselling programmes cost-effective. Early intervention in terms of education and counselling of high-risk groups has proven effective in other areas of medicine such as heart disease. Realising that becoming dependent upon drugs is related to biologically based processes would positively affect attitudes towards drug abusers and would encourage the development of novel pharmaceutical products for adjunctive use either in high-risk prophylactic counselling programmes or in drug abuse treatment centres.

9.8 Conclusions

Behavioural genetic studies are demonstrating that drug dependence is a complex biological process mediated by both genetic and environmental factors, as well as critical interactions between these two factors. For alcoholism the evidence is strong that for certain high-risk persons, alcohol dependence can develop early with only minimal environmental contribution, mostly in terms of access and peer pressure. For other drugs, recent animal studies are showing that certain strains are predisposed towards initiation and subsequent maintenance of drug self-administration, while others apparently do not initiate drug self-administration, even under favourable environmental conditions, such as ready access to drugs.

Experimentally, the integration of behavioural genetic methods with those of operant conditioning has great potential for increasing our understanding of the processes of drug dependence. The objectives of this integrative approach are to identify, at the molecular, cellular and behavioural levels, those factors that maintain drug-seeking behaviour. Issues in dependence processes, such as the biochemical sites of drug reinforcement, the relationship between drug preference and operant responding for drugs, and the commonality of self-administration behaviour across drugs, can be most effectively addressed using genetically defined animals within self-administration paradigms. Thus, genetic factors are being shown to play a critical role in drug dependence and the use and study of genetic models in this area will not only improve our understanding of these genetic contributions to dependence, but, via the powerful approaches of behavioural genetic models, will ultimately aid in our overall understanding of the serious problem of drug dependence.

References

Abbott, F.V., Melzack, R. & Leber, B.F. (1982) *Pharmacol. Biochem. Behav.* **17**, 1213–1219.

Abbott, F.V., Franklin, K.B.J. & Leber, B.F. (1986) *Life Sci.* **39**, 2017–2024.

Altshuler, H.L., Weaver, S. & Phillips, P. (1975) *Life Sci.* **17**, 883–890.

Basbaum, A.I. & Fields, H.L. (1984) *Annu. Rev. Neurosci.* **7**, 309–338.

Belknap, J.K. (1980) In *Alcohol Tolerance and Dependence* (eds Rigter, H. & Crabbe, J.C.), pp 157–180. New York, Elsevier/North-Holland Biomedical Press.

Belknap, J.K., Haltli, N., Goebel, D. & Lame, M. (1982) *Proc. West. Pharmacol. Soc.* **25**, 299–302.

Belknap, J.K., Noordewier, B. & Lame, M. (1989) *Physiol. Behav.* **46**, 69–74.

Bohman, M., Sigvardsson, S. & Cloninger, C.R. (1981) *Arch. Gen. Psychiatry* **38**, 965–969.

Boyer, C.S., Ross, D. & Peterson, D.R. (1988) *J. Biochem. Toxicol.* **3**, 295–307.

Broadhurst, P.L. (1979) *Drugs and the Inheritance of Behavior: A Survey of Comparative Pharmacogenetics.* New York and London, Plenum Press.

Cadoret, R.J. & Gath, A. (1978) *Br. J. Psychiatry* **132**, 252–258.

Cadoret, R.J., Troughton, E., O'Gorman, T.W. & Heywood, E. (1986) *Arch. Gen Psychiatry* **43**, 1131–1136.

Calligaro, D.O. & Eldefrawi, M.E. (1987) *J. Pharmacol. Exp. Ther.* **243**, 61–67.

Carney, J.M., Cheng, M.-S., Wu, C. & Seale, T.W. (1991) *Adv. Alcohol Subst. Abuse* (in press).

Carroll, M.E. & Meisch, R.A. (1984) In *Advances in Behavioural Pharmacology*, vol. 4 (eds Thompson, T., Dews, P.B. & Barret, J.E.), pp 47–88. New York, Academic Press.

Carroll, M.E., Pederson, M.C. & Harrison, R.G. (1986) *Pharmacol. Biochem. Behav.* **24**, 1095–1099.

Carroll, M.E., Lac, S.T., Asencio, M. & Kragh, R. (1990) *Psychopharmacology* **100**, 293–300.

Cazala, P., Darracq, C. & Saint-Marc, M. (1987) *Brain Res.* **416**, 283–288.

Chan, A.W.K. (1976) *Life Sci.* **19**, 587–604.

Cloninger, C.R., Bohman, M. & Sigvardsson, S. (1981) *Arch. Gen. Psychiatry* **38**, 861–868.

Collins, A.C. (1981) In *Development of Animal Models as Pharmacogenetic Tools* (eds McClearn, G.E., Deitrich, R.A. & Erwin, V.G.), pp 161–170. National Institute on Alcohol Abuse and Alcoholism, Research Monograph No. 6. Rockville, Maryland, DHHS Publication No. (ADM) 81-1133.

Crabbe, J.C. & Belknap, J.K. (1980) *Subst. Alcohol Actions Misuse* **1**, 385–413.

Crabbe, J.C., Jarvik, L.F., Liston, E.H. & Jenden, D.J. (1983) *Acta Genet. Med. Gemellol. (Roma)* **32**, 139–149.

Davis, W.M. & Smith, S.G. (1975) *J. Pharm. Pharmacol.* **27**, 540–542.

de la Garza, R. & Johanson, C.E. (1982) *Pharmacol. Biochem. Behav.* **17**, 1295–1299.

deWit, H. & Wise, R.A. (1977) *Can. J. Psychol.* **31**, 195–203.

Dymshitz, J. & Lieblich, I. (1987) *Psychopharmacology* **92**, 473–477.

Eidelberg, E., Erspamer, R., Kreinick, C.J. & Harris, J. (1975) *Eur. J. Pharmacol.* **32**, 329–336.

Elmer, G.I., Meisch, R.A. & George, F.R. (1986) *Pharmacol. Biochem. Behav.* **24**, 1417–1421.

Elmer, G.I., Meisch, R.A. & George, F.R. (1987a) *Alcohol* **4**, 63–68.

Elmer, G.I., Meisch, R.A. & George, F.R. (1987b) *Behav. Genet.* **17**, 439–451.

Elmer, G.I., Meisch, R.A., Goldberg, S.R. & George, F.R. (1988) *Psychopharmacology* **96**, 431–436.

Elmer, G.I., Meisch, R.A., Goldberg, S.R. & George, F.R. (1990) *J. Pharmacol. Exp. Ther.* **254**, 1054–1062.

Eriksson, K. (1968) *Science* **159**, 739–741.

Eriksson, K. (1972) *Ann. N.Y. Acad. Sci.* **197**, 32–41.

Eriksson, K. & Kianmaa, K. (1971) *Ann. Med. Exp. Fenn.* **49**, 73–78.

Eriksson, K. & Rusi, M. (1981) In *Development of Animal Models as Pharmacogenetic Tools* (eds McClearn, G.E., Deitrich, R.A. & Erwin, V.G.), pp 87–117. National Institute on Alcohol Abuse and Alcoholism, Research Monograph No. 6. Rockville, Maryland, DHHS Publication No. (ADM) 81-1133.

Erwin, V.G., Heston, D.W., McClearn, G.E. & Deitrich, R.A. (1976) *Pharmacol. Biochem. Behav.* **4**, 679–683.

Erwin, V.G., McClearn, G.E. & Deitrich, R.A. (1980) *Pharmacol. Biochem. Behav.* **13**, 297–302.

Ettenberg, A., Pettit, H.O., Bloom, F.E. & Koob, G.F. (1982) *Psychopharmacology* **78**, 204–209.

Forgie, M.L., Beyerstein, B.L. & Alexander, B.K. (1988) *Psychopharmacology* **95**, 237–244.

Franklin, K.B.J. & Abbot, F.V. (1989) In *Neuromethods*, vol. 13 (eds Boulton, A.A., Baker, G.B. & Greenshaw, A.J.), pp 145–216. Clifton, New Jersey, Humana Press.

Fuller, J.L. (1980) In *Animal Models in Alcohol Research* (eds Eriksson, K., Sinclair, J.D. & Kiianmaa, K.), pp 57–62. London, Academic Press.

George, F.R. (1987) *Pharmacol. Biochem. Behav.* **27**, 379–384.

George, F.R. (1988) *Alcoholism: Clin. Exp. Res.* **12**, 86–90.

George, F.R. (1989) *Psychopharmacology* **99**, 147–150.

George, F.R. (1990) *Alcohol* **7**, 207–211.
George, F.R. & Goldberg, S.R. (1988) In *Mechanisms of Cocaine Abuse and Toxicity* (eds Clouet, D., Asghar, K. & Brown, R.), pp 239–249. National Institute on Drug Abuse Monograph, 88.
George, F.R. & Goldberg, S.R. (1989) *Trends Pharmacol. Sci.* **10**, 78–83.
George, F.R. & Meisch, R.A. (1984) *Behav. Genet.* **17**, 439–451.
George, F.R. & Ritz, M.C. (1990) *Psychopharmacology* **101**, 18–24.
George, F.R., Porrino, L.J., Ritz, M.C. & Goldberg, S.R. (1991) *Psychopharmacology* (in press).
Goeders, N.E. & Smith, J.E. (1983) *Science* **221**, 773–775.
Goeders, N.E., Dworkin, S.I. & Smith, J.E. (1986) *Pharmacol. Biochem. Behav.* **24**, 1429–1440.
Goldberg, S.R., Morse, W.H. & Goldberg, D.M. (1976) *J. Pharmacol. Exp. Ther.* **199**, 278–286.
Goodwin, D.W., Schulsinger, F. & Hermansen, L. (1973) *Arch. Gen. Psychiatry* **28**, 238–243.
Goudie, A.J., Leathley, M., McNally, J. & West, C.R. (1989) *Drug Dev. Res.* **16**, 123–131.
Gurling, H.M.D., Murray, R.M. & Clifford, C.A. (1981) *Twin Research 3: Epidemiological and Clinical Studies.* New York, Alan R. Liss, Inc.
Hadaway, P.F., Alexander, B.K., Coambs, R.B. & Beyerstein, B. (1979) *Psychopharmacology* **66**, 87–91.
Hilakivi, L., Eriksson, C.J.P., Sarviharju, M. & Sinclair, J.D. (1984) *Alcohol* **1**, 71–75.
Horowitz, G.P. (1976) *Behav. Genet.* **6**, 109–110.
Horowitz, G.P. (1981) In *Development of Animal Models as Pharmacogenetic Tools*, pp 209–231. NIAAA Research Monograph 6.
Horowitz, G.P., Whitney, G., Smith, J.C. & Stephan, F.K. (1977) *Psychopharmacology* **52**, 119–122.
Hrubec, Z. & Omenn, G.S. (1981) *Alcoholism: Clin. Exp. Res.* **5**, 207–215.
Jatlow, P., Barash, P.G., Van Dyke, C., Radding, J. & Byck, R. (1979) *Anesth. Analg.* **58**, 235–238.
Judson, B.A. & Goldstein, A. (1978) *J. Pharmacol. Exp. Ther.* **206**, 56–60.
Kennedy, L.T. & Hanbauer, I. (1983) *J. Neurochem.* **41**, 172–178.
Kleven, M.S., Anthony, E.W., Goldberg, L.I. & Woolverton, W.L. (1988) *Psychopharmacology* **95**, 427–429.
Koob, G.F., Le, H.T. & Creese, I. (1987) *Neurosci. Lett.* **79**, 315–320.
Lecesse, A.P. & Lyness, W.H. (1984) *Brain Res.* **303**, 153–162.
Li, T.-K. & Lumeng, L. (1984) *Alcoholism: Clin. Exp. Res.* **8**, 485–486.
Li, T.-K., Lumeng, L., McBride, W.J. & Waller, M.B. (1979) *Drug Alcohol Depend.* **4**, 45–60.
Li, T.-K., Lumeng, L., McBride, W.J. & Waller, M.B. (1981) In *Development of Animal Models as Pharmacogenetic Tools* (eds McClearn, G.E., Dietrich, R.A. & Erwin, V.G.), pp 171–191. National Institute on Alcohol Abuse and Alcoholism, Research Monograph No. 6. Rockville, Maryland, DHHS Publication No. (ADM) 81-1133.
London, E.D., Dent, G.W., George, F.R. & Goldberg, S.R. (1991) Submitted.
Lyness, W.H. (1983) *Subst. Alcohol Actions Misuse* **4**, 305–312.
Martin-Iverson, M.T., Szostak, C. & Fibiger, H.C. (1986) *Psychopharmacology* **88**, 310–314.
McClearn, G.E. & DeFries, J.C. (1973) *Introduction to Behavior Genetics*. San Francisco, W.H. Freeman and Company.

McClearn, G.E. & Kakihana, R. (1981) In *Development of Animal Models as Pharmacogenetic Tools* (eds McClearn, G.E., Deitrich, R.A. & Erwin, V.G.), pp 147–160. National Institute on Alcohol Abuse and Alcoholism, Research Monograph No. 6. Rockville, Maryland, DHHS Publication No. (ADM) 81-1133.
McClearn, G.E. & Rodgers, D.A. (1959) *Q. J. Stud. Alcohol.* **20**, 691–695.
McClearn, G.E. & Rodgers, D.A. (1961) *J. Comp. Physiol. Psychiatry* **54**, 116–119.
Meisch, R.A. (1984) In *Research Advances in Alcohol and Drug Problems*, vol. 8 (eds Smart, R.G., Cappell, H.D., Glaser, F.B., Israel, Y., Kalant, H., Popham, R.E., Schmidt, W. & Sellers, E.M.), pp 23–45. New York, Plenum Press.
Melchior, C.L. & Myers, R.D. (1976) *Pharmacol. Biochem. Behav.* **5**, 63–72.
Nichols, J.R. & Hsiao, S. (1967) *Science* **157**, 561–563.
Oliverio, A. & Castellano, C. (1974) *Psychopharmacology* **39**, 13–22.
Oliverio, A., Castellano, C. & Eleftheriou, B.E. (1975) *Psychopharmacology* **42**, 219–224.
Pedersen, N. (1981) In *Twin Research 3: Epidemiological and Clinical Studies*, pp 53–59. New York, Alan R. Liss, Inc.
Pickens, R.W. & Svikus, D.S. (1991) *Adv. Alcohol Subst. Abuse* (in press).
Porrino, L.J., Ritz, M.C., Sharpe, L.G., Goodman, N.L., Kuhar, M.J. & Goldberg, S.R. (1989) *Life Sci.* **45**, 1529–1535.
Post, R.M., Contel, N.R. & Gold, P. (1982) *Life Sci.* **31**, 2745–2750.
Reith, M.E.A., Shershen, H. & Lajtha, A. (1980) *Life Sci.* **27**, 1055–1062.
Richter, C.P. & Campbell, K.H. (1940) *Science* **91**, 507–508.
Risner, M.E. & Jones, B.E. (1976) *Pharmacol. Biochem. Behav.* **5**, 477–482.
Ritz, M.C. & Kuhar, M.J. (1989) *J. Pharmacol. Exp. Ther.* **248**, 1010–1017.
Ritz, M.C., George, F.R., deFriebre, C. & Meisch, R.A. (1986) *Pharmacol. Biochem. Behav.* **24**, 1089–1094.
Ritz, M.C., Lamb, R.J., Goldberg, S.R. & Kuhar, M.J. (1987) *Science* **237**, 1219–1223.
Ritz, M.C., George, F.R. & Meisch, R.A. (1989a) *Alcohol* **6**, 227–233.
Ritz, M.C., George, F.R. & Meisch, R.A. (1989b) *Alcohol* **6**, 235–239.
Rodgers, D.A. & McClearn, G.E. (1962) *Q. J. Stud. Alcohol* **23**, 26–33.
Roe, A. (1944) *Q. J. Stud. Alcohol* **5**, 378–393.
Ruth, J.A., Ullman, E.A. & Collins, A.C. (1988) *Pharmacol. Biochem. Behav.* **29**, 157–162.
Satinder, K.P. (1977) *Pharmacol. Biochem. Behav.* **7**, 43–49.
Schuster, L., Yu, G. & Bates, A. (1977) *Psychopharmacology* **52**, 185–190.
Seale, T.W. & Carney, J.M. (1991) *Adv. Alcohol Subst. Abuse* (in press).
Sharkey, J., Glen, K.A., Wolf, S.A. & Kuhar, M.J. (1988a) *Eur. J. Pharmacol.* **149**, 171–174.
Sharkey, J., Ritz, M.C., Schendon, J.A., Hanson, R.C. & Kuhar, M.J. (1988b) *J. Pharmacol. Exp. Ther.* **246**, 1048–1052.
Shields, J. (1962) *Monozygotic Twins Brought Up Apart and Reared Together.* London, Oxford University Press.
Shoemaker, H., Pimoule, C., Arbilla, S., Scatton, B., Javoy-Agid, F. & Langer, S.Z. (1985) *Nauyn-Schmiedeberg's Arch. Pharmacol.* **329**, 227–235.
Smith, F.L., Yu, D.S.L., Smith, D.G., Lecesse, A.P. & Lyness, W.H. (1986) *Pharmacol. Biochem. Behav.* **25**, 849–855.
Spuhler, K. & Deitrich, R. (1984) *Alcoholism: Clin. Exp. Res.* **8**, 480–484.
Stolerman, I.P. & D'Mello, G.D. (1984) In *Advances in Behavioural Pharmacology*, vol. 4 (eds Thompson, T., Dews, P.B. & Barret, J.E.), pp 47–88. New York, Academic Press.
Suzuki, T., George, F.R. & Meisch, R.A. (1988) *J. Pharmacol. Exp. Ther.* **245**, 164–170.

Suzuki, T., Siiozaki, Y. & Misawa, M. (1989) *Jpn. J. Alcohol Drug Depend.* **24**, 480–489.
Swerdlow, N.R., Gilbert, D. & Koob, G.F. (1989) In *Neuromethods: Psychopharmacology* (eds Boulton, A.A., Baker, G.B. & Greenshaw, A.J.), pp 399–446. Clifton, NJ, Humana Press.
Ternes, J.W., Ehrman, R. & O'Brien, C. (1983) *Behav. Neurosci.* **97**, 327–330.
Thompson, M.L., Schuster, L., Casey, E. & Kanel, G.C. (1984) *Biochem. Pharmacol.* **33**, 1299–1307.
Tyers, M.B. (1980) *Br. J. Pharmacol.* **69**, 503–512.
Waller, M.B., McBride, W.J., Gatto, G.J., Lumeng, L. & Li, T.-K. (1984) *Science* **225**, 78–80.
Weeks, J.R. (1962) *Science* **138**, 143–144.
Whitney, G. & Horowitz, G.P. (1978) *Behav. Genet.* **8**, 182.
Wilson, M.C. & Schuster, C.R. (1972) *Psychopharmacology* **26**, 115–126.
Woolverton, W.L. (1986) *Pharmacol. Biochem. Behav.* **24**, 531–535.
Woolverton, W.L. & Virus, R.M. (1989) *Pharmacol. Biochem. Behav.* **32**, 691–697.
Woolverton, W.L., Goldberg, L.I. & Ginos, J.Z. (1984) *J. Pharmacol. Exp. Ther.* **230**, 678–683.
Yanagita, T., Ishida, K. & Funamoto, H. (1970) *Jpn. J. Clin. Pharmacol.* **1**, 13–16.
Yokel, R.A. & Wise, R.A. (1975) *Science* **187**, 547–549.
Yokel, R.A. & Wise, R.A. (1976) *Psychopharmacology* **48**, 311–318.
Yokel, R.A. & Wise, R.A. (1978) *Psychopharmacology* **58**, 289–296.
Yu, D.S.L., Smith, F.L., Smith, D.G. & Lyness, W.H. (1986) *Life Sci.* **39**, 1383–1388.

Index